Recent Advances in
INFECTION

D. S. REEVES MB BS MRCPath
Consultant Medical Microbiologist, Southmead Hospital, Bristol
Honorary Consultant, Public Health Laboratory Service
Honorary Clinical Teacher, University of Bristol

A. M. GEDDES FRCP(Edin) MRCP(Lond)
Consultant Physician, East Birmingham Hospital
Honorary Senior Clinical Lecturer, University of Birmingham

SIR ROBERT WILLIAMS MD FRCP(Lond) FRCPath FFCM
Director, Public Health Laboratory Service

Recent Advances in
INFECTION

EDITED BY
DAVID REEVES

ALASDAIR GEDDES

Foreword by
Sir ROBERT WILLIAMS

NUMBER ONE

CHURCHILL LIVINGSTONE
EDINBURGH LONDON AND NEW YORK 1979

CHURCHILL LIVINGSTONE
Medical Division of Longman Group Limited

Distributed in the United States of America by
Longman Inc., 19 West 44th Street, New York,
N.Y. 10036, and by associated companies,
branches and representatives throughout
the world.

First published 1979

ISBN 0 443 01661 5

British Library Cataloguing in Publication Data
1
1. Communicable diseases
I. Reeves, David S   II. Geddes, Alasdair
McIntosh
616.9   RC111   78–40950

Printed in Great Britain by Bell & Bain, Glasgow

Foreword

Infection has not, in the last few years, advanced; but nor has it retreated sufficiently for anyone aware of the current situation to do anything but welcome the volume of essays that Dr Reeves and Dr Geddes have assembled. There have been real advances in the microbiology of infections, with the recognition, as pathogens, of whole groups of microbes that were either unknown or unregarded previously; and with the development of new techniques for more rapid or more precise diagnosis. There have been quite bewildering advances in the number and variety of antimicrobial drugs, and—perhaps of more fundamental importance—we are now seeing real advances in understanding of their pharmacology and pharmacokinetics; both are advances that call for guidance for practitioners from the experts. Indeed this last represents the other major advance: the growing appreciation of the importance of a real partnership of the practitioners at the bedside and the laboratory bench.

Dr Reeves and Dr Geddes have gathered together a team of those who have contributed to these advances: they concentrate principally on bacteria and bacterial infections, and they concentrate on the practical—not the practical of the cook-book but the practical of the best travel book: stimulating interest, enough guidelines to indicate how the interest can be pursued, and plenty of references to enable the interest to be fully developed and applied. Surely many individual infections will be compelled to retreat when the lessons of this volume are applied.

R.W.

Preface

Although great advances have been made in the diagnosis, treatment and prevention of disease, infections remain the most frequent cause of illness and death throughout the world. New problems continue to appear; increasing travel, particularly by air, has provided an easy and rapid route for the dissemination of infections, both of the 'common' bacteria, which have developed resistance to antibiotics, and of the classical contagions.

To combat this, a considerable amount of current research is directed at increasing our knowledge of the pathogenesis of infections as well as their clinical management, both by antibiotic and non-antibiotic therapy. Advances have been made for many infections and, coupled with increasing specialisation in laboratory medicine, it seemed appropriate to provide a volume entitled *Recent Advances in Infection* covering only infectious diseases and clinical microbiology with the exclusion of virology, which is dealt with in a separate book. These two books along with others in the 'Recent Advances' series replace the topics originally found in *Recent Advances in Clinical Pathology*.

Because clinical bacteriology has altered considerably in the past decade, becoming a more clinical speciality instead of being laboratory orientated, it was decided that the combination of an infectious diseases physician with a clinical microbiologist was the most suitable to edit the first volume of this new series. The wide range of topics covered by using contributions from clinicians, microbiologists, pharmacologists and other scientists, with their rational approach to diagnosis and treatment of infections, will, we hope, be both a reminder of the importance of interdisciplinary collaboration and reflection of the expanding interest in infections.

D.S.R.
A.M.G.

Bristol, 1979

Contributors

G. A. J. AYLIFFE BSc MD FRCPath
Member of Scientific Staff, Medical Research Council.
Consultant Microbiologist, Hospital Infection Research Laboratory, Dudley Road Hospital, Birmingham.

A. P. BALL BSc MB ChB MRCP(UK)
Senior Registrar in Medicine, Department of Communicable and Tropical Diseases, East Birmingham Hospital

B. S. DRASAR BSc PhD DSc MRCPath
Senior Lecturer in Bacteriology, Department of Medical Microbiology, London School of Hygiene and Tropical Medicine

E. G. V. EVANS BSc PhD MIBiol
Lecturer in Medical Mycology, University Departments of Microbiology and Dermatology, The General Infirmary, Leeds

R. J. FALLON BSc MD FRCPath FRCP(Glas)
Consultant in Laboratory Medicine, Ruchill Hospital, Glasgow
Honorary Lecturer in Bacteriology and Immunology, University of Glasgow

A. M. GEDDES FRCP(Edin) MRCP(Lond)
Consultant Physician, East Birmingham Hospital
Honorary Senior Clinical Lecturer, University of Birmingham

M. J. HUDSON BSc
Scientific Officer, Bacterial Metabolism Research Laboratory, Central Public Health Laboratory, London

D. M. JONES MD FRCPath DipBact
Director, Public Health Laboratory, Withington Hospital, Manchester

H. P. LAMBERT MA MD FRCP(Lond)
Professor of Microbial Diseases, University of London
Consultant Physician, St George's Hospital, London

G. E. MAWER PhD FRCP(Edin)
Professor of Clinical Pharmacology, Medical School, University of Manchester

S. W. B. NEWSOM MA MD FRCPath
Consultant Bacteriologist, Addenbrookes and Papworth Hospitals, Cambridge

IAN PHILLIPS MA MD BCh MRCP MRCPath
Professor of Medical Microbiology, St Thomas' Hospital Medical School,
University of London

A. V. REYNOLDS BTech
Lecturer, The Microbiology Section, The Department of Pharmaceutics, The
School of Pharmacy, University of London

G. L. RIDGWAY MD BSc MRCPath
Consultant Microbiologist, University College Hospital, London

J. T. SMITH BPharm PhD
Professor, The Microbiology Section, The Department of Pharmaceutics, The
School of Pharmacy, University of London

E. JOAN STOKES MB FRCP FRCPath
Consulting Microbiologist, University College Hospital, London
Member of the Advisory Committee for Microbiology Quality Control

A. T. WILLIS MD DSc PhD FRACP FRCPath FRCPA
Director, Public Health Laboratory, Luton
Consultant Microbiologist, Luton and Dunstable Hospital, Luton

Contents

1. Trends in resistance and their significance in primary pathogenic bacteria

Graham A. J. Ayliffe

Antimicrobial agents developed in recent years have mainly been modifications of existing compounds. Their advantages usually consist of improved absorption, increased antibacterial activity, or greater stability to inactivating enzymes. Since most of these compounds show some degree of cross-resistance with the parent compound, their value in overcoming problems of resistant strains is limited. Nevertheless, cross-resistance is often not complete and the new compounds, particularly cephalosporins and aminoglycosides, are sometimes useful. The main interests in antimicrobial resistance recently have been in the structure, mode of action and transfer mechanisms of resistance plasmids (or 'R' factors) and genes, and in the enzymic inactivation of penicillins, cephalosporins and aminoglycosides. These are related problems since the inactivating enzymes are usually plasmid controlled.

Transfer of antibiotic resistance by conjugation was first described by Japanese workers and this was soon followed by similar reports in other countries. The original Japanese report suggested that strains of *Shigella flexneri* acquired resistance to tetracycline, streptomycin, sulphonamide and chloramphenicol from *Escherichia coli* (e.g. Watanabe, 1963). 'R' factors are still found mainly in Enterobacteriaceae although it is now apparent that certain plasmids can be transferred to a variety of genera and species. Some of these possible transfers are between biologically unlikely organisms such as *E. coli* and *Neisseria gonorrhoeae*. Not only can plasmids be transferred to a number of different types of organisms, but resistant genes can be transposed from one plasmid to another (Datta, 1977). These elements are termed transposons and the first one described contained a gene controlling β lactamase, TEM, which is now known to be very widespread (Hedges and Jacob, 1974; Mathew and Hedges, 1976).

Most strains of salmonella or shigella have acquired resistance to several antibiotics and occasionally to six or more, but reports of 'R' factors in *Salmonella typhi* were uncommon until 1972. As new antibiotics were introduced, additional resistance determinants were added to existing plasmids. This was well demonstrated by Anderson (1968) in a study of *S. typhimurium* in man and animals over several years. He showed that the incidence of infection with certain strains, especially phage type 29, had increased since 1961. The strains were initially sensitive to antibiotics, but by 1965 were resistant to streptomycin, tetracycline, ampicillin and furazolidine; resistance to each agent corresponded to usage of the antibiotic concerned. Although salmonella strains are sometimes transferred directly to man, a greater risk is the silent transfer from animal to man of non-pathogenic intestinal organisms carrying 'R' factors. Resistant strains of *E. coli* and klebsiella can be isolated from most people in small numbers (Datta, 1969) and are transferred from mothers to babies at or soon after birth (Noy, Ayliffe and Linton, 1974). The continued presence of these strains, resistant to tetracycline, ampicillin, sulphonamide and occasionally chloramphenicol, means that selection may occur wherever one of these antibiotics is given. 'R' factors have in some ways had a much less dramatic effect on chemotherapy than was originally expected. Ampicillin is the most frequently used antibiotic, but the incidence of infection caused by resistant strains of E. coli has not increased much over 30 per cent in over 20 years (Ayliffe, 1975). Transfer of resistance by conjugation appears to be more efficient in vitro than in vivo and new strains of E. coli do not readily colonise the intestinal tract unless present in large numbers or are selected by an antibiotic (Smith, 1969; Anderson, Gillespie and Richmond, 1973). However, in parts of the world where antibiotic selective pressures in the general population are high, 'R' factors are almost certainly more frequent in intestinal non-pathogens than elsewhere. Resistance is thus more readily transferred to pathogens, as in the outbreaks of chloramphenicol-resistant shigella and S. typhi in Central America and the Far East. Chloramphenicol is broad-spectrum and relatively cheap and often used in these countries, but not in economically advanced countries because of its toxicity.

The incidence of multiple-resistant strains of Enterobacteriaceae varies considerably in different countries and different parts of the same country. A study of E. coli from urinary tract infections in laboratories of four towns in the United Kingdom showed marked difference in resistance of strains to sulphonamides and ampicillin. Sulphonamide resistance varied from 17.6 per cent in outpatients to 42 per cent in in-patients, and ampicillin-resistance varied between 17 and 40 per cent (Andrews et al, 1975). Similar differences with other organisms will be considered in this chapter. Plasmids are also present in gram-positive organisms, but resistance is transferred by transduction and not conjugation. This is a less efficient process, but has been described with Staphylococcus aureus in vivo as well as in vitro (Lacey, 1975).

Until the last few years, treatment of severe infections caused by certain pathogens was predictable and antibiotic sensitivity tests were often unnecessary: benzylpenicillin could reliably be used for pneumococcal infections, ampicillin for Haemophilus influenzae infections and chloramphenicol for typhoid fever. The emergence of resistant strains in these and other previously sensitive organisms may have an important influence on future therapy.

Earlier problems of resistance have been discussed elsewhere (Lowbury and Ayliffe, 1974) and recent reports of resistance in a few primary pathogens are discussed in this chapter. The distinction between primary and secondary pathogens is not always clear, but the organisms I have included can all cause infection in previously healthy individuals. The term antibiotic will also be used for all antimicrobial agents.

SPECIFIC ORGANISMS

Streptococcus pneumoniae (pneumococci)
Resistance to tetracycline has been recognised for some years and was first reported in Australia (Evans and Hansman, 1963). Strains were later reported in other

countries, but numbers remained low until an incidence of 23 per cent resistant strains was reported from Liverpool (Percival, Armstrong and Turner, 1969). A more recent multi-centre study in the United Kingdom showed that 13 per cent of 1528 strains were resistant. There was considerable variation between centres, rates varying between 2 and 32 per cent (Report, 1977). Resistant strains were more common in males and older patients, and in a study from the U.S.A. were mainly obtained from patients with chronic lung disease (Gopalakrishna and Lerner, 1973). It is obvious that tetracyclines should not be used for treating severe pneumococcal infections, unless the results of sensitivity tests are available. Erythromycin and lincomycin (or clindamycin) are commonly used in the treatment of upper respiratory tract infection. Strains resistant to both these antibiotics have been isolated, but the incidence has remained low (Dixon, 1967).

Although strains of pneumococci resistant to low levels of benzylpenicillin (MIC 0.6 μg/ml) were reported in Australia in 1967 (Hansman and Bullen, 1967) and occasionally since then in other countries (Dixon, 1974; Howes and Mitchell, 1976), they were not considered of great interest from the therapeutic aspect. This is still true in most countries, but recent evidence suggests that careful surveillance for significant penicillin resistance is now necessary. Strains of higher resistance (MIC 8 μg/ml) have been isolated from patients in hospitals in Durban and Johannesburg. In the Durban outbreak, pneumococci resistant to penicillin were isolated from five patients (Appelbaum et al, 1977). Three of the patients with meningitis were treated with penicillin G, chloramphenicol and other antibiotics, including kanamycin, but all died. The two other patients with less severe infections survived when treated with erythromycin, rifampicin, or high doses of ampicillin. The pneumococci were all serotype 57 (or 19A by the Danish method) and were resistant to benzylpenicillin, methicillin, carbenicillin, chloramphenicol, the aminoglycosides, and were partially sensitive to ampicillin and the cephalosporins. Strains were sensitive to erythromycin, tetracycline, clindamycin, vancomycin and cotrimoxazole. Another strain of pneumococcus, resistant to benzylpenicillin, erythromycin, clindamycin, tetracycline, chloramphenicol, cotrimoxazole and the aminoglycosides was recovered from patients and staff in a hospital in Johannesburg (Leading Article, 1977b). This strain was sensitive to rifampicin, vancomycin and partially sensitive to fusidic acid, but a patient recovered on treatment with cephalothin and ampicillin.

From May to November, 1977, resistant pneumococci were isolated from blood, CSF or pleural fluids of fifteen children in either Durban or Johannesburg and eight died. The infections occurred in children admitted to hospital for other conditions, indicating that the strains were hospital acquired. Prevalence studies in the hospitals of both towns showed carriers of multiple-resistant strains in 8/28 hospitals investigated. A number of different resistance patterns which included penicillin-resistance was also found (Koornhof et al, 1978). Staff in contact with carriers or infected patients were infrequently colonised (0.9 per cent of 434 sampled), and carriers were not present in the community apart from occasional family contacts. Since these organisms were readily transmissible and highly resistant, a programme of eradication was necessary. Carriers were isolated, and wards containing carriers or infected patients were closed to new admissions. Eradication of strains from carriers obviously presented some chemotherapeutic problems. Erythromycin was effective when strains were sensitive, and rifampicin and fusidic acid given for ten days cleared 63 per cent of the more resistant strains; rifampicin resistance occasionally emerged during treatment. A variety of other agents were tried with little success apart from intravenous vancomycin given for five days.

The treatment of patients infected with the highly resistant strains was also difficult, particularly in meningitis. Prediction of antibiotic sensitivity was not possible and these outbreaks demonstrate the necessity for rapid sensitivity tests. β lactamase has not been detected in these strains, neither has transferable resistance, but it seems likely from the resistance patterns that plasmids are involved.

Streptococcus pyogenes (Lancefield group A. β haemolytic streptococci)
In contrast to pneumococci, *Strep. pyogenes* has remained sensitive to benzylpenicillin. Failure in treatment is not due to resistance, but to other factors such as the destruction of penicillin by associated penicillinase-producing organisms. Penicillinase-resistant penicillins (e.g. flucloxacillin) are effective in preventing streptococcal infection in burns (Lowbury and Miller, 1964). Tetracycline-resistance was reported in 1954 (Lowbury and Cason, 1954) and although the incidence has increased (Emslie, 1974), a fall has since occurred in some areas (Robertson, 1968). A survey (Report, 1977) showed considerable variations in different parts of the United Kingdom ranging between 15 and 63 per cent. Resistant strains were commoner in the older age groups and in sites other than respiratory tract. Occasional severe infections, e.g. post puerperal sepsis, caused by *Strep. pyogenes* still occur and disastrous failures in therapy may happen if tetracycline is used instead of benzylpenicillin.

Erythromycin and lincomycin (or clindamycin) are often used for treating streptococcal infections. Most strains are sensitive to these agents, but resistant strains have occasionally been reported, usually in special units, e.g. burns (Kohn, Hewitt and Fraser, 1968; Lowbury and Kidson, 1968), and we have isolated strains resistant to both antibiotics in dermatological wards. Cross-resistance exists between the two antibiotics as in *Staph. aureus* and is of an unusual nature. In Canada the incidence of lincomycin and erythromycin resistant strains increased from 0.24 per cent of isolates in 1971 to 1.38 per cent in 1972 (Dixon and Lipinski, 1974). Resistance to both antibiotics was also rarely found in other β haemolytic streptococci (Groups B, C and G).

Haemophilus influenzae
Haemophilus influenzae type B is a common cause of meningitis in children and sometimes of other severe infections such as acute epiglottitis. Ampicillin or chloramphenicol is still the antibiotic of choice, but problems of resistance now complicate the accepted treatment. Surveys showed no evidence of ampicillin-resistance before 1974 (Finland et al, 1976; Williams and Andrews, 1974) and only one instance of chloramphenicol resistance (Barrett et al, 1972). Ampicillin-resistant strains were then reported in several countries and different areas of the same country in 1974 (Gunn et al, 1974; Clymo and Harper, 1974; Thomas et al, 1974; and many others). In some studies the incidence of resistant strains was as high as 10 per cent (Nelson, 1974). The most recent survey in the United

Kingdom showed an incidence of 1.5 per cent of 952 strains and the highest incidence of resistance was 4.0 per cent in two centres (Howard, 1977).

Resistance is apparently due to a TEM β lactamase which is commonly found in enterobacteriaceae (Williams, Kattan, and Cavanagh, 1974; Madeiros and O'Brien, 1975). Since ampicillin-resistant coliforms are commonly found in sputum, particularly in patients treated with ampicillin, transfer of resistance could have occurred from these organisms. The opportunity for transfer has been present for many years and a possible new transfer factor has emerged (Elwell et al, 1977b). Chloramphenicol is now less frequently used in the treatment of meningitis or acute epiglottitis because of potential toxicity, but it is effective and still preferred by some clinicians. It is apparently bactericidal against *H. influenzae* (Garrod, Lambert and O'Grady, 1973) and in vitro tests have shown it to be more active than ampicillin (Turk, 1977). Four infections caused by chloramphenicol resistant type B strains have been reported in the U.S.A. (Morbidity and Mortality Weekly Report, 1976b) and occasionally elsewhere (Manten, Van Klingeren and Dessens-Kroon, 1976), but resistance is still very rare.

Since strains resistant to ampicillin are now relatively common and chloramphenicol resistance is always a possibility, consideration must be given to the treatment of meningitis before the results of sensitivity tests are available (Fallon, 1976). Haemophilus strains should always be screened for resistance to these antibiotics. If resistant strains are occurring in a certain area, it may be necessary to start treatment with both ampicillin and chloramphenicol. Antagonism between these agents is possible, but is probably not of clinical importance. It has been suggested that ampicillin should be given 30 minutes before chloramphenicol and both in high dosage. However, in most countries at the present time, chloramphenicol alone will be effective. Rapid tests for β lactamase are now available (O'Callaghan et al, 1972; Shannon and Wise, 1977) and should enable ampicillin sensitivity results to be given within 24 hours of admitting the patient.

Of other possible agents, tetracycline resistance is common, but tetracycline, erythromycin and most of the cephalosporins are probably inadequate for treating meningitis reliably (Williams and Andrews, 1974). It is possible that one of the newer cephalosporins, such as cephamandole, might be useful for the treatment of infections caused by ampicillin-resistant strains, but this suggestion is based mainly on in vitro tests (Yourrassowski, Schoutens and Vanderlinden, 1976). Co-trimoxazole is the most likely alternative treatment to ampicillin or chloramphenicol (Smith, 1976), but has not yet been adequately compared with these agents.

Neisseria gonorrhoeae (gonococci)
Strains of low resistance to benzylpenicillin, i.e. MIC to 2 μg/ml, have been isolated since the 1950's (Reyn, Korner and Bentzon, 1958). These strains have been reported from all parts of the world, but most of the infections still respond to high doses of penicillin with probenecid. Resistance to other antibiotics including erythromycin, streptomycin, tetracycline and chloramphenicol have been reported (Maier, Beilstein and Zubrzycki, 1974) and appears to be of chromosomal origin. In 1976, strains of higher resistance to benzylpenicillin and containing a plasmid controlling β lactamase appeared. Initially they were isolated

in the U.S.A. from origins in the Far East (Morbidity and Mortality Weekly Report, 1976a), and about the same time they were reported in Liverpool, England (Percival et al, 1976; Turner, Ratcliffe and Anderson, 1976). Since then strains have been reported from the Ivory coast (Piot, 1977), Ghana (Phillips, 1976) and at least 14 other countries. There is evidence that the Far East strains differ from the African (Perine et al, 1977; Elwell et al, 1977a). The Far East organisms tend to be tetracycline-resistant and carry a plasmid with a molecular weight of 5.8×10^6 daltons coding for β lactamase production. The African strains are more sensitive to tetracycline and carry a smaller plasmid (3.2×10^6 daltons). There are also differences in nutritional requirements between the strains. In the Far East, the R plasmid has spread to a variety of strains and transmissibility seems to be higher than in African strains. In January, 1976, 5–7.5 per cent of strains isolated in Liverpool were β lactamase producers, but isolates of resistant strains fell almost to nil in 1977 (CDR 1977b). This reduction suggested a local epidemic controlled by good contact tracing and treatment, but it may also be partly due to the absence of a conjugative plasmid. The β lactamase has similar nucleotide sequences to the β lactamase from $H.$ $influenzae$ and the TEM lactamase of $E.$ $coli$ (Elwell et al, 1977a). The substrate profile of the β lactamase from the Liverpool strains is also similar to the TEM enzyme (Percival et al, 1976).

Transfer of resistance in gonococci seems to be due to conjugation (Kirven and Thornsberry, 1977), which is rather surprising. Although gonococci are gram-negative, they behave in many ways as gram-positive cocci and not as gram-negative bacilli, particularly in respect to antibiotic sensitivities. Gram-positive cocci tend to transfer plasmids infrequently and by transduction. The R factor may have been acquired from $E.$ $coli$ perhaps in ano-rectal lesions. The other possibility is that it was acquired from $H.$ $influenzae$ or ampicillin-resistant coliforms in oro-pharyngeal lesions. Other antibiotics are available for treating gonorrhoea, e.g. amingolycosides and spectinamycin (Wilkinson, 1977). Spectinamycin resistance has been described and its use should be kept whenever possible to the treatment of penicillin-resistant organisms. Some of the newer cephalosporins may also be useful, particularly cefuroxime (Phillips et al, 1976).

Neisseria meningitidis (meningococci)
Resistance to penicillin has not been reported in this organism, but the opportunity of acquiring a β lactamase plasmid is always present. This likelihood has increased with the appearance of ampicillin-resistant $H.$ $influenzae$ and particularly gonococci in oro-pharyngeal lesions. Good surveillance is necessary to detect resistant strains or some patients may well die in the future, due to inappropriate initial therapy. The incidence of sulphonamide-resistant strains also varies in different countries, as well as in different parts of the same country, and also with different strains of the organisms. Of 323 strains tested in England in 1976, 13 per cent showed an MIC of over 50 μg/ml (CDR, 1977a). Infections are usually treated with benzylpenicillin, but sulphonamides are still useful for treating carriers and contacts. Early identification of sulphonamide-resistant strains is, therefore, of some importance. Problems of meningococcal infections are dealt with in Chapter 5.

Staphylococcus aureus

The problem of multiple-resistant *Staph. aureus* decreased from the early 1960's following the introduction of methicillin and its later analogues. The reason for this decrease is not certain and improved hygienic measures may also have played a role. Resistance was reported almost as soon as methicillin was introduced (Jevons, 1961) and the resistant strains showed some cross-resistance with the cephalosporins (Barber and Waterworth, 1964). Outbreaks of infection with methicillin-resistant strains were later reported from many countries, e.g. Denmark, Switzerland, United Kingdom, Poland, France, but rarely in the U.S.A. (see Lowbury and Ayliffe, 1974). The incidence of methicillin-resistant infections appeared to reach a maximum in 1970–72 and has since fallen

Table 1.1 Cross-sectional surveys: use of antibiotics and resistance of *Staph. aureus* to cloxacillin

Year	Percentage of patients* treated with		Percentage of nasal carriers* of cloxacillin-resistant *Staph. aureus*
	tetracycline	cloxacillin	
1968	11.2	1.8	0.6
1970	8.5	2.7	2.6
1974	2.8	2.4	1.0
1976	0.6	5.1	0.4
1977	0.6	3.0	0.0

*1000–2000 patients a year

(Rosendal et al, 1977; Parker, M. T., personal communication) despite the continuing high use of penicillinase-resistant penicillins and cephalosporins. The reduced incidence has also been associated with a reduction in tetracycline-resistance and in the use of tetracycline (Parker et al, 1974; Mouton, Glerum and Van Loenen, 1976; Rosendal et al, 1977). A similar reduction in methicillin-resistant strains in patients noses was found in cross-sectional surveys of hospitals in Birmingham, England; resistant strains increased to over 2.0 per cent in 1970, falling to 0.3 per cent in 1972 and nil in 1977. The reduction in tetracycline usage and use of cloxacillin in a large general hospital is shown in Table 1.1, but this fall commenced before 1970 when the incidence of methicillin-resistance was at its highest. In the Birmingham Burns Unit, a decrease in methicillin-resistant strains has recently occurred on stopping erythromycin (Lowbury, personal communication). An association between the use of an antibiotic and resistance is well known, but the reduction in the incidence of resistant strains with increasing usage of an antibiotic as with methicillin (and its analogues) is an exception.

The mechanism of methicillin-resistance is also unusual and is detected either by growth at $30°C$ or on agar containing 5 per cent salt (Parker and Hewitt, 1970; Sabath, 1977). It has been suggested by some workers that in vitro resistance is not relevant to the clinical situation (Lacey, 1974). The small amount of clinical evidence available suggests that these strains are also resistant in vivo (Acar, Courvalin and Chabbert, 1971; Benner and Kayser, 1968) and this is supported by mouse protection experiments (Ayliffe, Andrews and Williams, 1974). Controlled clinical trials are not possible in severe infections, but resistant strains were removed from burns by treatment with oral flucloxacillin in doses of 250 mgm six hourly for five days; significantly fewer strains disappeared spontaneously in untreated controls (Lowbury, Lilly and Kidson, 1977). It seems likely that 'methicillin-resistant' strains are only slightly resistant and infections might respond to higher doses of the more active compounds, e.g. flucloxacillin and some of the cephalosporins. However, the practical problem is not great at present since 'resistant' strains are now infrequent, and alternative antibiotics are available.

A reduction in multiple resistant strains since 1959 was reported initially in Seattle (Plorde and Sherris, 1974), the reduced incidence in resistance involved penicillin, tetracycline, chloramphenicol, erythromycin and kanamycin. This reduction has more recently been reported from other countries (e.g. Rosendal et al, 1977) but not necessarily a corresponding reduction in penicillin-resistant strains in hospital (Parker et al, 1974). Penicillin-resistant strains have tended to increase in the community (Goldie, Alder and Gillespie, 1971), and all infections requiring chemotherapy should now be treated with a penicillinase-resistant penicillin if sensitivity tests are not available. Co-trimoxazole is not often used for treating staphylococcal infections but resistant strains have been reported (Chattopadhay, 1977). The reduction in infections caused by multiple-resistant strains has not occurred everywhere, and small outbreaks of highly resistant strains continue to appear, although less frequently than formerly. Methicillin-resistant strains are still present in the Birmingham Burns Unit and strains resistant to fusidic acid and lincomycin in a dermatological ward (Ayliffe et al, 1977). Novobiocin-resistance is still detected in some strains, although the antibiotic has not been used for a number of years.

Resistance of *Staph. aureus* is usually controlled by plasmids and transfer by transduction has been reported in vitro and in vivo (Lacey and Richmond, 1974). The evidence of in vivo transfer in patients is usually circumstantial, and depends on evidence of varying resistance patterns in related phage-types (Ayliffe, 1970; Noble, 1972; Lacey, 1975; Wyatt et al, 1977). This commonly occurs following the topical usage of antibiotics such as neomycin or gentamicin in dermatology patients. Gentamicin resistance in *Staph. aureus* has only emerged recently in the United Kingdom, although the antibiotic has been used for a number of years (Speller et al, 1976; Bint et al, 1977; Wyatt et al, 1977). A strain resistant to methicillin and gentamicin has also caused problems in a London hospital (Kensit and Shanson, 1976). Although parenteral gentamicin is not usually required for treating staphylococcal infections, it is a good antibiotic to keep in reserve, and is useful for preliminary treatment of severe infections before the causative organism is identified.

Intestinal pathogens
Since transferable resistance was initially detected in strains of *Sh. flexneri* in Japan, multi-resistant strains of shigella and salmonella have been reported from all over the world (see Lowbury and Ayliffe, 1974). *Sh. sonnei*, although usually causing mild infections, are often resistant to ampicillin and resistance is usually transferable (Davies, Farrant and Uttley, 1970; Ross, Cantoni and Khan, 1972; Gordon et al, 1975; Robinson, 1976). Resistance of shigella and salmonella to

ampicillin probably corresponds to the high usage of the antibiotic in some countries (Weissman, Gangarosa and Dupont, 1973; Neu et al, 1975; Byers, Dupont and Goldschmidt, 1976).

An extensive epidemic of chloramphenicol-resistant *Sh. dysenteriae* type 1 emerged in Central America in 1968. This organism had not been isolated in major outbreaks for several decades and the new epidemic was explosive with severe infections and a high mortality (Levine et al, 1970). The organisms were mainly sensitive to ampicillin, but resistant to tetracycline, streptomycin and sulphonamide in addition to chloramphenicol. A further possible connection with this epidemic was reported in the U.S.A. in family outbreaks of *Sh. flexneri* types 2A and 6. Infections were again severe and the organisms showed a similar antibiotic sensitivity pattern to the *Sh. dysenteriae* strains (Gangarosa et al, 1972). Chloramphenicol-resistant strains of *S. typhi* were occasionally reported in India and Africa, and resistance was sometimes transferable (see Lowbury and Ayliffe, 1974). Resistance in strains isolated in Kuwait in 1967 (Anderson and Smith, 1972) was transferable, and involved both ampicillin and chloramphenicol. Nevertheless, there was not much cause for general concern until the Mexico outbreak in 1972 (Gangarosa et al, 1972). This epidemic differed from others in its long duration, the large number of people infected (over 10 000) and its wide geographical extent. Resistance was transferable and the resistance pattern was the same as in the shigella strains of the previous epidemic. Although it seemed likely that the plasmid was the same one, later studies showed that it was not (Datta and Olarte, 1974). The 'R' factor in the Mexican *S. typhi* strain was identified as belonging to a plasmid compatibility group H which has been subdivided into H_1 and H_2 (Grindley, Humphreys and Anderson, 1973; Anderson, 1975). The plasmids are large (120×10^6 daltons) and the H_1 plasmids found in the *S. typhi* strains are rather unstable and are transferred at increased frequency at temperatures of 22–28°C. Transfer at lower temperatures than usual suggest that it could occur in the environment, such as sewage, and may be of relevance to the extensive spread of the disease (Smith, 1974). All the strains in the Mexican outbreak also showed a similar Vi phage type suggesting they arose from a single clone. Other outbreaks of chloramphenicol-resistant *S. typhi* containing the H_1R factor have been isolated in other parts of the world (Anderson, 1975). Typing has shown that a single but different clone was involved in strains from India (Paniker and Vimala, 1972), whereas strains from the Far East (Butler et al, 1973; Lampe, Mansuwan and Duangmani, 1974; Brown, Duong Hong Mo and Rhoades, 1975) were of different Vi phage types. As well as in *S. typhi*, H_1R factors have been found in strains of *S. typhimurium* isolated in the Far East and Europe. Strains were sensitive to chloramphenicol, but carried resistance determinants to ampicillin, tetracycline and often kanamycin. These studies suggest a widespread distribution of H_1R factors, indicating they are probably common in non-pathogenic intestinal organisms. Patients infected with chloramphenicol-resistant strains of *S. typhi* imported from endemic areas have been reported in the U.S.A., Canada, United Kingdom and other countries, but the Mexican epidemic has ceased and the chloramphenicol resistant R factor seems to have disappeared (Balows, 1977). This may be related to the possible instability of the R factor. The Mexican strains were ampicillin-sensitive, but resistance has emerged in patients (Cohen, 1973) in the U.S.A. and elsewhere. The hazard of major outbreaks of ampicillin and chloramphenicol resistant strains of *S. typhi* and *Sh. dysenteriae* is, therefore, no longer a theoretical possibility but a reality.

Typhoid fever can be treated effectively with other agents, particularly co-trimoxazole (Geddes and Goodall, 1972; Gilman et al, 1975). However, trimethoprim resistance may occur and has already been associated with an 'R' factor in enterobacteriaciae (Fleming, Datta and Gruneberg, 1972). Other anti-biotics may also be effective, e.g. mecillinam (Geddes and Clark, 1977), but loss of availability of chloramphenicol and ampicillin in the treatment of enteric fever could be a serious defect in our therapeutic resources.

Cholera is still endemic in some countries and spread outside these areas has often occurred in recent years. Although replacement of fluids is the mainstay of treatment, antibiotics are often necessary. The El Tor biotype was initially sensitive to antibiotics, but the incidence of infection with resistant strains has increased (O'Grady, Lewis and Pearson, 1976). A plasmid of compatibility group C with varying resistance patterns has been identified. The plasmid is found in a range of organisms, especially providencia (Hedges et al, 1977). The common pattern of resistance to streptomycin, tetracycline, chloramphenicol and sulphonamide is similar to that in many shigella and salmonella strains; resistance to ampicillin is uncommon.

Mycobacterium tuberculosis

Pulmonary tuberculosis is still a common disease in the world, and in some areas of Africa, India and the Far East an incidence of 200–250 cases per 100 000 population has been reported (Fox, 1977). The incidence has also increased in the United Kingdom due to importation by the immigrant population and about 450 new cases a year are detected in Birmingham, England (Morrison-Smith, 1975). Initial resistance to the commonly used drugs has not shown any major changes in recent years in most of the economically advanced countries and is about 4–6 per cent. It is much higher in some areas, e.g. 20–30 per cent in Hong Kong. The incidence of acquired resistance is falling in most advanced countries, but more slowly in many developing countries (Horne, 1969). However, the main reason for treatment failure is still incomplete or ineffective treatment and not the emergence of resistant strains.

Recent developments in treatment have been concerned mainly with shorter courses, less frequent administration of drugs, and new regimes involving rifampicin, pyrazinamide and ethambutol (Fox and Mitchison, 1975; Angel, 1977). The standard course of treatment consisting of streptomycin, isoniazid (INAH) and para-amino salicylic acid (PAS) for two years or more is still effective. Shorter courses should reduce costs and toxicity problems, but in particular will increase the likelihood of completion of courses. Relapses on 6-month courses with bac-tericidal drugs (rifampicin, streptomycin and pyrazinamide) are few, and in the short courses relapses are mainly due to sensitive organisms that have not been eradicated. In the E. African studies (East Africa/BMRC, 1974), 68/73 relapses were due to sensitive strains. Evidence from other countries confirm the efficiency of short courses of 6–12 months with varying drug combination regimes (Fox,

1977). It seems likely that a 9–12 month course would be preferable in the economically advanced countries since it is more reliable.

The efficacy of treatment and emergence of resistant strains is mainly assessed by sensitivity tests. Nevertheless, changes in treatment based on the results of sensitivity tests on initial isolates have to be carefully considered for several reasons.

1. Tests are not necessarily reliable and should be carried out only in specialised laboratories (Canetti et al, 1969).
2. Pre-existing mutants may be present in the early stages of an infection and may be eliminated at a later stage without changing the therapy (transitional resistance).
3. The second line drugs are often more toxic and usually more expensive.

In a study in Hong Kong (Hong Kong/BMRC, 1974), a comparison of patients treated without sensitivity testing with another series in which therapy was changed on the basis of sensitivity tests showed very little difference in failure rate. Initial resistance of organisms was high (20 per cent) in the study yet the proportion of patients failing due to pre-treatment drug resistance was small in both groups. In countries where initial resistance rates are low, the advantages of treating on the basis of sensitivity tests would be even less. However, the occasional patient might benefit since failure of treatment is likely to be much higher if the strain is resistant to two of the three drugs used in treatment.

The influence of initial drug resistance might be greater in shorter courses. In the East African studies (E. African/BMRC, 1974) initial resistance was fairly low (i.e. about 8.0 per cent resistant to one drug and 1.2 per cent resistant to two drugs) and the estimated failure rates probably due to resistant organisms was about 2 per cent. This was similar to the Hong Kong study using conventional treatment. The Hong Kong studies on short courses (Hong Kong/BMRC, 1975) showed a greater difference estimated at about 7–8 per cent failure due to resistant organisms. The initial resistance rate was much higher (21.2 per cent) but rifampicin was not included in the therapy. If these short courses are used, the selected regime should be based on initial resistance rates found in the population of the area concerned. If the initial resistance to standard drugs is high, rifampicin and pro-bably pyrazinamide should be included in regimes (Fox, 1977). Resistance to rifampicin emerging during treatment was reported in the early days of its use, but this appears to be rare even in countries where it is widely used (Acoccella, Hamilton-Miller and Brumfitt, 1977). It is rather an expensive drug and has some toxic side-effects which limit its usage at present; short courses of intermittent therapy or inclusion in the first part of a longer course is reasonably safe and will considerably decrease costs. Widespread uncontrolled use may be associated with increasing emergence of resistance and may reduce the value of one of the most effective drugs against tuberculosis. Wherever possible it should only be used in the treatment of tuberculosis (Morrison-Smith, 1975) and leprosy (Waters et al, 1978). Surveillance remains important even in countries where infections are in-frequent. Inadequate treatment of a patient may be associated with a number of secondary infections. This is particularly hazardous if the original strain is resistant to the standard drugs (Blakey, 1977).

CONCLUSIONS

A disturbing feature recently has been the emergence of significant resistance in strains which have previously been sensitive to an antibiotic for many years. Some of these resistant organisms such as penicillin-resistant pneumococci have so far remained localised in certain countries, and treatment still remains predictable in other parts of the world. Spread from country to country occurs with readily communicable organisms, such as penicillin-resistant gonococci, and careful surveillance is particularly necessary. With less communicable organisms, transfer by infected or colonised subjects is not a good explanation for simultaneous appearance of similar organisms in several different countries at the same time. For instance *Staph. aureus* acquires resistance to antibiotics rapidly, but resistance did not emerge to neomycin until about ten years after its introduction. Resistant strains were then reported at about the same time in several parts of the world including Australia, U.S.A. and Europe. A similar delay in emergence of resistance has occurred with gentamicin resistance. Methicillin-resistant *Staph. aureus* have been described in Enterobacteriaceae, *H. influenzae*, *N. gonorrhoeae* and *Ps.* and widespread use of penicillinase-resistant penicillins or cephalosporins. Although knowledge of mechanisms of resistance has considerably increased, the reason for differences in geographical behaviour are still uncertain.

Another source of anxiety is the possibility of an increase in readily transmissible R plasmids. The $H_1 R$ factor has been identified in strains of *S. typhi* in Mexico, India and the Far East as well as in *S. typhimurium*. R factors may also be associated with increased virulence as has been suggested in the South American outbreak of *Sh. dysenteriae*. A single type of plasmid or transposable gene has been described in enterobacteriaceae, *H. influenzae*, *N. gonorrhoeae* and *Ps. aeruginosa* (Datta, 1977), and could well spread to other important primary pathogens such as *N. meningitidis*, brucella or yersinia. The widespread appearance of the $H_1 R$ factor and the TEM gene or plasmid suggests that a large silent pool of similar R plasmids or transposons might be present in the normal flora of individuals throughout the world.

Since R plasmids are selected by antibiotics, the plasmid population is probably higher in developing countries. Whereas the occasional outbreak of typhoid or penicillin-resistant gonorrhoea in Europe or America is due to one strain and can be controlled, the resistant organisms in the developing countries tend to consist of a variety of different types.

On the credit side, resistance problems in *Staph. aureus* have not increased as predicted, and multiple and methicillin resistance has been decreasing. However, highly resistant strains still appear and could cause outbreaks in hospitals in the developing countries as occurred previously in Europe and U.S.A. in 1950–65. Resistance is not yet an important problem with most of the other primary pathogens, although tetracycline-resistance has been described in brucella and dapsone-resistance occurs in *M. leprae* (Waters et al, 1978).

As well as isolation and effective treatment of known patients infected with resistant strains, it is important to detect carriers or subclinical infections. The termination of the outbreak of infections caused by penicillinase-producing gonococci in the Liverpool area was an example of effective contact tracing and treatment of infections. Surveys in hospitals are still required to detect carriers of highly resistant *Staph. aureus* when an infection is first identified. Major outbreaks of *S. typhi* and severe dysentery or cholera occur in countries with poor hygienic standards, housing conditions and sewage disposal; improvements in these standards is obviously an urgent requirement. Unfortunately in many of these countries antibiotics are easily obtained without prescription and this accounts for the high rates of chloramphenicol resistance (Leading Article, 1975). World-wide agreement on the principles of antibiotic usage and their rational use would be a major step forward. Antibiotic treatment of most shigella or salmonella infections (apart from enteric fever) is usually unnecessary. Topical use of antibiotics is commonly associated with the emergence of resistance in *Staph. aureus* and gram-negative bacilli. Topical gentamicin should be avoided if possible since important systemic pathogens such as *Pseudomonas aeruginosa* may acquire resistance.

Most of the organisms are resistant because of the plasmids they carry. These plasmids are often unstable and may be lost, particularly if there is no antibiotic selective pressure to maintain them. Instead of concentrating on modifying existing antibiotics, it may be more advantageous in the long term to look for agents that will eliminate the plasmids from bacterial cells, or prevent their transfer from one organism to another.

The emergence of resistance to commonly used antibiotics in strains causing severe infections acquired in the community has accentuated the need for rapid detection of resistance. Infections by *H. influenzae*, *N. meningitidis* or *N. gonorrhoeae* can no longer be treated predictably. Although the incidence of resistant strains is generally low, failure to identify resistance may result in death from meningitis or pneumonia, or may allow an epidemic situation to develop without it being recognised at an early stage. Since β lactamase is often involved, interests in tests have been revived. β lactamase can be rapidly detected when the organism has grown after 18 hours incubation and a result should be available within 18–24 hours. Earlier detection during initial growth of the organism in the laboratory may also be possible. Surveillance for resistant strains is obviously important and isolations should be reported to a central agency such as the Communicable Diseases Surveillance Centre in the U.K. or Centre for Disease Control in the U.S.A.

Prevention of spread is also necessary. Although there is little disagreement about the isolation of a patient with typhoid, which is unlikely to spread in a hospital ward, it may be difficult to persuade clinicians to isolate patients with pneumococcal pneumonia. Nevertheless, the experience of the South African hospitals show that strains of resistant pneumococci can be readily transmissible. Patients carrying *S. aureus* resistant to methicillin, gentamicin, fusidic acid or lincomycin should also be isolated even in the absence of clinical infection. Although these resistant strains are still infrequent, hospitals should be provided with an isolation unit to accommodate such patients when they appear.

Antibiotic-resistant non-pathogens as well as pathogens in animals are another world-wide problem and the hazards have frequently been discussed by Anderson (1975) and others. Policies for the rational use of antibiotics in the treatment of infection in animals are as necessary as in humans, and antibiotics important for treating human infections should be excluded from animal feeds.

The principles of control of spread of resistant organisms are similar to those of any communicable disease, i.e. good surveillance, rapid detection, isolation of infected patients, good hygiene, treatment of carriers and possibly contacts, and possibly an antibiotic policy. (see Lowbury et al, 1975). The essential difference is a change of emphasis involving not only a consideration of transmissibility of organisms, but of antibiotic resistance patterns and the possibility of spread of plasmids or genes. The investigations of plasmid (or transposable gene) epidemics suggest a future requirement for new typing techniques (Chabbert and Roussel, 1977). The development of vaccines for the prevention of gonorrhoea (Leading Article 1977a), pneumococcal infections, and others should also help to reduce problems of resistant strains.

REFERENCES

Acar, J. F., Courvalin, P. & Chabbert, Y. A. (1971) Methicillin-resistant staphylococcaemia: Bacteriological failure of treatment with cephalosporins. Antimicrobial Agents and Chemotherapy, 1970. *American Society for Microbiology*, 280–285. Proceedings of 10th Interscience Conference on Antimicrobial Agents and Chemotherapy, Chicago, 1970, ed. Hobby, Gladys L.)

Acocella, G., Hamilton-Miller, J. M. T. & Brumfitt, W. (1977) Can rifampicin use be safely extended? *Lancet*, **2**, 740–742.

Anderson, E. S. (1968) Drug resistance in *Salmonella typhi murium* and its implications. *British Medical Journal*, **3**, 333–339.

Anderson, E. S. (1975) The problem and implications of chloramphenicol resistance in the typhoid bacillus. *Journal of Hygiene*, **74**, 289–299.

Anderson, E. S. & Smith, H. R. (1972) Chloramphenicol resistance in the typhoid bacillus. *British Medical Journal*, **3**, 329–331.

Anderson, J. D., Gillespie, W. A. & Richmond, M. H. (1973) Chemotherapy and antibiotic resistance transfer between enterobacteria in the human gastro-intestinal tract. *Journal of Medical Microbiology*, **6**, 461–473.

Andrews, J., Bywater, M. J., Emmerson, A. M., Keane, C., Reeves, D. S. & Wise, R. (1975) The prevalence of ampicillin, cephalosporin and sulphonamide resistance amongst urinary tract pathogens. *Scottish Medical Journal*, **20**, 232–235.

Angel, J. H. (1977) Short course chemotherapy in pulmonary tuberculosis. *Journal of Antimicrobial Chemotherapy*, **4**, 290–293.

Appelbaum, P. C., Bhamjee, A., Scragg, J. N., Hallett, A. E., Bowen, A. & Cooper, R. C. (1977) *Streptococcus pneumoniae* resistant to penicillin and chloramphenicol. *Lancet*, **2**, 995–997.

Ayliffe, G. A. J. (1970) Stability of neomycin resistance in *Staphylococcus aureus*. *Journal of Clinical Pathology*, **23**, 19–23.

Ayliffe, G. A. J. (1975) Antibiotic policies. *Journal of Antimicrobial Chemotherapy*, **1**, 255–257.

Ayliffe, G. A. J., Andrews, J. & Williams, J. D. (1974) Methicillin-resistant *Staph. aureus*. *Lancet*, **1**, 573.

Ayliffe, G. A. J., Green, W., Livingstone, R. & Lowbury, E. J. L. (1977) Antibiotic-resistant *Staphylococcus aureus* in dermatology and burn wards. *Journal of Clinical Pathology*, **30**, 40–44.

Balows, A. (1977) An overview of recent experiences with plasmid-mediated antibiotic-resistance or induced virulence in bacterial diseases. *Journal of Antimicrobial Chemotherapy*, **3**, Supplement C, 3–6.

Barber, M. & Waterworth, P. M. (1964) Penicillinase-resistant penicillins and cephalosporins. *British Medical Journal*, **2**, 344–349.

Barrett, F. F., Taber, L. H., Jones, J. F. & Thornsberry, C. (1972) A twelve year review of the antibiotic management of *Haemophilus influenzae* meningitis. *Journal of Paediatrics*, **81**, 370–377.

Benner, E. J. & Kayser, F. H. (1968) Growing clinical significance of methicillin-resistant *Staphylococcus aureus*. *Lancet*, **2**, 741–744.

Bint, A. J., George, R. H., Healing, D. E., Wise, R. & Davies, M. (1977) An outbreak of infection caused by a gentamicin-resistant *Staph. aureus*. *Journal of Clinical Pathology*, **30**, 165–167.

Blakey, D. L. (1977) Drug-resistant tuberculosis-Mississippi. *Morbidity and Mortality Weekly Report*, **26**, 417–418, 423.

Brown, J. D., Duong Hong Mo & Rhoades, E. R. (1975) Chloramphenicol-resistant *Salmonella typhi* in Saigon. *Journal of American Medical Association*, **231**, 162–166.

Butler, T., Link, N. N., Arnold, K. & Pollack, M. (1973) Chloramphenicol-resistant typhoid fever in Vietnam associated with an R factor. *Lancet*, **2**, 983–985.

Byers, P. A., Dupont, H. L. & Goldschmidt, M. C. (1976) Antimicrobial susceptibility of shigella isolated in Houston, Texas in 1974. *Antimicrobial Agents and Chemotherapy*, **9**, 281–291.

Canetti, G., Fox, W., Khomenko, A., Mahler, H. T., Menon, N. K., Mitchison, D. A., Rist, N. & Smelev, N. A. (1969) Advances in techniques in testing mycobacterial drug sensitivity and the use of sensitivity tests in tuberculosis control programmes. *Bulletin of World Health Organisation*, **41**, 21–43.

Chabbert, Y. A. & Roussel, A. (1977) Taxonomy and epidemiology of R plasmids as molecular species. *Journal of Antimicrobial Chemotherapy*, **3**, Supplement C, 25–33.

Chattopadhay, B. (1977) Co-trimoxazole-resistant *Staphylococcus aureus* in hospital practice. *Journal of Antimicrobial Chemotherapy*, **3**, 371–373.

Clymo, A. B. & Harper, I. A. (1974) Ampicillin-resistant *Haemophilus influenzae*. *Lancet*, **1**, 313.

Cohen, S. N. (1973) Chloramphenicol-ampicillin resistant *Salmonella typhi* in California. *Morbidity and Mortality Weekly Report*, **22**, 183.

Communicable Disease Report (1977a) Meningococcal meningitis. *British Medical Journal*, **1**, 1671.

Communicable Disease Report (1977b) Penicillinase-producing gonococci in Liverpool, 77/19.

Datta, N. (1969) Drug resistance and R factors in the bowel bacteria of London patients before and after admission to hospital. *British Medical Journal*, **2**, 407–411.

Datta, N. (1977) Classification of plasmids as an aid to understanding their epidemiology and evolution. *Journal of Antimicrobial Chemotherapy*, **3**, Supplement C, 19–23.

Datta, N. & Olarte, J. (1974) R factors in strains of *Salmonella typhi* and *Shigella dysenteriae* type 1 isolated during epidemics in Mexico. *Antimicrobial Agents and Chemotherapy*, **5**, 310–317.

Davies, J. R., Farrant, W. N. & Uttley, A. H. C. (1970) Antibiotic resistance of *Shigella sonnei*. *Lancet*, **2**, 1157–1159.

Dixon, J. M. S. (1967) Pneumococcus resistant to erythromycin and lincomycin. *Lancet*, **1**, 573.

Dixon, J. M. S. (1974) Pneumococcus with increased resistance to penicillin. *Lancet*, **2**, 474.

Dixon, J. M. S. & Lipinski, A. E. (1974) Infections with β-haemolytic streptococcus resistant to lincomycin and erythromycin and observations on zonal-pattern resistance to lincomycin. *Journal of Infectious Diseases*, **130**, 351–356.

East African/British Medical Research Council, 1974. Controlled clinical trial of four short-course (6 month) regimens of chemotherapy for treatment of pulmonary tuberculosis. *Lancet*, **2**, 236–240, 1100–1106.

Elwell, L. P., Roberts, M., Mayer, L. W. & Falkhow, S. (1977a) Plasmid-mediated beta-lactamase production in *Neisseria gonorrhoeae*. *Antimicrobial Agents and Chemotherapy*, **11**, 528–533.

Elwell, L. P., Saunders, J. R., Richmond, M. H. & Falkhow, S. (1977b) Relationships among some R plasmids found in *Haemophilus influenzae*. *Journal of Bacteriology*, **131**, 356–362.

Emslie, J. A. N. (1974) Tetracycline-resistant Group A streptococci. *British Medical Journal*, **3**, 467.

Evans, W. & Hansman, D. (1963). Tetracycline-resistant pneumococcus. *Lancet*, **i**, 451.

Fallon, R. J. (1976) *Haemophilus influenzae* meningitis. *Journal of Antimicrobial Chemotherapy*, **2**, 3.

Finland, M., Garner, C., Wilcox, C. & Sabath, L. D. (1976) Susceptibility of pneumococci and *Haemophilus influenzae* to antibacterial agents. *Antimicrobial Agents and Chemotherapy*, **9**, 274–287.

Fleming, M. P., Datta, N. & Gruneberg, R. N. (1972) Trimethoprim resistance determined by R factors. *British Medical Journal*, **1**, 726–728.

Fox, W. (1977) The modern management and therapy of pulmonary tuberculosis. *Proceedings of the Royal Society of Medicine*, **70**, 4–15.

Fox, W. & Mitchison, D. A. (1975) Short course chemotherapy for pulmonary tuberculosis. *American Review of Respiratory Disease*, **111**, 325–353.

Gangarosa, E. J., Bennett, J. V., Wyatt, C., Pierce, P. E., Olorte, J., Hernandes, P. M., Vasquez, V. & Bessudo, M. D. (1972) An epidemic associated episome? *Journal of Infectious Diseases*, **126**, 215–218.

Garrod, L. P., Lambert, H. P. & O'Grady, F. 'Antibiotic and Chemotherapy'. Edinburgh & London: Churchill Livingstone (1973).

Geddes, A. M. & Clarke, P. D. (1977) The treatment of enteric fever with mecillinam. *Journal of Antimicrobial Chemotherapy*, **3**, Supplement B, 101–102.

Geddes, A. M. & Goodall, J. A. D. (1972) Chloramphenicol resistance in the typhoid bacillus. *British Medical Journal*, **3**, 329–331.

Gilman, R. H., Terminel, M., Levine, M. M., Hermandez-Mendozoa, P., Calderone, E., Vasquez, V., Martinez, E., Snyder, M. J. & Homick, R. B. (1975) Comparison of trimethoprim-sulfamethoxazole and amoxycillin in therapy of chloramphenicol-resistant and chloramphenicol-sensitive typhoid fever. *Journal of Infectious Diseases*, **132**, 630–636.

Goldie, D. J., Alder, V. G. & Gillespie, W. A. (1971) Changes in the drug resistance of *Staphylococcus aureus* in a non hospital population during a 20 year period. *Journal of Clinical Pathology*, **24**, 44–47.

Gopalakrishna, K. V. & Lerner, P. I. (1973) Tetracycline-resistant pneumococci. Increasing incidence and cross-resistance to newer tetracyclines. *American Review of Respiratory Diseases*, **108**, 1007–1010.

Gordon, R. C., Thompson, T. R., Carlson, W., Dyke, J. W. & Stevens, L. I. (1975) Antimicrobial resistance of shigella isolated in Michigan. *Journal of American Medical Association*, **231**, 1159–1161.

Grindley, N. D. F., Humphreys, G. O. & Anderson, E. S. (1973) Molecular studies of R factor compatibility groups. *Journal of Bacteriology*, **115**, 387–398.

Gunn, B. A., Woodall, J. B., Jones, J. F. & Thornsberry, C. (1974) Ampicillin-resistant *Haemophilus influenzae*. *Lancet*, **2**, 845.

Hansman, D. & Bullen, M. M. (1967) A resistant pneumococcus. *Lancet*, **2**, 264–265.

Hedges, R. W. & Jacob, A. E. (1974) Transposition of ampicillin-resistance from RP4 to other replicons. *Molecular and General Genetics*, **132**, 31–40.

Hedges, R. W., Vialand, J. L., Pearson, N. J. & O'Grady, F. (1977) R plasmids from Asian strains of *Vibrio Cholerae*. *Antimicrobial Agents and Chemotherapy*, **11**, 585–588.

Hong Kong Tuberculosis Service/British Medical Research Council (1974) A study in Hong Kong to evaluate the role of pre-treatment susceptibility tests in the selection of regimens of chemotherapy for pulmonary tuberculosis. Second report. *Tubercle*, **55**, 169–192.

Hong Kong Tuberculosis Service/British Medical Research Council (1975) Controlled trial of 6 and 9 months regimens of daily and intermittent streptomycin plus ioniazid plus pyrazinamide for pulmonary tuberculosis in Hong Kong. *Tubercle*, **56**, 81–96.

Horne, N. W. (1969) Drug-resistant tuberculosis: a review of the world situation. *Tubercle*, **50**, Supplement 2–12.

Howard, A. J. (1977) Ampicillin-resistance in *Haemophilus influenzae*. *Journal of Antimicrobial Chemotherapy*, **3**, 535–537.

Howes, V. & Mitchell, R. G. (1976) Meningitis due to relatively penicillin-resistant pneumococcus. *British Medical Journal*, **1**, 996.

Jevons, M. P. (1961) 'Celbenin'-resistant staphylococci. *British Medical Journal*, **1**, 124–126.

Kensit, J. G. & Shanson, D. C. (1976) Gentamicin resistance in methicillin-sensitive and resistant *Staphylococcus aureus*. *Journal of Antimicrobial Chemotherapy*, **2**, 311–312.

Kirven, L. A., & Thornsberry, C. (1977). Transfer of Beta-lactamase genes of *Neisseria gonorrhoeae* by conjugation. *Antimicrobial Agents and Chemotherapy*, **11**, 1004–1006.

Kohn, J., Hewitt, J. H., Fraser, C. A. M. (1968) Group A streptococci resistant to lincomycin. *British Medical Journal*, **1**, 703.

Koornhof, H. J., Jacobs, M., Isaacson, M., Appelbaum, P., Miller, B., Stevenson, C. M., Freeman, I., Daude, A., Bothna, P., Geathaar, E. & Gilliland, J. (1978) *Morbidity and Mortality Weekly Report*, **271**, 7.

Lacey, R. W. (1974) Can methicillin-resistant strains of *Staphylococcus aureus* be treated with methicillin? *Lancet*, **1**, 88.

Lacey, R. W. (1975) Antibiotic-resistance plasmids of *Staphylococcus aureus*. *Bacteriological Reviews*, **39**, 1–32.

Lacey, R. W. & Richmond, M. H. (1974) The genetic basis of antibiotic resistance in *S. aureus*. The importance of gene transfer in the evolution of this organism in the hospital environment. *Annals of the New York Academy of Sciences*, **236**, 395–410.

Lampe, R. M., Mansuwan, D. & Duangmani, C. (1974) Chloramphenicol-resistant typhoid. *Lancet*, **i**, 623–624.

Leading Article (1975) Antibiotics at risk. *British Medical Journal*, **2**, 582.

Leading article (1977a) A vaccine against gonorrhoea. *British Medical Journal*, **3**, 917–918.

Leading article (1977b) Resistant pneumococci. *Lancet*, **2**, 804–805.

Levine, M. M., Dupond, H. L., Formals, B. & Gangarosa, E. J. (1970) Epidemic shiga dysentery in Central America. *Lancet*, **2**, 607–608.

Lowbury, E. J. L. & Ayliffe, G. A. J. (1974) Drug resistance in antimicrobial therapy. Springfield, Illinois: Charles C. Thomas.

Lowbury, E. J. L. & Cason, J. S. (1954) Aureomycin and erythromycin therapy for *Str. pyogenes* in burns. *British Medical Journal*, **2**, 914–915.

Lowbury, E. J. L. & Kidson, A. (1968) Group A streptococci resistant to lincomycin. *British Medical Journal*, **2**, 490–491.

Lowbury, E. J. L. & Miller, R. W. S. (1962) Treatment of infected burns with BRL 1621. *Lancet*, **2**, 640–641.

Lowbury, E. J. L., Ayliffe, G. A. J., Geddes, A. M. & Williams, J. D. (eds) (1975) *Control of Hospital Infection*. A practical handbook. London: Chapman & Hall.

Lowbury, E. J. L., Lilly, H. A. & Kidson, A. (1977) 'Methicillin'-resistant *Staphylococcus aureus*: reassessment by controlled trial in burns unit. *British Medical Journal*, **1**, 1054–1056.

Madeiros, A. A. & O'Brien, R. F. (1975) Ampicillin-resistant *Haemophilus influenzae*. *Lancet*, **1**, 716–718.

Maier, T. W., Beilstein, H. R. & Zubrzycki, L. (1974) Multiple antibiotic resistance in *Neisseria gonorrhoeae*. *Antimicrobial Agents and Chemotherapy*, **6**, 22–28.

Manten, A., Van-Klingeren, B. & Dessens-Kroon, M. (1976) Chloramphenicol resistance in *Haemophilus influenzae*. *Lancet*, **1**, 702.

Mathew, M. & Hedges, R. W. (1976) Analytical isoelectric focussing of R factor determined β lactamases: correlation with plasmid compatibility. *Journal of Bacteriology*, **125**, 713–718.

Morrison-Smith, J. (1975) Rifampicin in clinical use. *Journal of Antimicrobial Chemotherapy*, **1**, 353–354.

Morbidity and Mortality Weekly Report (1976a) Penicillinase-producing *Neisseria gonorrhoea*, **25**, 261.

Morbidity and Mortality Weekly Report (1976b) Chloramphenicol-resistant *Haemophilus influenzae*, **25**, 385–386.

Mouton, R. P., Glerum, J. H. & Van Loenen (1976) Relationship between antibiotic consumption and frequency of antibiotic resistance of four pathogens—a seven year survey. *Journal of Antimicrobial Chemotherapy*, **2**, 9–19.

Nelson, J. D. (1974) Should ampicillin be abandoned for treatment of *Haemophilus influenzae* disease. *Journal of the American Medical Association*, **229**, 322–323.

Neu, H. C., Cherubin, C. E., Longo, E. D., Flouton, B. & Winter, J. (1975) Antimicrobial resistance and R factor transfer among isolates of salmonella in the north-eastern United States: a comparison of human and animal isolates. *Journal of Infectious Diseases*, **132**, 617–622.

Noble, W. C. (1972) Loss of antibiotic-resistance in staphylococci from a skin hospital. *Lancet*, **1**, 929–931.

Noy, J. H., Ayliffe, G. A. J. & Linton, K. B. (1974) Antibiotic-resistant gram-negative bacilli in the faeces of neonates. *Journal of Medical Microbiology*, **7**, 509–520.

O'Callaghan, C. H., Morris, A. & Kirby, S. M. (1972) Novel method for the detection of beta-lactamase using a chromogenic cephalosporin substrate. *Antimicrobial Agents and Chemotherapy*, **1**, 283–288.

O'Grady, F., Lewis, M. J. & Pearson, N. J. (1976) Global surveillance of antibiotic sensitivity of *Vibrio cholerae*. *Bulletin of World Health Organisation*, **54**, 181–185.

Paniker, C. K. J. & Vimala, K. W. (1972) Transferable chloramphenicol resistance in *Salmonella typhi*. *Nature* (Lond.), **239**, 109–110.

Parker, M. T., Asheshov, E. H., Hewitt, J. H., Nakhla, L. S. & Brock, B. (1974) Endemic staphylococcal infections in hospitals. *Annals of the New York Academy of Sciences*, **236**, 466–484.

Parker, M. T. & Hewitt, J. H. (1970) Methicillin-resistance in *Staphylococcus aureus*, *Lancet*, **1**, 800–804.

Percival, A., Armstrong, C. & Turner, G. C. (1969). Increased incidence of tetracycline-resistant pneumococci in Liverpool in 1968. *Lancet*, **1**, 998–1000.

Percival, A., Corkhill, J. E., Arya, O. P., Rowlands, J., Alergamt, C. D., Rees, E. & Annels, E. H. (1976) Penicillinase-producing gonococci in Liverpool. *Lancet*, **2**, 1379–1382.

Perine, P. L., Thornsberry, C., Schalla, W., Biddle, J., Segal, M. S., Wong, K. H. & Thompson, S. E. (1977) Evidence of two distinct types of penicillinase-producing *Neisseria gonorrhoeae*. *Lancet*, **2**, 993–995.

Phillips, I. (1976) β lactamase producing penicillin-resistant gonococci. *Lancet*, **2**, 656–657.

Phillips, I., King, A., Warren, C. & Watts, B. (1976) The activity of penicillin and eight cephalosporins on *Neisseria gonorrhoeae*, **2**, 31–37.

Piot, P. (1977) Resistant gonococcus from the Ivory Coast. *Lancet*, **1**, 857.

Plorde, J. J. & Sherris, J. C. (1974) Staphylococcal resistance to antibiotics; origin, measurement and epidemiology. *Annals of the New York Academy of Sciences*, **236**, 413–434.

Report (1977) Tetracycline-resistance in pneumococci and Group A streptococci. *British Medical Journal*, **1**, 131–133.

Reyn, A., Korner, B. & Bentzon, M. W. (1968) Effect of penicillin, streptomycin and tetracycline on *N. gonorrhoaea* isolated in 1944 and 1957. *British Journal of Venereal Diseases*, **34**, 227–239.

Robertson, M. H. (1968) Tetracycline-resistant streptococci in south-west Essex: a continuous survey. *British Medical Journal*, **3**, 349–350.

Robinson, R. A. (1976) Antibiotic resistance of shigella in New Zealand. *New Zealand Medical Journal*, **83**, 81–82.

Rosendal, K., Jesson, O., Bentzon, M. W. & Bulow, P. (1977) Antibiotic policy and spread of *Staphylococcus aureus* in Danish hospitals, 1969–1974). *Acta pathologica scandinavica*, Section B, **85**, 143–152.

Ross, S., Cantroni, G. & Khan, W. (1972) Resistance of shigella to ampicillin and other antibiotics. Its clinical and epidemiological implications. *Journal of American Medical Association*, **221**, 45–47.

Sabath, L. D. (1977) Chemical and physical factors influencing methicillin resistance of *Staphylococcus aureus* and *Staphylococcus epidemidis*. *Journal of Antimicrobial Chemotherapy*, **3**, Supplement C, 47–51.

Shannon, A. & Wise, R. (1977) A comparison of three rapid methods for the detection of β lactamase activity in *Haemophilus influenzae*. *Journal of Clinical Pathology*, **30**, 1030–1032.

Smith, A. L. (1976) Antibiotics and invasive *Haemophilus influenzae*. *New England Journal of Medicine*, **294**, 1329–1331.

Smith, H. Williams (1969) Transfer of antibiotic resistance from animal and human strain of *Escherichia coli* to resident *E. coli* in the alimentary tract of man. *Lancet*, **1**, 1174–1176.

Smith, H. Williams (1974) Thermosensitive transfer factors in chloramphenicol-resistant strains of *Salmonella typhi*. *Lancet*, **2**, 281–282.

Speller, D. C. E., Stephens, M., Raghunath, D., Viant, A. C., Reeves, D. S., Wilkinson, P. J., Broughall, J. M. & Holt, H. A. (1976) Epidemic infection by a gentamicin-resistant *Staphylococcus aureus* in three hospitals. *Lancet*, **1**, 464–466.

Thomas, W. J., McReynolds, J. W., Mock, C. R. & Bailey, D. W. (1974) Ampicillin-resistant *Haemophilus influenzae*. *Lancet*, **1**, 313.

Turk, D. C. (1977) A comparison of chloramphenicol and ampicillin as bactericidal agents for *Haemophilus influenzae*. *Journal of Medical Microbiology*, **10**, 127–131.

Turner, G. C., Ratcliffe, J. G. & Anderson, D. (1976) Penicillinase-producing *Neisseria gonorrhoea*. *Lancet*, **2**, 793.

Watanabe, T. (1963) Infective heredity of multiple-drug resistance in bacteria. *Bacteriological Reviews*, **27**, 87–115.

Waters, M. F. R., Rees, R. J. W., Pearson, J. M. H., Laing, A. B. G., Helmy, H. S. & Gellia, R. H. (1978) Rifampicin for lepromatous leprosy: nine years experience. *British Medical Journal*, **1**, 133–136.

Weissman, J. B., Gangarosa, E. J. & Dupont, H. L. (1973) Changing needs in the antimicrobial therapy of shigellas. *Journal of Infectious Diseases*, **127**, 611–613.

Wilkinson, A. E. (1977) The sensitivity of gonococci to penicillin. *Journal of Antimicrobial Chemotherapy*, **3**, 197–198.

Williams, J. D. & Andrews, J. (1974) Sensitivity of *Haemophilus influenzae* to antibiotics. *British Medical Journal*, **1**, 134–137.

Williams, J. D., Kattan, S. & Cavanagh, P. (1974) Penicillinase-production in *Haemophilus influenzae*. *Lancet*, **2**, 103.

Wyatt, J. P., Ferguson, W. P., Wilson, T. S. & McCormick, E. (1977) Gentamicin-resistant *Staphylococcus aureus* associated with the use of topical gentamicin. *Journal of Antimicrobial Chemotherapy*, **3**, 213–217.

Yourrassowski, E., Schcutens, E. & Vanderlinden, M. P. (1976) Antibacterial activity of eight cephalosporins against *Haemophilus influenzae* and *Streptococcus pneumoniae*. *Journal of Antimicrobial Chemotherapy*, **2**, 55–59.

2. New antibiotics—a review

A. P. Ball and A. M. Geddes

INTRODUCTION

During the past ten years there have been relatively few major advances in the field of antibacterial chemotherapy. Most 'new' antibiotics have merely been chemical modifications of existing drugs produced with a view to improving microbiological activity, altering pharmacology or reducing toxicity.

The two major areas of interest in the treatment of bacterial infections are the problem of increasing bacterial resistance and new knowledge about adverse reactions. Bacterial resistance may be due to a number of factors. Transferable (plasmid-mediated) resistance is now well documented and there is increasing information about the importance of antibiotic-inactivating enzymes, particularly those which inactivate the beta-lactam antibiotics and the aminoglycosides.

The present paper reviews the major groups of antibiotics with particular reference to new agents introduced during the past five years.

THE PENICILLINS

The ampicillins

Ampicillin was the first penicillin claimed to be 'broad-spectrum', having activity against certain Gram-negative bacilli and also Gram-positive and Gram-negative cocci. Since it was introduced almost 15 years ago ampicillin has been extensively used, and abused, both in hospital and general practice. However, it is by no means the ideal antibiotic. It is not stable to beta-lactamases and has therefore no activity against penicillin-resistant *Staphylococcus aureus* and beta-lactamase producing *Escherichia coli* and is inactive against *Pseudomonas aeruginosa*. Ampicillin is not particularly well absorbed from the gut. Gastro-intestinal side effects, especially diarrhoea, are common and blood levels relatively low. The absorption of ampicillin is delayed when given with food in the stomach. Urinary excretion of ampicillin is less than 50 per cent of an oral dose.

Numerous chemical modifications have been made to ampicillin with the intention of improving absorption and/or widening its antibacterial spectrum. Ampicillin is a zwitterion, having an amino and a carboxyl group and it is therefore ionized at all pH's. It has been postulated that 'masking' one of these groups might make ampicillin more lipophilic and create a pH range at which the molecule was unionized, thus improving absorption, while modification of the molecule might prevent interaction with food, thus making it unnecessary to take the drug before meals. Amoxycillin and talampicillin were both introduced with the purpose of improving the absorption of ampicillin and also possibly reducing the incidence of side-effects.

The new penicillins which are substituted ampicillins, i.e. mezlocillin and its analogue azlocillin have altered the spectrum of ampicillin. These are particularly important because of their activity against *Ps. aeruginosa*.

To date, none of the ampicillin analogues are resistant to beta-lactamases. However, the introduction of the beta-lactamase inhibitor, sodium clavulanate may alter this situation if it proves possible to produce a safe and therapeutically active combination with ampicillin or one of its analogues. This would 'reclaim' many Gram-negative bacilli such as *E. coli* which have developed resistance to ampicillin through beta-lactamase production.

Amoxycillin

Amoxycillin is α-amino-p-hydroxy benzylpenicillin and differs from ampicillin by the substitution of a hydroxyl group on the benzene ring of the side chain. It is bactericidal and has a spectrum similar to that of ampicillin although it has been shown that lysis of bacteria is more rapid with amoxycillin than with ampicillin (Rolinson, Macdonald and Wilson, 1977).

The main advantage conferred by the hydroxyl group in amoxycillin is improved absorption following oral administration, which unlike that of ampicillin, is not affected by food in the stomach. Sutherland, Croydon and Rolinson (1972) found that serum levels of amoxycillin were twice those obtained with oral ampicillin, and that the protein binding of the two compounds was similar at 17 per cent. Zarowny et al (1974) reported that the serum elimination half-life was approximately one hour. The drug is excreted unchanged in the urine, predominantly by glomerular filtration, 65 per cent of an oral dose being recovered in the first six hours (Sutherland et al, 1972). In the elderly, the serum elimination half-life appears to be prolonged to up to 2.5 hours (Ball et al, 1978).

Amoxycillin is possibly to be preferred to ampicillin in acute exacerbations of chronic bronchitis (May and Ingold, 1972; May and Ingold, 1974) as sputum levels are higher. Pillay, Adams and North-Coombes (1975), in a series of adults, and Scragg (1976) in children, found it a satisfactory alternative to chloramphenicol in the oral therapy of typhoid fever. Gray (1975) has recently suggested that amoxycillin might be the oral drug of choice in bacterial endocarditis, but the significant proportion of staphylococci causing this disease in the 1970s argues against this proposal. However, in *Streptococcus faecalis* endocarditis, amoxycillin and gentamicin, which are synergistic in vitro, may be of value (Russell and Sutherland, 1975). Amoxycillin causes less diarrhoea than ampicillin. An injectable preparation of amoxycillin has recently become available.

Talampicillin

Talampicillin is the phthalidyl ester of ampicillin of which it is a 'pro-drug', the ester having no antibacterial activity. It is hydrolysed by esterases in the small intestinal wall, liberating ampicillin and phthaladehydic acid. This esterification of ampicillin almost doubles its absorption after oral administration. Leigh et al (1976) reported that talampicillin produced serum levels which were double those obtained following an equivalent oral dose of ampicillin. The biological availability of ampicillin is significantly greater with talampicillin tablets than with ampicillin capsules and it has been estimated that from 50 to 80 per cent of intact talampicillin is absorbed from the gut as compared with only 40–60 per cent of ampicillin (Jones, 1977). Cross-over studies on the absorption and excretion of ampicillin, talampicillin and amoxycillin have shown that the latter two antibiotics are twice as well absorbed from the gut as compared with ampicillin (Verbist, 1976). The absorption of the ester is delayed but not reduced by food in the stomach. No toxic effects have been reported from the ester moiety, which is metabolised in the liver and excreted in the urine. Knudsen and Harding (1975) found that the incidence of diarrhoea with talampicillin (4.3 per cent) was only half that reported with ampicillin. Leigh et al (1976) have related this reduction in diarrhoea to the fact that talampicillin has no antibacterial activity and therefore does not alter faecal flora. In their study the incidence of rash was similar to that with ampicillin.

In a study in general practice, Knudsen and Harding (1975) concluded that talampicillin was as effective as ampicillin in equivalent dosage. In view of the availability of amoxycillin the place of talampicillin in therapy remains uncertain.

Mezlocillin and azlocillin
Mezlocillin, a 'substituted ampicillin', is a semi-synthetic ureidopenicillin whose chemical structure is 6-(D-2(3-(methylsulphonyl)-2-oxo-imidazolidine-1-carboxamido)-2-phenyl-acetamido)-penicillanic acid. It has a broad spectrum of activity which includes 'problem' organisms such as *Klebsiella, Proteus, Serratia, Bacteroides fragilis, Strep. faecalis* and *Pseudomonas* species but is not stable to beta-lactamases (Bodey and Pan, 1977). It has greater activity than carbenicillin against *Esch. coli, Klebsiella spp., Serratia marcescens, Haemophilus influenzae* and *Ps. aeruginosa* and has a spectrum which is broader than that of carbenicillin, ampicillin and the cephalosporins. It is highly active against gonococci and meningococci and, indeed, is more active than benzylpenicillin against these organisms. Gonococci of intermediate (non beta-lactamase) resistance to penicillin are up to 16 times more sensitive to mezlocillin. Synergy has been demonstrated between mezlocillin and the aminoglycosides against certain Gram-negative bacilli.

Mezlocillin is not absorbed from the gastrointestinal tract but can be given by intramuscular or intravenous injection. Its toxicity will presumably be similar to that of the other penicillins.

Azlocillin is closely related to mezlocillin but has greater activity against *Ps. aeruginosa* (Stewart and Bodey, 1977), having a mode MIC of 4 mg/l compared with 8 to 16 mg/l for mezlocillin and 32 mg/l for carbenicillin (Wise, 1977). Azlocillin has activity against carbenicillin-resistant Pseudomonas strains.

The broad spectrum of activity of mezlocillin and azlocillin suggests that they may be useful in undiagnosed life-threatening infections, for example in neutropaenic patients, possibly in combination with an aminoglycoside or cefoxitin. A recent clinical trial supports this view (Ellis et al, 1978).

THE CARBENICILLINS

Ticarcillin
Ticarcillin, a thienyl analogue of carbenicillin, is alpha-carboxy-3-thienylmethyl penicillin, having, in common with carbenicillin, the alpha-carboxy group which

confers activity against *Pseudomonas aeruginosa*. It is also active against indole-positive *Proteus* spp., and *Serratia marcescens* although resistance in these organisms is now being observed (Neu and Garvey, 1975). Ticarcillin is approximately twice as active as carbenicillin against susceptible organisms.

After an intramuscular injection of 1 g peak blood levels of 30 mg/l are obtained, falling six hours later to 7 mg/l. The serum elimination half-life is approximately 1.4 hours (Neu and Garvey, 1975). These levels are adequate for the treatment of *E. coli* and *Proteus mirabilis* infections but not for those caused by *Ps. aeruginosa*. Therapeutic levels for the treatment of infections caused by the latter organism are reached after infusion of 3 to 5 g, and are improved by the simultaneous administration of probenicid. Parry and Neu (1976) investigated the pharmacokinetics of ticarcillin in patients with abnormal renal function, and showed a progressive non-linear prolongation of the serum elimination half-life with decreasing kidney function.

Ervin and Bullock (1976) treated a series of patients with serious Gram-negative sepsis with ticarcillin using an average daily dose of 250 mg/kg/day, and obtained a 70 per cent cure rate. However, some evidence of the development of resistance in vivo was encountered. Adverse reactions included eosinophilia and a bleeding tendency associated with platelet dysfunction. Schimpff et al (1976) treated 127 episodes of infection in neutropaenic patients with combinations of ticarcillin and cephalothin or gentamicin, and assessed both regimes as effective.

Ticarcillin will undoubtedly play a part in the management of serious Gram-negative sepsis in those countries in which it is marketed. It is not yet available in the U.K.

Oral carbenicillin derivatives
Carbenicillin which, prior to the introduction of ticarcillin, was the only penicillin with activity against *Ps. aeruginosa*, is not absorbed from the intestinal tract. However, esterification of carbenicillin has resulted in two compounds which are orally active—carindacillin and carfecillin.

Carindacillin
Carindacillin is the indanyl ester of carbenicillin, the properties of which formed the subject of a Symposium in 1973. The major features of this compound have been summarised in a Leading Article (1973). It is absorbed unchanged from the upper gastro-intestinal tract, and hydrolysed in the intestinal mucosa to carbenicillin and indanol, the latter compound being detoxicated in the liver. Five hundred mgs of carindacillin are equivalent to 382 mg of carbenicillin. Peak serum levels of 10 mg/l are obtained after 500 mg administered orally. This level is not adequate for the treatment of invasive *Ps. aeruginosa* infections, but the subsequent renal excretion of the drug by glomerular filtration results in urine levels of up to 1000 mg/l. This is sufficient for the therapy of lower urinary tract infections, which are the only indication for this drug.

Carfecillin
Carfecillin is the phenyl ester of carbenicillin and, during absorption from the gut, is hydrolysed to carbenicillin and phenol, the latter compound being detoxified

in the liver. Blood levels are not sufficient for the therapy of invasive *Ps. aeruginosa* infections, but urine concentrations are adequate for lower urinary tract infections caused by this organism (Wilkinson et al, 1975; Leigh and Simmons, 1976). Only 25 per cent of an oral dose of carfecillin is recoverable as carbenicillin from the urine. Leigh and Simmons (1976) suggested that in view of the possible induction of plasmid-mediated carbenicillin resistance amongst bowel organisms, the use of carfecillin should be limited to lower urinary tract infections. However, there is a view that the esters of carbenicillin should not be prescribed because of the risk of inducing carbenicillin-resistance in *Ps. aeruginosa* as a result of the relatively low serum and urine levels of the antibiotic.

A recent comparative study of carfecillin and carindacillin showed that both were effective in 70 per cent of patients suffering from urinary tract infections (Kahan-Coppens and Klastersky, 1978). However, in the carindacillin-treated group recurrence of infection was commoner, as were adverse reactions which were mainly nausea and vomiting (35 per cent as compared with 19 per cent). Upper gastro-intestinal side-effects occur with all esters of the semi-synthetic penicillins.

AMIDINO-PENICILLINS

Mecillinam

Mecillinam differs from the penicillins in the method by which the side-chain is attached at the 6-position of the 6-aminopenicillanic acid 'nucleus'. Whereas the penicillins have an amino group acylated with various carboxylic acids at this position mecillinam has a substituted amidino group (Lund and Tybring, 1972). It has been claimed therefore that mecillinam is the first member of a new group of antibiotics, the amidinopenicillanic acids (Leading Article, 1976). Mecillinam induces morphological changes in coliform organisms which differ from those produced by the penicillins suggesting that the mode of action of mecillinam is different from that of the penicillins. This has been confirmed by biochemical studies which indicate that, although mecillinam like the penicillins interferes with bacterial cell wall synthesis, the target of inhibition is different. Mecillinam interacts with penicillin-binding protein number two of the cell walls of Gram-negative bacilli producing osmotically-stable round cells (Spratt, 1977).

Mecillinam is less rapidly bactericidal than the penicillins (Greenwood and O'Grady, 1973), and is hydrolysed by beta-lactamases. It is active mainly against Gram-negative bacteria including some ampicillin-resistant *E. coli*, Salmonellae and Shigellae (Williams et al, 1976). It is considerably less active against Gram-positive cocci than the conventional penicillins. Mecillinam has been shown to have synergistic activity with ampicillin and certain cephalosporins.

Mecillinam is not absorbed from the gastro-intestinal tract and the pivaloyloxy-methyl ester, pivmecillinam, is used for oral therapy. This compound is well absorbed and hydrolysed by esterases in the intestinal wall to mecillinam. Williams et al (1976) obtained peak serum levels of 3 mg/l following 400 mg pivmecillinam given by mouth and calculated a serum elimination half-life of about one hour in adult volunteers. Urinary excretion was found to be 25 per cent of an oral dose in the first six hours. Urine levels of between 100 and 250 mg/l were obtained after an oral dose of 400 mg. The disposition characteristics of mecillinam may differ in the elderly, Ball et al (1977) having found prolongation of the serum elimination half-life to four hours in elderly patients.

Pivmecillinam (and mecillinam) have been used for the eradication of bacteriuria (Verrier-Jones and Asscher, 1975; Clarke et al, 1977) and in the management of enteric fever (Clarke et al, 1976). The latter study found mecillinam to be at least four times more active in vitro than ampicillin against *Salmonella typhi* and also demonstrated satisfactory biliary levels of the drug. The lability of mecillinam to beta-lactamases has led to an investigation of its activity in combination with other antibiotics (Neu, 1977; Gray, 1977) with variable results. Few adverse effects have been reported, gastro-intestinal disturbances and rashes being infrequent.

Mecillinam has recently been the subject of a major symposium (*J. Antimicrob. Chemotherapy*, Suppl. B, 1977).

Beta-lactamase inhibition

Sodium clavulanate
The sodium salt of clavulanic acid is Z-(2R, 5R-3(B-hydroxyethylidene)-7-oxo-1-azabicyclo (3,2,0) heptane-2-carboxylic acid. It is produced by *Streptomyces clavuligerus* and is a potent and irreversible progressive inhibitor of many beta-lactamase enzymes. The compound has only weak antibacterial activity but, when combined with penicillins, shows marked synergy against a wide range of bacteria. The most important property of sodium clavulanate is its ability to protect beta-lactam antibiotics from inactivation by beta-lactamase producing organisms (Brown et al, 1976; Reading and Cole, 1977).

Sodium clavulanate has been developed at a time when resistance to beta-lactam antibiotics is increasing. It has a broad spectrum of activity against most important beta-lactamases, inhibiting these enzymes at low concentrations. It is well absorbed after oral administration, and appears to have similar disposition characteristics to amoxycillin. Toxicity studies in man and animals have shown that diarrhoea may occur following large doses of clavulanic acid. However, in a study in progress, no disturbance of bowel function has been observed in 21 patients receiving a combination of sodium clavulanate 125 mgm and amoxycillin 250 mgm both given eight hourly for seven days. To date, this combination has been successfully used to treat three patients with urinary tract infections due to amoxycillin-resistant *E. coli* strains (Geddes and Ball, unpublished observation).

The development of sodium clavulanate is potentially an important advance in antimicrobial chemotherapy and the results of clinical trials with the compound are awaited. It is of interest that in vitro studies with a combination of sodium clavulanate and benzylpenicillin have shown that it is possible to reduce the MIC of penicillins for *Bacteroides fragilis* to clinically attainable levels (Wise, 1977).

THE CEPHALOSPORINS

A bewildering number of new cephalosporin antibiotics have been introduced since the early 1970s. Many of these compounds have little advantage over the 'first

Table 2.1 The cephalosporins and cefoxitin

Antibiotic	Dose Studied	Route of administration	Peak serum level	T½	Protein binding	Urine recovery	Bile excretion	Pain at site of injection	Nephrotoxicity
Cephaloridine	500 mg	Parenteral	22 mg/l	1.5 hrs	20%	80% (24 hrs)	+	±	++
Cefazolin	500 mg	Parenteral	22–35 mg/l	1.8–2 hrs	75%	60% (6 hrs)	++	±	Animal studies only
Cephalexin	500 mg	Oral	22 mg/l	1.2 hrs	15%	68% (12 hrs)	+	Oral	Not reported
Cefatrizine	500 mg	Oral	5.6 mg/l		Not reported	35% (12 hrs)		Oral	Not reported
	500 mg	Parenteral	12 mg/l	1.4 hrs		45% (12 hrs)		±	
Cephalothin	1 g	Parenteral	20 mg/l	0.5 hrs	70%	70% (24 hrs)	+	++	+
Cephacetrile	1 g	Parenteral	15–20 mg/l	0.75 hrs	35%	70% (6 hrs)	–?	++	Not reported
Cephapirin	1 g	Parenteral	15–20 mg/l	0.6 hrs	50%	70% (8 hrs)	–?	++	Not reported
Cefamandole	1 g	Parenteral	20 mg/l	0.6 hrs	75%	80% (24 hrs)	++	++	Not reported
Cefuroxime	500 mg	Parenteral	25 mg/l	1.2 hrs	33%	95% (total)	++	±	Not reported
Cefoxitin	500 mg	Parenteral	11 mg/l	0.75 hrs	75%	90–99% (total)	+	++	Not reported

generation' cephalosporins, namely, cephaloridine, cephalothin and cephalexin. This review will consider:

a. The cephalothin-like compounds: cephacetrile, cephanone and cephapirin,
b. Modified cephalosporins which have potential advantages over the presently available agents: cefazolin and cefatrizine,
c. The beta-lactamase resistant cephalosporins: cefamandole and cefuroxime, and
d. The cephamycin antibiotic cefoxitin.

This classification differs somewhat from the recent excellent review by O'Callaghan (1975).

Cephalothin-like cephalosporins

Cephacetrile, cephanone and cephapirin
These antibiotics are all closely related to cephalothin and do not appear to have significant advantages over the parent compound. Their antibacterial spectrum is similar, cephapirin being perhaps the least active. All must be given parenterally and intramuscular injection is painful. Cephanone produces the highest blood and urine levels, but is 90 per cent protein-bound and may not reach tissue compartments in adequate concentration (Regamey and Kirby, 1973). In clinical use these drugs have no advantages over cephalothin. Although nephrotoxicity has not been reported, eosinophilia is common with cephacetrile and cephapirin, while cephacetrile has caused neutropaenia and cephapirin therapy has been associated with the development of a positive Coombs test. Kucers and Bennett (1975) have extensively reviewed the literature on these agents.

Cefazolin and cefatrizine

Cefazolin has a spectrum of activity identical to that of cephalothin with which there is cross-resistance. It must be administered parenterally, intramuscular injection of 500 mg producing blood levels of 35 mg/l at one hour. It has a prolonged elimination half-life of 1.8 hours, and is 75 per cent protein-bound. Sixty per cent of the dose appears in the urine within six hours, almost complete recovery occurring within 24 hours. Satisfactory bile levels have been obtained (Ishiyama et al, 1971; Kirby and Regamey, 1973). Cefazolin has been used successfully in pneumonia, septicaemia, soft tissue infections, urinary tract infection and gonorrhoea (Symposium, 1973). Eosinophilia, drug fever, and transient elevation of hepatic enzymes have been noted (Ries et al, 1973). Renal tubular damage has been reported in animals, but not, as yet, in man (Appel and Neu, 1977).

Cefatrizine is a new oral cephalosporin which is more active than cephalexin against a range of Gram-positive and Gram-negative bacteria (Del Busto et al, 1976). After 500 mg given orally, peak levels of 5.6 mg/l have been reported. This is about one quarter of the concentration obtained after a similar dose of cephalexin. However, more recent work (D. S. Reeves, personal communication) has shown peak levels to be higher at 8.7 mg/l, the discrepancy being due to the fact that cefatrizine is unstable in serum. The drug may also be administered parenterally but produces blood levels considerably lower than with cefazolin. The mean serum elimination half-life is 1.4 hours. Urinary recovery is only about 45 per cent of the dose. Despite the lesser magnitude of the blood and urine levels of this drug as compared with similar agents, satisfactory therapeutic levels are obtained, exceeding the MICs of susceptible bacteria (Actor et al, 1976; Del Busto et al, 1976). The latter have used cefatrizine successfully in urinary tract infection and in pneumonia. The greater antibacterial activity of cefatrizine may outweigh its less satisfactory pharmacokinetic properties.

BETA-LACTAMASE RESISTANT CEPHALOSPORINS AND CEPHAMYCINS

Cefuroxime

Cefuroxime is stable to the action of many beta-lactamases and is active against organisms resistant to the 'first generation' cephalosporins. It is highly active against *Neisseria gonorrhoeae, Neisseria meningitidis,* and *Haemophilus influenzae* (O'Callaghan et al, 1976; Eykyn et al, 1976). Cefuroxime must be administered parenterally. After 500 mg and 750 mg given by intramuscular injection, peak serum levels of 24.8 mg/l and 27.0 mg/l have been obtained (Daikos et al, 1977). The mean serum elimination half-life is 1.2 hours and urinary recovery is of the order of 95 per cent of the dose, equal proportions of the drug being excreted by glomerular filtration and tubular secretion (Foord, 1976). Cefuroxime is excreted in bile (Ball et al, 1978), but levels obtained are much lower than those in blood. Clinical information is as yet insufficient to assess the value of this cephalosporin. Although *N. meningitidis* is highly sensitive there seems no indication to use the drug in meningitis caused by this organism which, to date, remains sensitive to penicillin. However, if clinical trials confirm the potential of cefuroxime against *N. gonorrhoeae* it may find a place in the treatment of gonorrhoea. Fowler (1977), has reported that a single 1 g intramuscular dose of cefuroxime produces a 98 per cent cure rate in uncomplicated gonorrhoea although post-gonococcal urethritis was common in male patients. Cefuroxime, in view of its high activity against *H. influenzae,* may be of value in chest infections, particularly for the treatment of exacerbations of chronic bronchitis. Its activity against ampicillin-resistant strains of *H. influenzae* is important. Daikos and his colleagues (1977) have treated 41 patients suffering from various infections with cefuroxime. Twenty-nine were cured and nine improved following therapy. There were no serious adverse reactions in this series.

Cefamandole

Cefamandole has an antibacterial spectrum similar to that of cefuroxime, although it is less active against gonococci (Eykyn et al, 1976). Its main advantage over 'first-generation' cephalosporins is that it is active against beta-lactamase producing cephalothin-resistant *E. coli* (Bodey and Weaver, 1976) and *Staph. aureus* strains (Russel, 1975). Cefamandole is not absorbed from the gastro-intestinal tract, and 1 gram intramuscularly produces peak levels of the order of 20 mg/l. It has a short serum half-life (0.6 hours) and 80 per cent of the dose is recoverable in the urine within 24 hours (Fong et al, 1976). Cefamandole is not removed from the blood by either peritoneal or haemodialysis (Ahern et al, 1976; Appel et al, 1976). Waterman et al (1976) have shown adequate penetration into bile and interstitial fluid. This drug has been used successfully in Gram-negative bacillary pneumonia, although transient hepatic enzyme derangement and one episode of rash have been reported (Minor et al, 1976).

Cefoxitin

Cefoxitin is a semisynthetic derivative of cephamycin C. The cephamycins are differentiated from the cephalosporins by modifications at the 3 (3-carbamoyl), and 7 (7-alphamethoxy) positions on the 7-ACA nucleus. These changes confer stability to beta-lactamases. Kosmidis et al (1973), found cefoxitin to be more active than the 'first-generation' cephalosporins against most Gram-negative bacteria, particularly indole-positive *Proteus* spp. *Ps. aeruginosa* is uniformly resistant, but most *B. fragilis* strains are sensitive. Unlike the cephalosporins, cefoxitin is active against some strains of *Serratia marcescens* (Neu, 1974; Gray, McGhie and Ball, 1977). However, Gram-positive cocci are considerably less sensitive to cefoxitin than to cephalothin.

Cefoxitin must be administered by injection. Kosmidis et al (1973) found peak serum levels after 500 mg intramuscularly of 10–11 mg/l, approximately twice those obtained after an equivalent dose of cephalothin. The serum elimination half-life is 0.75 hours, and urinary recovery over 12 hours is 90–99 per cent of the dose as unchanged drug. Geddes et al (1977) reported that serum levels of cefoxitin 5 minutes after a dose of 2 grams given intravenously ranged from 130 to 340 mg/l (mean 229 mg/l). A breast milk level 2 hours after a 1 g dose was 5.6 mg/l, while bile levels following a 2 g dose exceeded 200 mg/l.

In a clinical study, Geddes et al (1977) found that cefoxitin was effective in a variety of serious infections caused by Gram-negative organisms. The activity of this drug against *E. coli* and *B. fragilis*, the most important pathogens in peritonitis, suggested that cefoxitin might be of value in abdominal sepsis. Geddes and Wilcox (1977) successfully treated a group of patients suffering from intra-abdominal sepsis with cefoxitin. Almost half of these patients were also septicaemic.

Unwanted effects of cefoxitin are minimal, nephrotoxicity, in particular, not having been reported. However, intrasmucular injection is painful.

Modification of the cephamycin molecule will undoubtedly produce further compounds related to cefoxitin. The stability of these compounds to beta-lactamases is likely to be a major advantage.

THE AMINOGLYCOSIDE ANTIBIOTICS

In a recent editorial, Neu (1976) posed the question 'Do we need new amino-glycosides?' The answer is not clear as geographical areas of increasing gentamicin-resistance co-exist with areas where resistance is not yet a problem (Meyer et al, 1976). Improvement in the activity of certain aminoglycosides against some organisms, e.g. tobramycin against *Ps. aeruginosa*, stability to amino-glycoside-inactivating enzymes as with amikacin, and reduced toxicity as with netilmicin, are some of the factors which must be considered when attempting to answer the question.

Tobramycin

Tobramycin is the sixth component of a complex of antibiotics, nebramycin, produced by *Streptomyces tenebrarius*. The literature on this antibiotic has recently been reviewed by Neu (1976). Tobramycin is more active than gentamicin against *Ps. aeruginosa* (Waterworth, 1972; Draser et al, 1976), but is somewhat less active against other Gram-negative bacilli. Some *Serratia* spp. and *Providencia* spp. are sensitive. *Proteus rettgeri* is invariably resistant (Britt et al, 1972). Tobramycin is inactivated by the enzymes responsible for gentamicin inactivation, but cross-resistance is not complete.

Tobramycin is not significantly absorbed from the gastro-intestinal tract. After 1 mg/kg intramuscularly, peak serum levels of 4 to 6 mg/l may be expected. Naber et al (1973) found the serum elimination half-life to be three hours, but subsequent studies, reviewed by Neu (1976), suggest a figure of two hours. Pechere and Dugal (1976) demonstrated a linear relationship between elimination half-life and serum creatinine in renal impairment. Kaplan et al (1973) showed a prolongation of the elimination half-life in neonates related to post-natal age, but this did not lead to the accumulation of the drug. Naber et al (1973) found tobramycin to be excreted by glomular filtration, 60 per cent of a dose being recovered in 6 hours after administration, urine levels averaging 125 mg/l. Tobramycin crosses the placenta, but does not penetrate the blood-brain barrier to any extent. It is removed from the body during haemodialysis, Lockwood and Bower (1973) demonstrating a 70 per cent fall in serum concentration during a 12 hour dialysis period.

Extensive clinical experience has established tobramycin as a useful addition to the aminoglycosides, principally for *Ps. aeruginosa* infections. Blair et al (1975) found tobramycin as effective as gentamicin in equivalent dosage in serious infection caused by this organism, but suggested that increase in dosage may be necessary over the 2.7–5.6 mg/kg/day that they employed. Other investigators have obtained better cure rates than the latter authors, especially in septicaemia, but in most patients more than one drug was prescribed. Transient and, in a few cases, lasting eradication of *Ps. aeruginosa* from the sputum of children with cystic fibrosis has been obtained with tobramycin (Hoff et al, 1974; McCrae et al, 1976). Tobramycin has also been used effectively in pseudomonas pyelonephritis, endocarditis, osteomyelitis and infection of burns (Bendush and Weber, 1976; Neu, 1976).

Ototoxicity due to tobramycin may involve the auditory or vestibular components of the eighth cranial nerve. A recent survey reported 21 cases of ototoxicity amongst 3506 patients receiving tobramycin, in four of whom damage was irreversible (Neu and Bendush, 1976). Associated factors were renal impairment, high total dose, and previous or concurrent exposure to other ototoxic agents. Wilson and Ramsden (1977) have demonstrated reversible acute effects on cochlear function when serum levels rise above 8–10 mg/l, but the relation of this to eighth nerve damage is uncertain. Bendush and Weber (1976) found nephrotoxicity in 1.5 per cent of a large number of patients. Combination with cephalosporins is unwise in view of the possibility of enhanced nephrotoxicity.

Sissomicin

Sissomicin is a gentamicin C_{1a} related aminoglycoside produced by *Micromonospora inyoensis*. Its spectrum of activity is similar to that of gentamicin and tobramycin, and cross-resistance is not infrequent due to overlap of amino-glycoside-inactivating enzymes.

Sissomicin is not absorbed from the gastro-intestinal tract and after intra-muscular dosage of 1 mg/kg peak serum levels of 3 mg/l are obtained (Meyers et al, 1976). Pechere et al (1976) calculated a serum elimination half-life of two hours in subjects with normal renal function and showed linear prolonga-tion of this parameter in relation to decreasing creatinine clearance and increasing serum creatinine.

No clinical studies with sissomicin have been reported. Animal toxicity appears to parallel that of gentamicin. Sissomicin does not appear to have any advantage over gentamicin.

Netilmicin

Netilmicin is 1-N-ethyl sissomicin, having a close resemblance to gentamicin C_{1a}, and is derived from *Micromonospora inyoensis*. The spectrum of activity is similar to that of gentamicin, but it is active against gentamicin-resistant organisms and, in general, is more active than sissomicin and tobramycin (Meyer et al 1976b). It is slightly less active than amikacin against *Ps. aeruginosa*. Kabins et al (1976) found most of their *Serratia* isolates to be sensitive, but other authors (Fu and Neu, 1976) found many strains to be resistant. Staphylococci are highly sensitive. Kabins et al (1976) have indicated that netilmicin is stable to adenylylases, but is inactivated by some acetylases.

Miller et al (1976) have shown the pharmacology of netilmicin in animals to be similar to that of gentamicin. However, netilmicin was considerably less toxic in chronic ototoxicity tests in cats, and Luft et al (1976) found the nephrotoxicity of netilmicin in rats to be much less than from gentamicin. Preliminary studies of netilmicin in human infections indicate that it is as effective as the other aminoglycosides (Edelstein and Meyer, 1978). If the apparent lesser toxicity of netilmicin is confirmed in man this agent would represent a valuable addition to the aminoglycosides. It is, however, important that toxicity studies in animals should be interpreted with caution as the results in humans may differ considerably.

Amikacin

Amikacin is an aminoglycoside antibiotic derived from kanamycin A which is resistant to degradation by eight of the nine characterized aminoglycoside-inactivating enzymes, including the six which inactivate gentamicin by acetyla-tion or adenylation. The only enzyme capable of modifying amikacin is the one which acetylates the 6-amino group (AAC-6′). Reynolds et al (1974) found it to be the most active compound against a range of organisms resistant to one or more of the other aminoglycosides. Meyer et al (1976) reported that it was more active against *Ps. aeruginosa* than tobramycin, sissomicin or netilmicin, although Drasar et al (1976) found tobramycin to be most effective in vitro against U.K. isolates. Meyer et al (1975) have shown amikacin to be effective against gentamicin-resistant *S. marcescens*.

Amikacin is not absorbed from the gastro-intestinal tract. After an intra-muscular dosage of 500 mg, peak serum concentrations of 20 mg/l occur at one hour, the serum elimination half-life being 2.3 hours. Eighty per cent of the dose is excreted, by glomular filtration, into the urine (Cabana and Taggart, 1973). Howard and McCracken (1975) obtained peak serum levels in neonates of 20 mg/l following 7.5 mg/kg intramuscularly, and showed a prolongation of the half-life inversely related to post-natal age, as they have previously demonstrated with other aminoglycosides.

Amikacin has been used successfully in hospital-acquired *Proteus rettgeri* urinary tract infections (Sharp et al, 1974), in serious invasive Gram-negative infections (Tally et al, 1975), in opportunistic infection in patients suffering from cancer (Feld et al, 1977) and in paediatric practice (Howard et al, 1976). Black et al (1976) demonstrated high tone hearing loss, correlating with large doses and the resultant higher than average peak and trough serum levels. Feld et al (1977) noted evidence of nephrotoxicity in 20 per cent of their patients.

Amikacin, by virtue of its resistance to most aminoglycoside-inactivating enzymes, represents an advance over previous aminoglycosides, but at present should be reserved for the management of serious infections caused by gentamicin-resistant organisms. It should not be used for the treatment of infections caused by gentamicin-sensitive organisms as it has no advantage over gentamicin in these infections, and costs three times as much.

CLINDAMYCIN AND PSEUDOMEMBRANOUS COLITIS

Clindamycin is of proven value in the management of acute and chronic bone and joint infection (Geddes et al, 1977), in serious staphylococcal sepsis, and in the management of anaerobic infection caused by *B. fragilis*, fusobacteria, eubacteria and anaerobic streptococci (Keusch and Present, 1976). It has, however, been incriminated as the commonest cause of antibiotic-associated pseudomembraneous colitis, a serious bowel condition, the pathology of which has recently been reviewed (Leading Article, 1977).

Clindamycin-associated colitis affects the large bowel and is characterised by diarrhoea, often with blood and tenesmus, and in severe cases dehydration, prostration and circulatory collapse. Acute toxic dilatation of the colon may occur, and fatalities have been recorded, especially in elderly patients. In an extensive review, Keusch and Present (1976) studied 1000 patients receiving clindamycin, 7 per cent of whom developed diarrhoea. Fifty per cent of these developed diarrhoea within two days of commencing therapy, and 80 per cent settled within two weeks of the onset. Females outnumbered males by 2 to 1. Endoscopy was not performed in most of the affected patients. Tedesco, Barton and Alpers (1974), found that 10 per cent of a group of prospectively studied patients receiving clindamycin had sigmoidoscopic changes suggestive of colitis, including the pathognomonic pseudomembraneous plaques. Our personal experience in this hospital with a large number of patients treated with clindamycin, some for prolonged periods, suggest that the incidence of colitis is about 1 per cent (Finch, Phillips and Geddes, 1975).

The pathogenesis of the condition remains uncertain. However, Larson and his colleagues (1977) have recently found a heat-labile toxin in the faeces of patients with antibiotic-associated colitis which workers in the United States (Rifkin et al,

1977) suggest may be produced by *Clostridium sordellii*. Antigenic cross reactivity occurs between this organism and *Cl. difficile* which has now been implicated as a possible cause of the condition. Vancomycin is recommended for its treatment.

METRONIDAZOLE

The activity of metronidazole against anaerobic organisms has been recognised since the early 1960s when it was first used for the treatment of Vincent's angina. However, only recently has interest in serious infections caused by non-sporing anaerobic bacteria established this drug as a potent antibacterial agent. Its activity extends throughout the obligate anaerobic species including *Bacteroides* spp., fuso-bacteria, and clostridia, and includes many, but not all, of the anaerobic strepto-cocci (Ingham et al, 1975a). It is also highly active against the anaerobic protozoa including *Entamoeba histolytica* and *Giardia lamblia*. The development of resistance amongst sensitive species exposed to metronidazole is rare, indeed the sensitivity of most anaerobes after many years of use of the drug has not changed appreciably and resistance has not been induced in vitro. The drug acts by interfering with RNA and DNA polymerases. Its bactericidal effect on anaerobic organisms is probably due to reduction of the 5-nitro group on the molecule to a hydroxylamine group, which then binds to DNA, thus blocking cell division (Ings et al, 1974).

Metronidazole is well absorbed after oral or rectal administration (Willis et al, 1976), 200–400 mg producing peak serum levels of 5–10 mg/l within two hours. The serum elimination half-life is six hours, 40 per cent of the drug being metabolised to inactive breakdown products which are then excreted in the urine, together with the unchanged fraction. Metronidazole penetrates into the cerebro-spinal fluid and enters breast milk in variable concentration. A parenteral preparation produces sustained high levels when administered intravenously (Selkon et al, 1975). The pharmacology has been reviewed by Ingham et al (1975a) and Hamilton-Miller (1975).

Metronidazole is now recommended for the treatment of a variety of infections caused by anaerobic organisms. In surgical patients a considerable reduction in post-operative sepsis and wound infection has been claimed using metronidazole prophylaxis for patients undergoing gynaecological surgery (Study Group, 1975), appendicectomy (Willis et al, 1976), and elective colonic surgery (Willis et al, 1977). In all of these studies anaerobic infections occurring in the control group were successfully treated with metronidazole. Anaerobic pulmonary infection (Tally et al, 1975), brain abscess, septicaemia (Ingham et al, 1975b), and severe periodontal infection have all been successfully treated with this drug. Eykyn and Phillips (1976) have recently reported their experience of metronidazole therapy in 50 patients suffering from anaerobic infections. Metronidazole is of established value in the management of trichomoniasis, giardiasis and amoebiasis.

Metronidazole has relatively few unwanted effects of which mild gastrointestinal intolerance is the most common. A reversible neutropaenia and a peripheral sensory neuropathy (Bradley et al, 1977) may rarely occur. Metronidazole has a disulfiram-like (Antabuse) effect when alcohol is taken simultaneously. Metroni-dazole can cause fragmentation of mammalian DNA and, particularly in the United States, this has led to anxiety regarding the long-term effects of the drug.

In anaerobic sepsis the dose of metronidazole is 500 mg 6–8 hourly. Doses of up to 1 gram have been administered both orally and rectally but appear unnecessary in practice. If a pulmonary or cerebral abscess is being treated, benzyl penicillin, to which *Bacteroides* spp., other than *B. fragilis*, and other oral anaerobes are sensitive, should be given simultaneously.

RIFAMPICIN

Medical opinion in many countries has restricted the use of rifampicin to certain well-defined indications with the purpose of preventing the emergence of resistance to the drug. Rifampicin is fundamental to the recently introduced short-course treatment regimes for tuberculosis and is the only agent which is *bactericidal* against *Mycobacterium leprae*. However, this restriction has been questioned (Leading Article, 1976), and it has been suggested that resistance in mycobacteria would not increase if rifampicin were used for the treatment of non-mycobacterial infections (Acocella, Hamilton-Miller and Brumfitt, 1977). Before such evidence leads to the extended use of the drug it is pertinent to consider whether there is any requirement for rifampicin in the therapy of non-tuberculous bacterial infections.

In vitro, rifampicin is highly active against Gram-positive and Gram-negative cocci including penicillin-resistant *Staph. aureus*, but is less active against most Gram-negative bacilli. *Proteus* spp. and *Klebsiellae* are variably sensitive, as are *Ps. aeruginosa*, *H. influenzae* and *Bacteroides spp.* In combination, rifampicin and colistin (Traub and Kleber, 1975), and rifampicin and trimethoprim (Hamilton-Miller, Kerry and Brumfitt, 1977), are synergistic against *S. marcescens*. In vivo, rifampicin has been used with success in the single dose therapy of gonorrhoea (Cobbold et al, 1968), and also in the prophylaxis of meningococcal disease (Devine et al, 1973). However, it has not been shown to be effective in exacerbations of chronic bronchitis due to *H. influenzae* (Citron and May, 1969) or in urinary tract infections (Murdoch et al, 1969).

Rifampicin has an impressive list of side effects with five different adverse reaction syndromes including drug hypersensitivity, liver and renal damage, thrombocytopaenia and also interaction with other drugs due to induction of liver enzymes.

Rifampicin is of value in the limited application of meningococcal prophylaxis and the treatment of carriers, and also possibly in aminoglycoside-resistant *Serratia* infection. It is a readily diffusable antibiotic, penetrating well into bacterial cells. It is lipid soluble and may be of use in the treatment of bacterial endocarditis occurring following prosthetic heart valve replacement.

SPECTINOMYCIN

Spectinomycin is an aminocyclitol antibiotic produced by *Streptomyces spectabilis* and is related structurally to the aminoglycosides. It is not absorbed from the gastrointestinal tract. Following intramuscular injection of 2 g peak blood levels of 100 mg/l are obtained. Excretion is by glomerular filtration.

Although active against many bacteria its use has been almost entirely restricted to gonorrhoea. A single dose of 2 grams is effective in most cases of uncomplicated ano-genital gonorrhoea, although pharyngitis responds less well. Spectinomycin has an effect on *Treponema pallidum* and may, therefore, mask concomitant syphilis. It is ineffective in non-gonococcal urethritis, as the most frequent cause, chlamydiae, are resistant.

McCormack and Finland (1976) in a recent review suggest that spectinomycin should be reserved for uncomplicated gonorrhoea which has failed to respond to other agents. Rapid emergence of bacterial resistance in vivo may limit its usefulness.

CINOXACIN

Cinoxacin is a synthetic organic acid, which is closely related to nalidixic acid and oxolinic acid. It has a similar range of activity against Gram-negative bacteria, but is more active, being effective against some strains of *E. coli* which are resistant to nalidixic acid (Greenwood, 1978).

Cinoxacin is well absorbed after oral administration and, after a 500 mg dose produces peak serum levels of 15 mg/l, and urine levels of 400–750 mg/l. These are higher than those obtained with a similar dose of nalidixic acid. Cinoxacin penetrates into prostatic tissue and renal parenchymal levels exceed those in serum (Anderson, Mardh and Colleen, 1978). The serum elimination half-life of 1.5 hours is prolonged by probenecid (Rodriguez, Madsen and Welling, 1978). In renal failure elimination is delayed, the half-life and creatinine clearance being inversely related.

Cinoxacin causes drowsiness in some patients, but otherwise is free of adverse effects in normal dosage (500 mg 12 hourly). Preliminary studies have shown that it is at least as effective as nalidixic acid, co-trimoxazole and nitrofurantoin in uncomplicated urinary tract infection.

COMMENT

Most of the drugs which have been discussed in this paper are pharmaceutical variants of existing agents which have been 'refined' with the intention of producing microbiological, pharmacological or toxicological improvement. By no means all of the antibiotics are of clinical importance. Some, however, do have significant advantage over previously available drugs.

Microbiologically improved antibiotics

Ticarcillin, tobramycin and azlocillin are notable for their activity against *Ps. aeruginosa*. It is, however, important to remember that, in general, pseudomonas infections are uncommon. Mezlocillin, which also has activity against *Ps. aeruginosa*, has the added advantage of being more active against gonococci and meningococci than benzylpenicillin. Mecillinam is the most active antibiotic in vitro against *Salmonella* species but in vivo does not appear to have any advantage over chloramphenicol or co-trimoxazole in the treatment of typhoid fever. This finding is important as it illustrates the problems of correlating laboratory findings with clinical results.

The development of new cephalosporins, such as cefuroxime, and the cephamycin cefoxitin which are stable to beta-lactamases is an important achievement and further advances in this field are anticipated. Similarly, amikacin's resistance to eight of the nine aminoglycoside-inactivating enzymes makes it a significant addition to the aminoglycoside group of antibiotics. In this context it is important to remember that amikacin is less active than gentamicin against gentamicin-sensitive organisms, microbiological activity thus being sacrificed at the expense of enzyme stability.

Apart from mecillinam very few of the new antibiotics have a novel action.

Pharmaceutically improved antibiotics

The pharmaceutically improved 'ampicillins', amoxycillin and talampicillin are of interest but doubt still exists as to their clinical superiority over ampicillin and as to which of the two drugs is best. There is also uncertainty as to the place of carfecillin and carindacillin in the therapy of infections and some would doubt whether they should be used at all. The clinical significance of the different protein-binding capacities of related antibiotics such as the various cephalosporins remains uncertain and further studies of this problem are needed.

Toxicologically improved antibiotics

Antibiotics are fortunately relatively non-toxic drugs. However, the ototoxicity and nephrotoxicity of the aminoglycosides is of clinical importance and the suggestion that netilmicin might be less ototoxic stimulated considerable interest. This hypothesis was based on animal studies and it seems likely, from so far unpublished human investigations, that netilmicin will not prove to be less ototoxic than gentamicin and may be more nephrotoxic. This illustrates the difficulties of comparing human and animal toxicological data. More information is becoming available on antibiotic-associated colitis but, so far, this condition has not been completely elucidated, particularly with regard to its prevention.

New concepts in antibiotic therapy

The discovery of sodium clavulanate, a beta-lactamase inhibiting drug, is an important development and points the way to a new method of tackling bacterial resistance. Finally, it is extremely important to remember that many problems in infection are related to poor host response rather than to a lack of available antibiotics and research in chemotherapy must therefore be combined with investigations of methods of improving host responses, especially in patients with compromised defence mechanisms.

REFERENCES

The Penicillins
Amoxycillin
Ball, A. P., Barford, A. V., Gilbert, J., Johnson, T. & Mitchard, M. (1978) Prolonged serum elimination half-life of amoxycillin in the elderly. *Journal of Antimicrobial Therapy*, **4,** 385–386.
Gray, I. R. (1975) The choice of antibiotic for treating infective endocarditis. *Quarterly Journal of Medicine*, **45,** 449–458.
May, J. R. & Ingold, A. (1972) Amoxycillin in the treatment of chronic non-tuberculous bronchial infections. *British Journal of Diseases of the Chest*, **66,** 185–191.
May, J. R. & Ingold, A. (1974) Amoxycillin in the treatment of infections of the lower respiratory tract. *Journal of Infectious Diseases* (Suppl.), **129,** 189–193.

Pillay, N., Adams, E. B. & North-Coombes, D. (1975) Comparative trial of amoxycillin and chloramphenicol in the treatment of typhoid fever in adults. *Lancet*, **2**, 333–334.

Rolinson, G. N., Macdonald, A. C. & Wilson, D. A. (1977) Bactericidal action of beta-lactam antibiotics on *Escherichia coli* with particular reference to ampicillin and amoxycillin. *Journal of Antimicrobial Chemotherapy*, **3**, 541–553.

Russel, E. J. & Sutherland, R. (1975) Activity of amoxycillin against enterococci and synergism with aminoglycoside antibiotics. *Journal of Medical Microbiology*, **8**, 1–10.

Scragg, J. N. (1976) Further experience with amoxycillin in typhoid fever in children. *British Medical Journal*, **2**, 1031–1033.

Sutherland, R., Croydon, E. A. P. & Rolinson, G. N. (1972) Amoxycillin: a new semi-synthetic penicillin. *British Medical Journal*, **3**, 13–16.

Zarowny, D., Ogilvie, R., Tamblyn, D., McLeod, C. & Ruedy, J. (1974) Pharmacokinetics of amoxycillin. *Clinical Pharmacology and Therapeutics*, **16**, 1045–1051.

Talampicillin

Jones, K. H. (1977) Bioavailability of talampicillin. *British Medical Journal*, **3**, 232–233.

Knudsen, E. T. & Harding, J. W. (1975) A multicentre trial of talampicillin and ampicillin in general practice. *British Journal of Clinical Practice*, **29**, 255–266.

Leigh, D. A., Reeves, D. S., Simmons, K., Thomas, A. L. & Wilkinson, P. J. (1976) Talampicillin: a new derivative of ampicillin. *British Medical Journal*, **1**, 1378–1380.

Verbist, L. (1976) Triple crossover study on absorption and excretion of ampicillin, talampicillin and amoxycillin. *Antimicrobial Agents and Chemotherapy*, **10**, 173–175.

Ticarcillin

Ervin, F. R. & Bullock, W. E. (1976) Clinical and pharmacological studies of ticarcillin in Gram-negative infections. *Antimicrobial Agents and Chemotherapy*, **9**, 94–101.

Neu, H. C. & Garvey, G. J. (1975) Comparative in vitro activity and clinical pharmacology of ticarcillin and carbenicillin. *Antimicrobial Agents and Chemotherapy*, **8**, 457–462.

Parry, M. F. & Neu, H. C. (1976) Pharmacokinetics of ticarcillin in patients with abnormal renal function. *Journal of Infectious Diseases*, **133**, 46–49.

Schimpff, S. C., Landesman, S., Hahn, D. M., Standiford, H. C., Fortner, C. L., Young, V. M. & Wiernik, P. M. (1976) Ticarcillin in combination with cephalothin or gentamicin as empiric antibiotic therapy in granulocytopaenic cancer patients. *Antimicrobial Agents and Chemotherapy*, **10**, 837–844.

Oral carbenicillin derivatives

Kahan-Coppens, L. & Klastersky, J. (1978) Comparative study of carfecillin and indanyl carbenicillin in patients with complicated urinary tract infections. *Current Chemotherapy*, eds. Siegenthaler & Lüthy. American Society for Microbiology, Washington, pp. 591–593.

Leading Article (1973) An oral carbenicillin. *British Medical Journal*, **3**, 555–556.

Leigh, D. A. & Simmons, K. (1976) The treatment of simple and complicated urinary tract infections with carfecillin: a new oral ester of carbenicillin. *Journal of Antimicrobial Chemotherapy*, **2**, 293–298.

Symposium on Carindacillin (1973) *Journal of Infectious Diseases*, **127**, (Suppl. May) Whole Issue.

Wilkinson, P. J., Reeves, D. S., Wise, R. & Allen, J. T. (1975) Volunteer and clinical studies with carfecillin: a new orally administered ester of carbenicillin. *British Medical Journal*, **2**, 250–252.

Mezlocillin/Azlocillin

Bodey, G. P. & Pan, T. (1977) Mezlocillin: in vitro studies of a new broad-spectrum penicillin. *Antimicrobial Agents and Chemotherapy*, **11**, 74–79.

Ellis, C. J., Geddes, A. M., Davey, P. G., Wise, R., Andrews, J. & Grimley, R. P. (1978) Mezlocillin and azlocillin: an evaluation of two new β-lactam antibiotics. *Journal of Antimicrobial Chemotherapy* (in press).

Stewart, D. & Bodey, G. P. (1977) Azlocillin: *in vitro* studies of a new semisynthetic penicillin. *Antimicrobial Agents and Chemotherapy*, **11**, 865–870.

Wise, R. (1977) Personal communication.

Mecillinam

Ball, A. P., Viswan, A. L., Mitchard, M. & Wise, R. (1977) Plasma concentrations and excretion of mecillinam after oral administration of pivmecillinam in elderly patients. *Journal of Antimicrobial Chemotherapy*, **4**, 241–246.

Clarke, P. D., Geddes, A. M., McGhie, D. & Wall, J. C. (1976) Mecillinam: a new antibiotic for enteric fever. *British Medical Journal*, **2**, 14–15.

Clarke, P. D., Geddes, A. M., McGhie, D. & Wall, J. C. (1977) Pivmecillinam in urinary tract infections: a correlation of urinary bactericidal activity with clinical efficacy. *Journal of Antimicrobial Chemotherapy*, **3**, 169–174.

Gray, J. (1977) Synergy and mecillinam. *Journal of Antimicrobial Chemotherapy*, **3**, 531–532.

Greenwood, D. & O'Grady, F. (1973) FL1060: a new beta-lactam antibiotic with novel properties. *Journal of Clinical Pathology*, **26**, 1–6.

Leading Article (1976) Mecillinam. *Lancet*, **2**, 503–505.

Lund, F. & Tybring, L. (1972) 6 beta-amidino penicillanic acids—a new group of antibiotics. *Nature New Biology*, **236**, 135–137.

Neu, H. C. (1977) Mecillinam—an amidino penicillin which acts synergistically with other beta-lactam compounds. *Journal of Antimicrobial Chemotherapy*, **3**, (Suppl. B), 43–52.

Spratt, B. G. (1977) The mechanism of action of mecillinam. *Journal of Antimicrobial Chemotherapy*, **3**, (Suppl. B), 13–19.

Symposium (1977) Mecillinam. *Journal of Antimicrobial Chemotherapy*, **3**, (Suppl. B), whole issue.

Verrier-Jones, E. R. & Asscher, A. W. (1975) Treatment of recurrent bacteriuria with pivmecillinam (FL1039). *Journal of Antimicrobial Chemotherapy*, **1**, 193–196.

Williams, J. D., Andrews, J., Mitchard, M. & Kendall, M. J. (1976) Bacteriology and pharmacokinetics of the new amidino penicillin-mecillinam. *Journal of Antimicrobial Chemotherapy*, **2**, 61–69.

Sodium clavulanate

Brown, A. G., Butterworth, D., Cole, M., Hanscomb, G., Hood, G. D., Reading, C. & Rolinson, G. N. (1976) Naturally occurring β-lactamase inhibitors with antibacterial activity. *Journal of Antibiotics*, **29**, 668–669.

Reading, C. & Cole, M. (1977) Clavulanic acid: a β-lactamase-inhibiting β-lactam from *Streptomyces clavuligerus*. *Antimicrobial Agents and Chemotherapy*, **11**, 852–857.

Wise, R. (1977) Clavulanic acid and susceptibility of bacteroides fragilis to penicillin. *Lancet*, **2**, 145.

The Cephalosporins

O'Callaghan, C. H. (1975) Classification of cephalosporins by their antibacterial activity and pharmacokinetic properties. *Journal of Antimicrobial Chemotherapy*, **1**, (Suppl.), 1–12.

Cephalothin-like cephalosporins

Kucers, A. & Bennet, N. McK. (1975) The use of antibiotics. 2nd edition. London: William Heinemann Medical Books Ltd.

Regamy, C. & Kirby, W. M. M. (1973). Pharmacokinetics of cephanone in healthy adult volunteers. *Antimicrobial Agents and Chemotherapy*, **4**, 589–592.

Cefazolin and Cefatrizine

Actor, P., Pitkin, D. H., Lucyszyn, G., Weisbach, J. & Bran, J. L. (1976) Cefatrizine (SKF60771), a new oral cephalosporin: serum levels and urinary recovery in humans after oral or intramuscular administration—comparative study with cephalexin and cefazolin. *Antimicrobial Agents and Chemotherapy*, **9**, 800–803.

Appel, G. B. & Neu, H. C. (1977) The nephrotoxicity of antimicrobial agents. *New England Journal of Medicine*, **296**, 663–670.

Del Busto, R., Haas, E., Madhavan, T., Burch, K., Cox, C., Fisher, E., Quinn, E. & Pohlod, D. (1976) In vitro and clinical studies of cefatrizine, a new semisynthetic cephalosporin. *Antimicrobial Agents and Chemotherapy*, **9**, 397–405.

Ishiyama, S., Nakayama, I., Iwamoto, H., Iwai, S., Okui, M. & Matsubara, T. (1971) Absorption, tissue concentration and organ distribution of cefazolin. *Antimicrobial Agents and Chemotherapy*, 1970, p. 476.

Kirby, W. M. M. & Regamey, C. (1973) Pharmacokinetics of cefazolin compared with four other cephalosporins. *Journal of Infectious Diseases*, **128**, (Suppl.), 341–346.

Ries, K., Levison, M. E. & Kaye, D. (1973) Clinical and in vitro evaluation of cefazolin, a new cephalosporin antibiotic. *Antimicrobial Agents and Chemotherapy*, **3**, 168–174.

Symposium: Cefazolin (1973) *Journal of Infectious Diseases*, **128**, (Suppl.), Whole issue.

Beta-lactamase resistant cephalosporins and cephamycins cefamandole and cefuroxime

Ahern, M. J., Finkelstein, F. O. & Andriole, V. T. (1976) Pharmacokinetics of cefamandole in patients undergoing haemodialysis and peritoneal dialysis. *Antimicrobial Agents and Chemotherapy*, **10**, 457–461.

Appel, G. B., Neu, H. C., Parry, M. F., Goldberger, M. J. & Jacob, G. B. (1976) Pharmacokinetics of cefamandole in the presence of renal failure and in patients undergoing haemodialysis. *Antimicrobial Agents and Chemotherapy*, **10**, 623–625.

Ball, A. P., Brookes, G. R., Farrell, I. D., Geddes, A. M. & Gould, I. (1978) Studies with cefuroxime: a new β-lactamase resistant cephalosporin. *Chemotherapy (Basle)*. In press.

Bodey, G. P. & Weaver, S. (1976) In vitro studies of cefamandole. *Antimicrobial Agents and Chemotherapy*, **9**, 452–457.

Daikos, G. K., Kosmidis, J. C., Stathakis, Ch. & Giamarellou, H. (1977) Cefuroxime: antimicrobial activity, human pharmacokinetics and therapeutic efficacy. *Journal of Antimicrobial Chemotherapy*, **3**, 555–562.

Eykyn, S. J., Jenkins, C., King, A. & Phillips, I. (1976) Anti-bacterial activity of cefuroxime, a new cephalosporin antibiotic, compared with that of cephaloridine, cephalothin and cefamandole. *Antimicrobial Agents and Chemotherapy*, **9**, 690–695.

Fong, I. W., Ralph, E. D., Engelking, E. R. & Kirby, W. M. M. (1976) Clinical pharmacology of cefamandole as compared with cephalothin. *Antimicrobial Agents and Chemotherapy*, **9**, 65–69.

Foord, R. D. (1976) Cefuroxime: human pharmacokinetics. *Antimicrobial Agents and Chemotherapy*, **9**, 741–747.

Fowler, W. (1977) Experiences in the treatment of gonorrhoea. *Proceedings of International Conference on Cefuroxime*, Amsterdam, 1977.

Minor, M. R., Sande, M. A., Dilworth, J. A. & Mandell, G. L. (1976) Cefamandole treatment of pulmonary infection caused by gram-negative rods. *Journal of Antimicrobial Chemotherapy*, **2**, 49–53.

O'Callaghan, C. H., Sykes, R. B., Griffiths, A. & Thornton, J. E. (1976) Cefuroxime, a new cephalosporin antibiotic: activity in vitro. *Antimicrobial Agents and Chemotherapy*, **9**, 511–519.

Russel, A. D. (1975) The antibacterial activity of a new cephalosporin, cefamandole. *Journal of Antimicrobial Chemotherapy*, **1**, 97–101.

Waterman, N. G., Eickenberger, H. U. & Scharfenberger, L. (1976) Concentration of cefamandole in serum interstitial fluid, bile and urine. *Antimicrobial Agents and Chemotherapy*, **10**, 733–735.

Cefoxitin

Geddes, A. M., Schnurr, L. P., Ball, A. P., McGhie, D., Brooks, G. R., Wise, R. & Andrews, J. (1977) Cefoxitin: a hospital study. *British Medical Journal*, **1**, 1126–1128.

Geddes, A. M. & Wilcox, R. M. L. (1978) Treatment of abdominal sepsis with cefoxitin. *Current Chemotherapy*, American Society for Microbiology, Washington, pp. 299–300.

Gray, J., McGhie, D. & Ball, A. P. (1978) Serratia marcescens: antibacterial sensitivity and synergy. *Current Chemotherapy*, American Society for Microbiology, Washington, pp. 434–436.

Kosmidis, J., Hamilton-Miller, J. M. T., Gilchrist, J. N. G., Kerry, D. W. & Brumfitt, W. (1973) Cefoxitin, a new semisynthetic cephamycin: an in vitro and in vivo comparison with cephalothin. *British Medical Journal*, **4**, 653–655.

Neu, H. C. (1974) Cefoxitin, a semisynthetic cephamycin antibiotic: antibacterial spectrum and resistance to hydrolysis by Gram-negative beta-lactamases. *Antimicrobial Agents and Chemotherapy*, **6**, 170–176.

The Aminoglycoside Antibiotics

Meyer, R. D., Halter, J., Lewis, R. P. & White, M. (1976a) Gentamicin-resistant Pseudomonas aeruginosa and Serratia marcescens in a general hospital. *Lancet*, **1**, 580–583.

Neu, H. C. (1976) Aminoglycosides: do we need new agents? *Drugs*, **12**, 161–165.

Tobramycin

Bendush, C. L. & Weber, R. (1976) Tobramycin sulfate: a summary of worldwide experience from clinical trials. *Journal of Infectious Diseases*, **134**, (Suppl. Aug.), 219–234.

Blair, D. C., Fekety, F. R., Bruce, B., Silva, J. & Archer, G. (1975) Therapy of Pseudomonas aeruginosa infections with tobramycin. *Antimicrobial Agents and Chemotherapy*, **8**, 22–29.

Britt, M. R., Garibaldi, R. A., Wilfert, J. N. & Smith, C. B. (1972) In vitro activity of tobramycin and gentamicin. *Antimicrobial Agents and Chemotherapy*, **2**, 236–241.

Drasar, F. A., Farrell, W., Maskell, J. & Williams, J. D. (1976) Tobramycin, amikacin, sisomicin and gentamicin resistant Gram-negative rods. *British Medical Journal*, **2**, 1284–1287.

Hoff, G. E., Schiotz, P. O. & Paulsen, J. (1974) Tobramycin treatment of Pseudomonas aeruginosa infections in cystic fibrosis. *Scandinavian Journal of Infectious Diseases*, **6**, 333–337.

Kaplan, J. M., McCracken, G. H., Thomas, M. L., Horton, L. J. & Davis, N. (1973) Clinical pharmacology of tobramycin in newborns. *American Journal of Diseases of the Child*, **125**, 656–660.

Lockwood, W. R. & Bower, J. D. (1973) Tobramycin and gentamicin concentrations in the serum of normal and anephric patients. *Antimicrobial Agents and Chemotherapy*, **3**, 125–129.

McCrae, W. M., Raeburn, J. A. & Hanson, E. J. (1976) Tobramycin therapy of infections due to Pseudomonas aeruginosa in patients with cystic fibrosis: effect of dosage and concentration of antibiotic in sputum. *Journal of Infectious Diseases*, **134**, (Suppl. Aug.), 191–193.

Naber, K. G., Westenfelder, S. R. & Madsen, P. O. (1973) Pharmacokinetics of the aminoglycoside antibiotics in humans. *Antimicrobial Agents and Chemotherapy*, **3**, 469–473.

Neu, H. C. (1976) Tobramycin: an overview. *Journal of Infectious Diseases*, **134**, (Suppl. Aug.), 3–19.

Neu, H. C. & Bendush, C. L. (1976) Ototoxicity of tobramycin: a clinical overview. *Journal of Infectious Diseases*, **134**, (Suppl. Aug.), 206–218.

Pechere, J-C. & Dugal, R. (1976) Pharmacokinetics of intravenously administered tobramycin in normal volunteers and in renal-impaired and haemodialysed patients. *Journal of Infectious Diseases*, **134**, (Suppl. Aug.), 118–124.

Waterworth, P. M. (1972) The in vitro activity of tobramycin compared with that of other aminoglycosides. *Journal of Clinical Pathology*, **25**, 979–983.

Wilson, P. & Ramsden, R. J. (1977) Immediate effects of tobramycin on human cochlea and correlation with serum tobramycin levels. *British Medical Journal*, **1**, 259–261.

Sissomicin

Meyers, B. R., Hirschman, S. Z., Yancovitz, S. & Ribner, B. (1976) Pharmacokinetic parameters of sissomicin. *Antimicrobial Agents and Chemotherapy*, **10**, 25–27.

Pechere, J-C., Pechere, M-M. & Dugal, R. (1976) Clinical pharmacokinetics of sissomicin: dosage schedules in renal-impaired patients. *Antimicrobial Agents and Chemotherapy*, **9**, 761–765.

Netilmicin

Edelstein, P. H. & Meyer, R. D. (1978) Netilmicin therapy of serious Gram-negative bacillary infections. *Current Chemotherapy*, American Society for Microbiology, Washington, pp. 982–984.

Fu, K. P. & Neu, H. C. (1976) In vitro study of netilmicin compared with other aminoglycosides. *Antimicrobial Agents and Chemotherapy*, **10**, 526–534.

Kabins, S. A., Nathan, C. & Cohen, S. (1976) In vitro comparison of netilmicin, a semisynthetic derivative of sissomicin, and four other aminoglycoside antibiotics. *Antimicrobial Agents and Chemotherapy*, **10**, 139–145.

Luft, F. C., Yum, M. N. & Kleit, S. A. (1976) Comparative nephrotoxicities of netilmicin and gentamicin in rats. *Antimicrobial Agents and Chemotherapy*, **10**, 845–849.

Meyer, R. D., Kaans, L. L. & Pasiecznik, K. A. (1976b) In vitro susceptibility of gentamicin-resistant Enterobacteriaceae and Pseudomonas aeruginosa to netilmicin and selected aminoglycoside antibiotics. *Antimicrobial Agents and Chemotherapy*, **10**, 677–681.

Miller, G. H., Arcieri, G., Weinstein, M. J. & Waitz, J. A. (1976) Biological Activity of netilmicin, a broad spectrum semisynthetic aminoglycoside antibiotic. *Antimicrobial Agents and Chemotherapy*, **10**, 827–836.

Amikacin

Black, R. E., Lau, W. K., Weinstein, R. J., Young, L. S. & Hewitt, W. L. (1976) Ototoxicity of amikacin. *Antimicrobial Agents and Chemotherapy*, **9**, 956–961.

Cabana, B. E. & Taggart, J. G. (1973) Comparative pharmacokinetics of BB-K8 and kanamycin in dogs and humans. *Antimicrobial Agents and Chemotherapy*, **3**, 478–483.

Draser, F. A., Farrell, W., Maskell, J. & Williams, J. D. (1976) Tobramycin, amikacin, sissomicin and gentamicin resistant Gram-negative rods. *British Medical Journal*, **2**, 1284–1287.

Feld, R., Valdivieso, M., Bodey, G. P. & Rodriguez, V. (1977) Comparison of amikacin and tobramycin in the treatment of infection in patients with cancer. *Journal of Infectious Diseases*, **135**, 61–66.

Howard, J. B. & McCracken, G. H. (1975) Pharmacological evaluation of amikacin in neonates. *Antimicrobial Agents and Chemotherapy*, **8**, 86–90.

Howard, J. B., McCracken, G. H., Trujillo, H. & Mohs, E. (1976) Amikacin in newborn infants: comparative pharmacology with kanamycin and clinical efficacy in 45 neonates with bacterial diseases. *Antimicrobial Agents and Chemotherapy*, **10**, 205–210.

Meyer, R. D., Lewis, R. P., Carmalt, E. D. & Finegold, S. M. (1975) Amikacin therapy for serious gram-negative bacillary infections. *Annals of Internal Medicine*, **83**, 790–800.

Meyer, R. D., Halter, J., Lewis, R. P. & White, M. (1976) Gentamicin-resistant *Pseudomonas aeruginosa* and *Serratia marcescens* in a general hospital. *Lancet*, **1**, 580–583.

Reynolds, A. V., Hamilton-Miller, J. M. T. & Brumfitt, W. (1974) Newer aminoglycosides—amikacin and tobramycin: an in vitro comparison with kanamycin and gentamicin. *British Medical Journal*, **3**, 778–780.

Sharp, A. V., Saenz, C. A. & Martin, R. R. (1974) Amikacin (BB-K8) treatment of multiple-drug-resistant Proteus infections. *Antimicrobial Agents and Chemotherapy*, **5**, 435–438.

Tally, F. P., Louie, T. J., Weinstein, W. M., Bartlett, J. G. & Gorbach, S. L. (1975) Amikacin therapy for severe Gram-negative sepsis: emphasis on infections with gentamicin resistant organisms. *Annals of Internal Medicine*, **83**, 484–488.

Clindamycin and Pseudomembraneous Colitis

Finch, R. G., Phillips, I. & Geddes, A. M. (1975) A clinical, microbiological and toxicological assessment of clindamycin phosphate. *Journal of Antimicrobial Chemotherapy*, **1**, 297–303.

Geddes, A. M., Dwyer, N. StJ., Ball, A. P. & Amos, R. S. (1977) Clindamycin in bone and joint infections. *Journal of Antimicrobial Chemotherapy*, **3**, 501–507.

Keusch, G. T. & Present, D. H. (1976) Summary of a workshop on clindamycin colitis. *Journal of Infectious Diseases*, **133**, 578–587.

Larson, H. E., Parry, J. V., Price, A. B., Davies, D. R., Dolby, J. & Tyrrell, D. A. J. (1977) Undescribed toxin in pseudomembranous colitis. *British Medical Journal*, **1**, 1246–1248.

Leading Article (1977) Pseudomembraneous enterocolitis. *Lancet*, **1**, 839–840.

Rifkin, G. D., Fekety, F. R., Silva, J. & Sack, R. B. (1977) Antibiotic-induced colitis: implications of a toxin neutralised by *Clostridium sordellii* antitoxin. *Lancet*, **11,** 1103–1106.

Tedesco, F. J., Barton, R. W. & Alpers, D. H. (1974) Clindamycin-associated colitis: a prospective study. *Annals of Internal Medicine*, **81,** 429–433.

Metronidazole

Bradley, W. G., Karlsson, I. J. & Rassol, C. G. (1977) Metronidazole neuropathy. *British Medical Journal*, **3,** 610–611.

Eykyn, S. J. & Phillips, I. (1976) Metronidazole and anaerobic sepsis. *British Medical Journal*, **2,** 1418–1421.

Hamilton-Miller, J. M. T. (1975) Antimicrobial agents acting against anaerobes. *Journal of Antimicrobial Chemotherapy*, **1,** 273–289.

Ingham, H. R., Selkon, J. B. & Hale, J. H. (1975a) The antibacterial activity of metronidazole. *Journal of Antimicrobial Chemotherapy*, **1,** 355–361.

Ingham, H. R., Rich, G. E., Selkon, J. B., Hale, J. H., Roxby, C. M., Betty, M. J., Johnson, R. W. G. & Uldall, P. R. (1975b) Treatment with metronidazole of three patients with serious infections due to *Bacteroides fragilis*. *Journal of Antimicrobial Chemotherapy*, **1,** 235–242.

Ings, R. M. J., McFadzean, J. A. & Ormerod, W. E. (1974) The mode of action of metronidazole in *Trichomonas vaginalis* and other micro-organisms. *Biochemical Pathology*, **23,** 1421–1429.

Selkon, J. B., Hale, J. H. & Ingham, H. R. (1975) Metronidazole in the treatment of anaerobic infection in man. *Chemotherapy* (Proceedings of the 9th International Congress of Chemotherapy, London, 1975), pp. 277–281. Eds. Williams, J. D. & Geddes, A. M. New York and London: Plenum Press.

Study Group (1975) An evaluation of metronidazole in the prophylaxis and treatment of anaerobic infections in surgical patients. *Journal of Antimicrobial Chemotherapy*, **1,** 393–401.

Tally, F. P., Sutter, V. L. & Finegold, S. M. (1975) Treatment of anaerobic infections with metronidazole. *Antimicrobial Agents and Chemotherapy*, **7,** 672–675.

Willis, A. T., Ferguson, I. R., Jones, P. H., Phillips, K. D., Tearle, P. V., Berry, R. B., Fiddian, R. V., Graham, D. F., Harland, D. H. C., Innes, D. B., Mee, U. M., Rothwell-Jackson, R. L., Sutch, I., Kilbey, C. & Edwards, D. (1976) Metronidazole in prevention and treatment of *Bacteroides* infections after appendicectomy. *British Medical Journal*, **1,** 318–321.

Willis, A. T., Ferguson, I. R., Jones, P. H., Phillips, K. D., Tearle, P. V., Hughes, D. F. R., Fiddian, R. V., Graham, D. F., Harland, D. H. C., Knight, D., Mee, U. M., Pashby, N., Rothwell-Jackson, R. L., Sachdeva, A. K., Sutch, I., Kilbey, C. & Edwards, D. (1977) Metronidazole in prevention and treatment of *Bacteroides* infections in elective colonic surgery. *British Medical Journal*, **1,** 607–610.

Rifampicin

Acocella, G., Hamilton-Miller, J. M. T. & Brumfitt, W. (1977) Can rifampicin use be safely extended. *Lancet*, **1,** 740–741.

Citron, K. M. & May, J. R. (1969) Rifamycin antibiotics in chronic purulent bronchitis. *Lancet*, **2,** 989–983.

Cobbold, R. J. C., Morris, G. D. & Willcox, R. R. (1968) Treatment of gonorrhoea with single oral doses of rifampicin. *British Medical Journal*, **4,** 681–682.

Devine, L. F., Pollard, R. B., Krumpe, P. E., Hoy, E. S., Mammen, R. E., Miller, C. H. & Peckinpaugh, R. O. (1973) Field trial of the efficacy of a previously proposed regimen using minocycline and rifampicin sequentially for the elimination of meningococci from healthy carriers. *American Journal of Epidemiology*, **97,** 394–401.

Hamilton-Miller, J. M. T., Kerry, D. W. & Brumfitt, W. (1977) The use of antibiotic combinations in the treatment of Serratia marcescens infections. *Journal of Antimicrobial Chemotherapy*, **3,** 193–194.

Leading Article (1976) Rifampicin: for tuberculosis only? *Lancet*, **1,** 290–291.

Murdoch, J.McC., Spiers, C. F., Wright, N. & Wallace, E. T. (1969) Rifampicin. *Lancet*, **1,** 1094.

Traub, W. H. & Kleber, I. (1975) In vitro additive effect of polymyxin B and rifampicin against Serratia marcescens. *Antimicrobial Agents and Chemotherapy*, **7,** 874–876.

Spectinomycin

McCormack, W. M. & Finland, M. (1976) Spectinomycin. *Annals of Internal Medicine*, **84,** 712–716.

Cinoxacin

Anderson, K. E., Mardh, P. A. & Colleen, S. (1978) Studies on the antibacterial activity and tissue distribution of cinoxacin. *Current Chemotherapy*, American Society for Microbiology, Washington. pp. 690–691.

Greenwood, D. (1978) The activity of cinoxacin against *Escherichia coli*. *Current Chemotherapy*, American Society for Microbiology, Washington. pp. 686–688.

Rodriguez, N., Madsen, P. O. & Welling, P. G. (1978) Pharmacokinetics of cinoxacin following intravenous infusion. *Current Chemotherapy*, American Society for Microbiology, Washington. pp. 692–693.

3. Spiral organisms in intestinal disease

B. S. Drasar and M. J. Hudson

INTRODUCTION

Anaerobic spiral bacteria and campylobacters are common inhabitants of the gastrointestinal tract of both animals and man. Although neither group of organisms has been considered to be a common cause of disease in man they are clearly associated with several animal diseases. Reports of human disease due to campylobacters, such as *Campylobacter (Vibrio) fetus*, were confined to cases of neonatal meningitis and bacteraemia in the compromised adult. The recent report of Skirrow (1977), however, suggests that campylobacters are a major identifiable cause of diarrhoea in man.

Spiral bacteria exist as normal components of the luminal and mucosal flora of a large number of animal species and in a wide variety of niches within the gastrointestinal tract. The morphological distinctions between spirochaetes, spirilla and campylobacters are far from clear. Spiral forms of campylobacters are common while aberrent spirilla may look like vibrios. The subject of host-spirochaete associations in animals and man has been reviewed by Harris and Kinyon (1974), Takeuchi et al (1974) and Rosebury (1962). Recent studies of several animal diseases have suggested that both spiral bacteria and campylobacters may be involved in the genesis of certain enteropathies in animals. Bearing in mind the valuable contribution of studies concerning the enteropathogenicity of *Escherichia coli* in piglets and calves to our understanding of *E. coli* diarrhoea in man, we consider it to be a suitable time to re-examine the role of spiral and curved bacteria in the genesis of intestinal disease in animals and man.

Although both spiral bacteria and campylobacters require specialised techniques for isolation and cultivation, they are sufficiently distinct as morphological types within the intestinal flora to have been widely studied by light and electron microscopy. The relative abundance of these organisms within the intestinal microflora varies widely between species, probably between individuals of a species and certainly according to site within the intestinal tract. Neither group commonly exist as homogenous populations, but usually form close symbiotic relationships with other bacteria. Some spiral bacteria even appear to possess the special ability to associate intimately and specifically with the host mucosal epithelium in a tolerated and apparently non-destructive manner. The factors controlling the stability of microbial inter-relationships, both within the indigenous microflora and between flora and host, is of paramount importance in the understanding of the genesis of intestinal disease.

It is beyond the scope of this review to discuss the biology and ecology of all gastrointestinal curved rods and spiral bacteria, and we will not include the oral and ano-genital spirochaetes and the anaerobic curved rods (*Selenomonas* spp.,

Butyrivibrio spp., etc.). Our intention is to discuss some general aspects of the biology and ecology of anaerobic spiral bacteria and campylobacters within the human and animal intestine, concentrating attention on associations between these bacteria and certain specific enteropathies.

INTESTINAL SPIROCHAETES AND CAMPYLOBACTERS

The taxonomy of campylobacters has been clarified in the recent edition of Bergey's manual (Smibert, 1974). Although morphologically similar to the classical vibrios (of which the type species is *Vibrio cholerae*) their requirement for reduced oxygen tension and their markedly different range of DNA base ratios shows them to comprise a distinct genus *Campylobacter* (Sebald and Véron, 1963). Campylobacters are oxidase positive and do not attack sugars. The genus is broadly divisible into two groups based on catalase production and nitrite reduction. Subsequent speciation is determined according to biochemical profile and growth response in the presence of glycine, bile, high NaCl concentration or at various temperatures.

Bergey's classification does not recognise the validity of *C. coli* and *C. jejuni* species proposed by Véron and Chatelain (1973) and states that these may be synonymous with *C. fetus* subspecies *jejuni*. These two 'species' are, for the convenience of this review, referred to as the *C. coli–C. jejuni* group of campylobacters. The clarification of the taxonomy of these important intestinal campylobacters must await future critical comparative studies on representative strains. The differential characteristics of campylobacters are shown in Table 3.1.

The taxonomy of the intestinal spiral bacteria is confused due to the few isolated strains available for comparative study. Thus many classification systems for these organisms have relied on microscopical or ultrastructural appearance unsupported by in vitro studies. We use the term spirochaetes to include an heterogeneous group of bacteria including treponemes, borrelia, spiral bacteria without axial filaments, and anaerobic spirilla. The interested reader is referred to Smibert (1974 and 1976) for such biochemical characterisation that exists concerning treponemes but the lack of variety of intestinal isolates available for comparison does not permit a systematic approach to the classification of intestinal spirochaetes.

Because of their distinctive motility and morphology, intestinal spirochaetes are easily examined in wet preparations using either critical phase contrast or darkfield light microscopy. The greater resolving power of the electron microscope, both transmission (TEM) and scanning (SEM) techniques, has allowed a much more precise examination of the spirochaetes present in the intestinal flora. In the absence of suitable isolation techniques electron microscopy provides the main characters used in comparative classification (Hovind-Hougen, 1976). Ultrastructural differences between spirochaetes will not necessarily correspond to biotypes, but the arrangements of axial filaments, flagellae, cytoplasmic granulation and inclusions and overall cell morphology and dimensions may be used to type particular organisms within a particular microhabitat.

Immunofluorescent staining techniques have been used successfully by several investigators to demonstrate spirochaetes and campylobacters present in intestinal material. This may be performed by an indirect fluorescent-labelled antibody test

(FAT) using convalescent sera from diseased animals or specific hyperimmune sera raised against a particular organism. The latter method has been used in studies on the sequential colonisation of the intestine of young mice (Davis, McAllister and Savage, 1973).

It should be recognised that some spiral bacteria observed in the intestine may be pleomorphic or bizarre forms of bacteria of other genera.

Table 3.1   Differential characteristics of campylobacters. (After Smibert, 1974)

	Catalase	NO_3 Redn	NO_2 Redn	H_2S in TSI	H_2S from cysteine	Growth in 1% glycine	Growth at 25°C	Growth at 42°C
C. sputorum								
ss. sputorum	−	+	+	+	+	+	+	−
ss. bubulus	−	+	+	+	+	+	V	V
ss. mucosalis	−	+	+	+	+	−	V	V
C. fetus								
ss. fetus	+	+	−	−	−	−	+	−
ss. intestinalis	+	+	−	−	+	+	+	−
ss. jejuni*	+	+	−	−	+	+	−	+
C. faecalis	+	+	−	+	+	+	−	+

(*C. coli-C. jejuni group)—Veron and Chatelain (1973)
V = variable

Isolation and cultivation techniques
Both campylobacters and spirochaetes are fastidious in their requirements for a defined oxygen tension. Campylobacters are microaerophilic, requiring between 2 and 5 per cent oxygen atmosphere enriched with at least 10 per cent CO_2 for optimal growth. They do not grow aerobically and generally grow poorly under anaerobic conditions. The intestinal spirochaetes are all obligate anaerobes and require rich media which is thoroughly deoxygenated and maintained in an oxygen-free condition. At least 10 per cent CO_2 is used in oxygen-free hydrogen or nitrogen as a gas phase for such cultures.

The less stringent conditions necessary for the isolation and cultivation of campylobacters are generally available in the routine laboratory. Cultures may be incubated in an ordinary 'anaerobe jar', without catalyst, after evacuation and replacement of the air with a suitable gas mixture. Alternatively, the inclusion of 0.25 to 0.45 per cent agar into broth media is sufficient to form an oxygen gradient within the depth of the medium and inoculated campylobacters will grow just below the surface in such media incubated in air. Campylobacters grow well on media such as tryptone blood agar, trypticase-soy agar or brain-heart infusion agar. Although they require neither blood nor serum for growth it is usual to use an agar medium supplemented with 5 to 10 per cent blood for primary isolation.

The conditions of strict anaerobiosis necessary for the isolation and subsequent cultivation of intestinal spirochaetes require more sophisticated techniques. Spirochaetes are nutritionally fastidious and require complex media containing added vitamins and co-factors, and chemical reducing agents. Strains vary in their requirement for whole blood, serum, rumen fluid supplements or fermentable carbohydrates.

Obligate anaerobes are at their most oxygen sensitive during initial isolation and tend to become relatively tolerant to brief exposure to oxygen on subsequent passage in vitro. Therefore it is at this stage that the specimen should be least exposed to air. Such exposure can be minimised by the use of pre-reduced and anaerobically sterilised media and the modified 'Hungate' technique (Holdeman and Moore, 1975) or by the use of more conventional media manipulated within an anaerobic chamber (Drasar, 1974).

Selective isolation techniques from intestinal samples
The isolation of fastidious organisms, particularly, as a minor component of a particular bacterial population, may be aided by the use of selective techniques. Both the physical fractionation of the flora by membrane filtration and the inclusion of antimicrobial agents in the media have been employed. The active motility and small cell dimensions of spirochaetes and campylobacters enable them to pass through the pores of membrane filters, either under pressure or by active migration. The faecal or mucosal homogenate is suspended in a suitably anaerobic broth, coarsely filtered or centrifuged to remove debris and filtered through membrane filters with a pore size between 0.65 μ and 0.30 μ. Alternatively it may be filtered through progressively smaller pore sizes from 1.2 μ down to 0.30 μ. Filtrates are then inoculated into or onto suitable media. Sterile membrane filters may be placed onto the surface of an agar medium and the suspension inoculated directly onto the top of the filter and retained there within a ring of petroleum jelly. After incubation for at least 48 hours suspicious surface growth and underlying agar medium is examined by light microscopy and spirochaetes subcultured. Some spirochaetes do not readily grow in broth culture and others will not produce surface growth on agar media in the absence of suitably anaerobic conditions. Solid, semi-solid and broth media should therefore be used for subculture of isolates.

Smibert (in Holdeman and Moore, 1975) suggests the following agents to be generally suitable for inclusion in media selective for spirochaetes: polymyxin B (800 units/ml), nalidixic acid (800 units/ml), cycloserine (100 μg/ml), nitrofurazone (200 μg/ml) and any sulphonamide (500 μg/ml). The inclusion of spectinomycin (400 μg/ml) in media may be used for the selective isolation of *Treponema hyodysenteriae* from normal and dysenteric pig faeces (Songer, Kinyon and Harris, 1976).

Campylobacters are generally resistant to novobiocin (2 μg/ml) and bacitracin (2 units/ml) and these agents may be used as selective agents (Holdeman and Moore, 1975). *C. sputorum* subspecies *mucosalis* may be isolated on a medium containing novobiocin 5 μg/ml and brilliant green 1 :60 000 (Lawson and Rowlands, 1974). Skirrow (1977) describes a medium for the selective isolation of *C. coli-C. jejuni* group by direct inoculation of faeces onto a medium containing vancomycin (10 μg/ml), polymyxin B (2.5 units/ml) and trimethoprim (5 μg/ml). Tanner and Bullin (1977) described the enrichment of low numbers of *C. coli-C. jejuni* by microaerophilic incubation in peptone broth at pH 8.4.

Other selective techniques may be used, for example, incubation temperatures other than 37°C. Skirrow (1977) suggests the incubation of cultures at 43°C as an aid to the selective isolation of *C. coli-C. jejuni*. Similarly, incubation at 25°C would favour the growth of *C. fetus* subspecies *intestinalis*. Kinyon, Harris and Glock (1977) reported that incubation of cultures for the isolation of *T. hyodysenteriae* at 42°C allows these organisms to outgrow other microbes present in faeces. The combination of antimicrobial agent and temperatures act in concert to produce good selective conditions.

Campylobacters and proliferative enteropathies of the pig

Porcine intestinal adenomatosis (PIA) is an infectious disease of weaned pigs characterised by adenomatous proliferations of the intestinal mucosa. The lesion, which is generally confined to ileum, caecum and colon, resembles a transient neoplasm and indeed metastatic spread to the mesenteric lymph nodes has been described. The condition will resolve without treatment and may not produce any obvious pathological signs, the most usual manifestation being reduction of growth rate and general loss of condition of individual pigs within a herd.

Aetiological studies
Rowland and Lawson (1974) demonstrated the specific fluorescence of particulate inclusions within the apical cytoplasm of affected mucosa when convalescent serum from a case of PIA was used in an indirect FAT. Electron microscopy showed the presence of large numbers of vibrio-like bacteria lying within the cytoplasm of affected cells, not subjected to phagocytosis or pinocytosis and apparently dividing. Further bacteriological studies resulted in the consistent isolation of between 10^5 and 10^8 catalase-negative microaerophilic vibrios per gram of affected mucosa, sometimes in association with lesser numbers of *C. coli* (Lawson and Rowland, 1974). This new campylobacter, subsequently named *C. sputorum* subspecies *mucosalis* was found only in PIA tissue, and antisera prepared against these organisms can be used to demonstrate specific cytoplasmic fluorescence by indirect FAT on affected tissue. *C. sputorum* subspecies *mucosalis* may also be demonstrated in or isolated from the intestinal lesions of pigs suffering from a number of other proliferative enteropathies, such as Regional Ileitis (RI), Necrotic enteritis (NE) and proliferative haemorrhagic enteropathy (PHE) (Rowland and Lawson, 1975a; 1976; Love, Love and Edwards, 1977). Such conditions are often associated with PIA within a herd of pigs and represent the more serious manifestations of proliferative disease. Cultural, serological and biochemical comparison of *C. sputorum* subspecies *mucosalis* with other campylobacters and *C. coli* show that this organism to be easily distinguishable by catalase reaction, cultural characteristics and serologically (Lawson, Rowland and Wooding, 1974; Lawson, Rowland and Roberts, 1975).

Transmission studies
The consistent finding of *C. sputorum* subspecies *mucosalis* in association with PIA, and in the epidemiologically related conditions RI, PHE, NE and the presence of elevated specific serum immunoglobulins to this organism strongly suggest that the campylobacter plays an important role in the aetiology of these adenomatous proliferations. Although transmission between pig is presumably by faecal contamination, experimental evidence is lacking. *C. sputorum* subspecies *mucosalis* may be isolated from the buccal cavity of pigs within a PIA herd and

may act as a reservoir of infectious material (Lawson, Rowland and Roberts, 1975). Recently Roberts, Rowland and Lawson (1977) have described the transmission of PIA and NE to experimental piglets given a 'cocktail' of a homogenate of adenomatous mucosa (containing *C. sputorum* subspecies *mucosalis*), pure cultures of the campylobacter, powdered chalk and a drug to slow gut motility. Without the tissue homogenate, however, the campylobacter was unable to initiate lesions.

Further studies are required to determine the factors necessary for cellular invasion by *C. sputorum* subspecies *mucosalis* and the genesis of adenomatous proliferative disease, and to clarify the role of *C. coli* in these conditions.

Relevance to human disease
Porcine adenomatous enteropathies may prove to be useful models of several human intestinal diseases including large bowel cancer, Crohn's disease and α-chain disease with intestinal lymphoma. The porcine intestine shares many common features with that of man and may be more relevant to the experimental study of human disease than is the bowel of the rat, rabbit or mouse. We have already noted that PIA appears to be a transient neoplasm with a rare capability of metastatic spread. Colorectal carcinoma in man arises from a pre-existing adenomatous polyp but the factors controlling the transformation to carcinoma are unknown. PIA, readily transmissible under controlled conditions, might be used to study these changes.

Regional ileitis (RI) of pigs is an obstructive ileitis manifesting as 'hosepipe bowel' with mucosal atrophy, muscular hypertrophy and proliferations of granulation tissue. These pathological features are also present in Crohn's disease in man. Recent evidence for the transmissibility of Crohn's disease (Cave, Mitchell and Brooke, 1975) suggests a microbial aetiology although the infectious agent has not been identified. An understanding of the mechanism by which *C. sputorum* subspecies *mucosalis* might initiate granulomatous changes within the intestinal mucosa and submucosa would be a valuable contribution to our understanding of the genesis of Crohn's disease.

Alpha-chain disease is an immunoproliferative disorder of the small intestine of man which eventually develops into frankly neoplastic lymphoma (WHO Study Group, 1976). It is characterised by massive plasma cell infiltration and an immunological disorder which is associated with high serum levels of virtually complete α-chain protein (heavy chain) of immunoglobulin A. There is good evidence that if treated early enough, the premalignant immunoproliferative disease can show complete regression following prolonged antibiotic therapy, suggesting that this disorder might also be associated with a microbial aetiology. PIA might serve as a most useful model for the study of microbial stimulation of the intestinal mucosa into a proliferative disorder.

Campylobacter enteritis in man

Although diarrhoea and abdominal pain are common features of campylobacter bacteraemia, these organisms are not readily isolated from microaerophilic stool culture because of overgrowth with normal faecal flora. Skirrow (1977) extending earlier observations of increased incidence of campylobacters in some patients with diarrhoea, examined stool specimens of patients of all ages presenting with diarrhoea using either membrane filtration (0.65 μ pore size) or a selective medium incubated at 43°C. Of 803 specimens, 7.1 per cent yielded campylobacters fitting the description of the *C. coli-C. jejuni* group and in 6.7 per cent these organisms were present as the sole 'pathogen'. The incidence of all other pathogens isolated (including Salmonellae, Shigellae, enteropathogenic *E. coli*, etc.) was 6.2 per cent. Furthermore, 31 of 38 patients had specific serum agglutinins to their own campylobacters, and in several patients a rising titre was observed. Recent studies using the same techniques have found campylobacters to be the single most common pathogen associated with diarrhoea (Table 3.2).

Table 3.2   Percentage isolations of campylobacters and other enteric pathogens from faeces

Reference	Patients with (+) without (−) diarrhoea	Campylobacter isolates	Total other bacterial pathogens and parasites
Skirrow (1977)	+	7.1 (6.7)*	6.2
	−	0	0
Dale (1977)	+	7.6 (ND)**	4.8
	−	0.2	ND
Tanner & Bullin (1977)	+	5.8 (ND)	ND
	−	0.8	ND
Pearson et al (1977)	+	4.2 (ND)	4.4
	−	0.2	ND
Telfer, Brunton & Heggie (1977)	+	8.7 (7.1)	15.8
	−	0	0
Bruce, Zochowski & Ferguson (1977)	+	13.9 (12.1)	12.9
	−	0.6	1.9

*Figures in parenthesis refer to campylobacters isolates as sole pathogen.
**ND = No data available.

Although most cases resolve rapidly and uneventfully, chemotherapy may be indicated in serious or debilitating cases. Skirrow (1977) suggests that a macrolide antibiotic, and in particular erythromycin, is probably the drug of choice although *C. coli-C. jejuni* are also sensitive to the aminoglycosides and tetracyclines.

It has been suggested that poultry, living or dead, may be the most important vector of campylobacter enteritis but further epidemiological studies are required to elucidate the environmental sources responsible. There is no doubt that poultry carry campylobacters intestinally and dogs may also suffer from campylobacter diarrhoea and particular human cases can be assigned to both sources.

The use of an incubation temperature of 43°C, of course, selects organisms of the *C. coli-C. jejuni* group. It might also be valuable to incubate at 25°C to select for other campylobacters from human faeces, in particular *C. fetus* subspecies *intestinalis* which is also present in the avian intestine.

Although routine examinations for campylobacter is a recent inovation, the Public Health Laboratory Service of the U.K., currently receives more than 500 notifications per month of campylobacter-associated enteritis and this must represent but a proportion of cases present in the population as a whole. We must await isolation data from other countries and of sources of infection to confirm that this is not simply a disease of North-West Europe and also to determine how great a risk to public health it may be, although there are already indications that this is not so (Butzler, 1973; Hallet et al, 1977).

Swine dysentery

Swine dysentery is an infectious mucohaemorrhagic diarrhoea of pigs and is an economically important disease associated with modern techniques of intensive pig rearing. Within a herd morbidity is high and in the absence of adequate treatment, high mortality occurs.

Lesions are commonly confined to the colonic and caecal mucosa, but may extend above the ileocaecal valve and throughout the colorectum. The lesion is characterised by oedema of the mucosa with copious mucus production and haemorrhage. Severely affected animals show extensive ulceration, a necrotic fibrinous pseudomembrane and sloughing of the mucosa. The condition is transmissible by feeding susceptible pigs with colonic contents, mucosa or faeces from affected pigs.

Infectious agents

In the 50 years following the original description of the disease the aetiological agent was considered to be a microaerophilic vibrio, *Campylobacter coli* although transmission experiments with this organism were not uniformly successful, and the organism is non-pathogenic for germ-free pigs (see Harris, 1974). Moreover, *C. coli* may be recovered from the faeces of both normal and dysenteric pigs and such isolates are indistinguishable both biochemically and by the electrophoretic comparison of several cell protein preparations (Morris and Park, 1973). *C. coli*, however, is often more numerous in the faeces of dysenteric pigs than in healthy pigs and the possibility exists that in terms of the disease in the field it may play an important role in determining the severity of the disease.

A number of morphological types of spirochaete are present in the colonic contents of both normal and dysenteric pigs (see Harris and Kinyon, 1974). Taylor and Blakemore (1971) examined the mucosa of early lesions of swine dysentery by TEM and noticed that the cellular invasion by a particular morphological type of spirochaete was associated with the earliest signs of cell damage. The spirochaete present in dysenteric lesions and faeces is large by comparison with most pig spirochaetes and has a characteristic serpentine motility. The spirochaete was cultured from dysenteric faeces by Taylor and Alexander (1971) in the U.K. and Harris et al (1972) independently in the U.S.A., and shown to be capable of producing typical swine dysentery when fed to pigs. The spirochaete, named *Treponema hyodysenteriae*, may be isolated from 0.65 μ filtrates of faeces or mucosal homogenate inoculated onto pre-reduced blood agar and incubated anaerobically. After 48 to 72 hours growth appears as a faint area of surface growth associated with complete haemolysis of the medium.

T. hyodysenteriae is an oxygen tolerant anaerobe, approximately 8 μ long and 0.35 μ in diameter, with between seven and nine axial filaments arising from each end of the cell and overlapping in the centre resulting in a 7-14-7 or 9-18-9 arrangement. It has been isolated from swine dysentery material in many countries (see Harris, 1974 and Kinyon, Harris and Glock, 1977) and the consistent reproduction of the disease in conventional pigs suggests a primary aetiological role in swine dysentery. This organism is capable of producing swine dysentery in pigs which are demonstrably free of *C. coli*.

Pathogenesis of T. hyodysenteriae dysentery

T. hyodysenteriae, alone or in combination with certain other bacteria such as *C. coli*, *E. coli*, *Megasphaera elsdenii* and others, is incapable of penetrating the intestinal mucosa and producing lesions in germ-free pigs, suggesting that a synergistic flora is necessary for initiation of mucosal invasion.

Alexander and co-workers reasoned that other bacteria present on the mucosa of the colon might be involved in initiating penetration of *T. hyodysenteriae* and isolated and compared the predominant flora of the colonic mucosa of normal pigs with that of very early lesions of swine dysentery (Alexander, Wellstead and Hudson, 1976). The predominant normal flora of normal conventional pigs comprised two species of *Lactobacillus*, *M. elsdenii* and *Sel. ruminantium*. In early lesions these were replaced by *T. hyodysenteriae*, and two previously undescribed anaerobes, a *Fusobacterium* spp. and an obligately anaerobic spiral bacteria resembling *Spirillum* spp. (probably belonging to the new genus *Anaerobiospirillum*, Davis et al, 1976). Penetration by *T. hyodysenteriae* was not observed in gnotobiotic pigs inoculated with dysenteric, normal, or both flora although the presence of the *Fusobacterium* spp. and anaerobic spirillum favoured colonisation of the mucosa by *T. hyodysenteriae*.

Meyer et al (1975), described the production of lesions of swine dysentery in germ-free pigs given *T. hyodysenteriae* in combination with four Gram-negative anaerobic bacteria, probably bacteroides and fusobacteria, which alone were nonpathogenic. Further studies are necessary to determine which combination of individual isolates are capable of initiating the penetration of the mucosa by the spirochaete.

Alexander et al (1976) isolated and compared the flora of early experimentally induced dysentery in Primary SPF pigs with that previously isolated from conventional pigs. These pigs were hysterectomy-derived and reared in a clean environment from which they acquired an intestinal flora which was different from that of conventional pigs, including the absence of the anaerobic *Spirillum* spp. and *C. coli*. The two isolates most commonly present in both SPF and conventional dysentery flora were *B. vulgatus* and *F. necrophorum*, similar groups of bacteria to those used by Meyer et al (1975). Preliminary results from experiments in both the U.K. and U.S.A. suggest that lesions resembling those of swine dysentery are produced in germ-free pigs inoculated with these two isolates and *T. hyodysenteriae* (Alexander, T. J. L. and Lysons, R. J., Personal Communication, 1977).

Recently *T. hyodysenteriae* has been shown to be capable of producing lesions in the caecum of experimentally inoculated guinea-pigs (Joens et al, 1976) which may prove to be a most useful model for studies on swine dysentery.

Field cases of dysentery show raised antibody titres to both *T. hyodysenteriae* and *C. coli* but may or may not be resistant to further infection. Similar partial protection can be induced by both oral and parenteral immunisation with laboratory attenuated *T. hyodysenteriae* (Hudson et al, 1976). It would be of interest to examine the role of locally synthesised immunoglobulins on the ability of *T. hyodysenteriae* to attach and penetrate the mucosa.

Certain other spirochaetes, morphologically and serologically related to *T. hyodysenteriae*, are present in the intestine of pigs and may proliferate on the mucosal surface in enteropathies other than swine dysentery and possibly result in erroneous diagnosis (Hudson, Alexander and Lysons, 1976). Such colo-caecal spirochaetoses occur with several diarrhoeic conditions, such as post weaning scour, colibacillosis and also in gastric ulceration and porcine intestinal adenomatosis (Taylor, D. J., Personal communication, 1977).

Spirochaetosis of the human colorectal mucosa

Although the role of *T. hyodysenteriae* in swine dysentery is well established, the role of spirochaetes in human intestinal disease remains far from clear. There are a few suggestive reports, but whether these represent a largely unrecognised enteropathy or merely the result of normal flora overgrowth in disadvantaged host intestine is not clear. The reports are often conflicting in their findings and the lack of isolation data is especially troubling.

Shera (1962) described a specific lesion of the recto-sigmoid said to be associated with vitamin C deficiency and altered bowel habit. A fuso-spirochaetal flora was present in these 'strawberry lesions' resembling those seen in Vincent's stomatitis (which was also present in the majority of patients). Treatment with organic arsenicals resulted in the resolution of both lesions and diarrhoea. Hurst and Vollum (1943) had found a similar flora associated with extensive colorectal ulceration in a patient who responded to treatment with organic arsenicals. These authors suggested that the lesions observed in their patients were definitely correlated with intestinal symptoms.

Harland and Lee (1967) found a correlation between spirochaetal infestation of the intestinal mucosa and gastrointestinal disturbance in a review of biopsies from the recto-sigmoid of patients presenting for investigation. Nine per cent of biopsies had a strongly basophilic brush-border visible by light microscopy which by TEM proved to be an homogenous layer of spirochaetes uniformly oriented parallel to the long axis of the cells and lying in between the microvilli. In subsequent studies, however, in which spirochaetosis of the mucosa was observed in 6.7 per cent of unselected rectal biopsies and 7.8 per cent of appendices obtained at surgery, a correlation between mucosal inflammation, intestinal disturbance and spirochaetes on the mucosa could not be demonstrated (Lee et al, 1971).

A similar massive spirochaetal colonisation of the colo-rectal mucosa has been observed in 28 per cent of Rhesus monkeys examined by TEM without any obvious signs of intestinal disturbance. In most of these animals the infestation was restricted to the colon although involvement of rectum and caecum may occur. When these workers examined human large bowel tissue by similar methods, spirochaetosis of the mucosa was found in only 1.9 per cent of 210 unselected large bowel specimens, and 2.1 per cent of 388 appendices (Takeuchi et al, 1974). These authors found no correlation between spirochaetal infestation and intestinal disturbance or disease. The presence of infestation in both monkey and man is evident in conventional histological sections as a strongly basophilic brush border and examination by TEM or SEM reveals massive colonisation by uniformly orientated spiral bacteria lying between the microvilli. The appearance of the condition is indistinguishable in either primate and two spiral bacteria can be distinguished. The predominant type is a typical treponeme with two to six spirals, 3 to 6 μ long by 0.2 to 0.4 μ wide, and has a 4-8-4 or 6-12-6 arrangement of axial filaments. This conforms with the description of *T. vincentii* on morphological grounds. The second organism is a spiral bacteria of similar dimensions but without axial filaments and with a single polar flagellum at each end, a description which does not conform to any cultivated bacteria.

Gad et al (1977) have recently reported the association of colorectal spirochaetosis, demonstrated by SEM, and long standing diarrhoea in four patients which resolved after eradication of the infestation with either doxycycline or neomycin.

A fresh approach to the investigation is overdue, using the recent innovations in isolation techniques for spirochaetes, to try to cultivate intestinal spirochaetes from the human bowel mucosa.

CONCLUSIONS

This brief examination of some of the animal diseases involving spiral bacteria illustrates the diversity of their pathological activity. Perhaps the application of the insight gained will illuminate some of the problems of intestinal disease in man. Indeed, the success of the studies on campylobacter enteritis gives us every ground for hope.

REFERENCES

Alexander, T. J. L., Wellstead, P. D. & Hudson, M. J. (1976) Studies of bacteria other than *Treponema hyodysenteriae* which may contribute to the lesion of swine dysentery. *Proc. Ann. Meeting Int. Pig. Vet Soc.* Abst. L.1.

Bruce, D., Zochowski, W. & Ferguson, I. R. (1977) Campylobacter enteritis. *Brit. Med. J.*, **ii**, 1219.

Butzler, J.-P. (1973) Related vibrios in Africa. *Lancet*, **ii**, 858.

Cave, D. R., Mitchell, D. N. & Brooke, B. N. (1975) Experimental animal studies of the etiology and pathogenesis of Crohn's disease. *Gastroenterology*, **69**, 618–624.

Dale, B. (1977) Campylobacter enteritis. *Brit. Med. J.*, **ii**, 318.

Davis, C. P., McAllister, J. S. & Savage, D. C. (1973) Microbial colonisation of the intestinal epithelium of suckling mice. *Infect. Immun.*, **7**, 666–672.

Davis, C. P., Cleven, D., Brown, J. & Balish, E. (1976) *Anaerobiospirillum*, a new genus of spiral-shaped bacteria. *Int. J. Syst. Bact.*, **26**, 498–504.

Drasar, B. S. (1974) The isolation and identification of non-sporing anaerobic bacteria. In *Infections with nonsporing anaerobic bacteria*, pp. 20–35. Eds. Philips, I. & Sussman, M. Edinburgh, London and New York: Churchill Livingstone.

Gad, A., Willen, R., Furugard, K., Fors, B. & Hradsky, M. (1977) Intestinal spirochaetosis as a cause of longstanding diarrhoea. *Upsala J. Med. Sci.*, **82**, 49–54.

Hallett, A. F., Botha, P. L. & Logan, A. (1977) Isolation of *Campylobacter fetus* from recent cases of human vibriosis. *J. Hyg. Camb.*, **79**, 381–389.

Harland, W. A., Lee, F. D. (1967) Intestinal spirochaetosis. *Lancet*, **iii**, 718–719.

Harris, D. L. (1974) Current status of research on swine dysentery. *Am. J. Vet. Res.*, **164**, 809–812.

Harris, D. L. & Kinyon, J. M. (1974) Significance of anaerobic spirochaetes in the intestines of animals. *Am. J. Clin. Nutr.*, **27**, 1297–1304.

Harris, D. L., Glock, R. D., Christensen, C. R. & Kinyon, J. M. (1972) Swine dysentery I inoculation of pigs with *Treponema hyodysenteriae* (new species) and reproduction of the disease. *Vet. Med. Small Anim. Clin.*, **67**, 61–64.

Holdeman, L. V. & Moore, W. E. C. (1975) *Anaerobic Laboratory Manual*, 3rd Edition. Virginia Polytechnic Institute and State University.

Hovind-Hougen, K. (1976) Determination by means of electron microscopy of morphological criteria of value for classification of some spirochaetes in particular treponemes. *Acta. Path. Microbiol. Scand. B. Suppl 255.*

Hudson, M. J., Alexander, T. J. L. & Lysons, R. J. (1976) Diagnosis of swine dysentery: spirochaetes which may be confused with *Treponema hyodysenteriae. Vet. Red.,* **99,** 498–500.

Hudson, M. J., Alexander, T. J. L., Lysons, R. J. & Prescott, J. F. (1976) Swine dysentery: protection of pigs by oral and parenteral immunisation with attenuated *Treponema hyodysenteriae. Res. Vet. Sci.,* **21,** 366–367.

Hurst, Sir A, & Vollum, R. L. (1943) Ulcerative colitis caused by Vincent's organisms. *Guy's Hosp. Rep.,* **92,** 118–120.

Kinyon, J. M., Harris, D. L. & Glock, R. D. (1977) Enteropathogenicity of various isolates of *Treponema hyodysenteriae. Infect. Immun.,* **15,** 638–646.

Joens, L. A., Songer, J. G., Harris, D. L. & Glock, R. D. (1976) Production of lesions resembling those of swine dysentery in guinea pigs with pure cultures of *Treponema hyodysenteriae.* Annual Meeting American Society of Microbiology (Abstract B15), p. 13.

Lawson, E. H. K. & Rowland, A. C. (1974) Intestinal adenomatosis in the pig: a bacteriological study. *Res. Vet. Sci.,* **17,** 331–336.

Lawson, G. H. K., Rowland, A. C. & Roberts, L. (1975) Isolation of *Campylobacter sputorum* subsp. *mucosalis* from oral cavity of pigs. *Vet. Rec.,* **97,** 308.

Lawson, G. H. K., Rowland, A. C. & Wooding, P. (1975) The characterisation of *Campylobacter sputorum* subsp. *mucosalis* isolated from pigs. *Res. Vet. Sci.,* **18,** 121–126.

Lawson, G. H. K., Rowland, A. C. & Roberts, L. (1976) Studies on *Campylobacter sputorum* subsp. *mucosalis. J. Med. Microbiol,* **9,** 163–191.

Lee, F. D., Kraszewski, A., Gordon, J., Howie, J. E. R., McSeverey, D. & Harland, W. A. (1971) Intestinal spirochaetosis. *Gut,* **12,** 126–133.

Love, R. J., Love, D. N. & Edwards, M. J. (1977) Proliferative haemorrhagic enteropathy in pigs. *Vet. Rec.,* **100,** 65–68.

Meyer, R. C., Simon, J. & Byerly, C. S. (1974 & 1975) The etiology of swine dysentery: 1. Oral inoculation of germ-free swine with *Treponema hyodysenteriae* and *Vibrio coli.* 2. Effect of a known microbial flora, weaning and diet on disease production in gnotobiotic and conventional swine. 3. The role of selected Gram-negative anaerobes. *Vet. Path.* (1974) **11,** 515–526[1], **11,** 527–534[2], (1975) **12,** 46–54[3].

Morris, J. A. & Park, R. W. A. (1973) A comparison using gel electrophoresis of cell proteins of campylobacters (vibrios) associated with infertility, abortion and swine dysentery. *J. Gen. Microbiol.,* **78,** 165–178.

Pearson, A. D., Suckling, W. G., Ricciardi, I. D., Knill, M. & Ware, E. (1977) Campylobacter-associated diarrhoea in Southampton. *Brit. Med. J.,* **2,** 955–956.

Roberts, L., Lawson, G. H. K. & Rowland, A. C. (1977) Porcine intestinal adenomatosis associated with serologically distinct *Campylobacter sputorum* subsp. *mucosalis. Res. Vet. Sci.,* **23,** 257–258.

Roberts, L., Rowland, A. C. & Lawson, G. H. K. (1977) Experimental reproduction of porcine intestinal adenomatosis and necrotic enteritis. *Vet. Rec.,* **100,** 12–13.

Rosebury, T. D. (1962) Micro-organisms indigenous to man. New York: McGraw-Hill Book Co.

Rowland, A. C. & Lawson, G. H. K. (1974) Intestinal adenomatosis in the pig: immunofluorescent and electron microscopic studies. *Res. Vet. Sci.,* **17,** 323–330.

Rowland, A. C. & Lawson, G. H. K. (1975) Porcine intestinal adenomatosis: a possible relationship with necrotic enteritis, regional ileitis and proliferative haemorrhagic enteropathy. *Vet. Rec.,* **97,** 178–180.

Sebald, M. & Véron, M. (1963) Tenur en bases de l'adu et classification des vibrions. *Annales de l'Institut Pasteur,* **105,** 897–910.

Shera, A. G. (1962) Specific granular lesions associated with intestinal spirochaetosis. *Brit. J. Surg.,* **50,** 68–77.

Skirrow, M. B. (1977) Campylobacter enteritis: a 'new' disease. *Brit. Med. J.,* **2,** 9–11.

Smibert, R. M. (1974) Genus *Treponema,* pp. 175–184, Genus *Campylobacter,* pp. 207–212. In *Bergey's Manual of Determinative Bacteriology,* 8th edition, eds. Buchanan, R. E. & Gibbons, N. E. Baltimore: Williams and Wilkins Co.

Smibert, R. M. (1976) 1. Cultivation, composition and physiology of avirulent treponemes. 2. Classification of non-pathogenic treponemes, *Borrelia* and *Spirochaeta.* In *The Biology of Parasitic Spirochaetes,* ed. Johnson, R. C., pp. 49–56[1], 121–131[2]. New York, San Francisco and London: Academic Press.

Songer, J. G., Kinyon, J. M. & Harris, D. L. (1976) Selective medium for the isolation of *Treponema hyodysenteriae. J. Clin. Microbiol.,* **4,** 57–60.

Takeuchi, A., Jervis, H. R., Nakazawa, H. & Robinson, D. M. (1974) Spiral-shaped organisms on the surface colonic epithelium of the monkey and man. *Am. J. Clin. Nutr.,* **27,** 1287–1296.

Tanner, E. I. & Bullin, C. H. (1977) Campylobacter enteritis. *Brit. Med. J.*, **2,** 579.

Taylor, D. J. & Alexander, T. J. L. (1971) The production of dysentery in swine by feeding cultures containing a spirochaete. *Br. Vet. J.*, **127,** lviii–lxi.

Taylor, D. J. & Blakemore, W. F. (1971) Spirochaetal invasion of the colonic epithelium in swine dysentery. *Res. Vet. Sci.*, **12,** 177–179.

Telfer-Brunton, W. A. & Heggie, D. (1977) Campylobacter-associated diarrhoea in Edinburgh. *Brit. Med. J.*, **2,** 956.

Veron, M. & Chatelain, R. (1973) Taxonomic study of the genus *Campylobacter*, Sebald and Véron and designation of the neotype strain for type species, *Campylobacter fetus* (Smith and Taylor) Sebald and Véron. *Int. J. System. Bact.*, **23,** 124–134.

WHO Study Group (1976) Alpha-chain disease and related small-intestinal lymphoma. *Bull. World Health Organization*, **54,** 615–624.

4. Diagnosis of systemic fungal infections

E. G. V. Evans

Progress in the diagnosis of systemic mycoses over the last few years has been steady rather than spectacular and further improvements are necessary.

Diagnosis of systemic mycoses on clinical grounds alone is seldom possible. Traditionally it has relied upon the demonstration of fungi in tissue by culture and histology but this is not always successful. Nowadays serology is proving to be an increasingly useful adjunct to diagnosis.

Fungal infections are now accorded greater recognition by clinicians and laboratory workers and this improved awareness has, in itself, considerably increased the chances of diagnosis of a systemic mycosis. The increase in interest is due in large part to a rise in the incidence of opportunistic fungal infections. These infections are rapidly fulminating, frequently fatal, and are unfortunately among the most difficult to diagnose. The availability of new antifungal agents and better methods for administration of amphotericin B has increased the chances of successful treatment, providing a diagnosis is made sufficiently early. This has provided a further stimulus for the development of rapid and reliable diagnostic methods.

The established criteria used for the diagnosis of systemic mycoses are comprehensively described in text-books, such as those by Conant et al (1971), Rippon (1974) and Emmons et al (1977), and basic details are therefore omitted from this chapter.

OCCURRENCE OF SYSTEMIC MYCOSES

It is worthwhile reviewing briefly the more recent literature with particular reference to the opportunistic infections, as an awareness of the situations under which an infection may arise increases the likelihood of diagnosis and, moreover, these articles frequently deal with aspects of diagnosis. It is not intended to present an exhaustive list but rather a selection of references to provide those interested with a source of more detailed information.

The features of the diseases caused by *Histoplasma capsulatum*, *Coccidioides immitis*, *Blastomyces dermatitidis* and *Paracoccidioides brasiliensis* are well documented. Their importance, primarily as respiratory pathogens, is underlined by the fact that several large congresses have been held to discuss histoplasmosis (Ajello, Chick and Furcolow, 1971), coccidioidomycosis, and paracoccidioidomycosis (Pan American Health Organisation, 1972). The proceedings of the most recent on histoplasmosis and coccidioidomycosis are to be published shortly. There are also worthwhile reviews of African histoplasmosis (Vanbreuseghem, 1976) and paracoccidioidomycosis (Giraldo et al, 1976).

Opportunistic fungal infections have received the most attention over the past few years and they too have been the subject of an international meeting (Chick, Balows and Furcolow, 1975). Aspergillosis, candidiasis, cryptococcosis and phycomycosis are the most frequently encountered opportunistic infections, although it must be recognised that almost any species of fungus is capable of causing disease in a compromised host and, furthermore, that diseases such as coccidioidomycosis and histoplasmosis can appear as 'opportunistic infections' in these patients. The factors that predispose to these infections are complex and a good overview of the conditions under which they arise is given by Louria (1974). In general, they are those which lower host resistance or provide more favourable conditions for the growth of the fungus; the risk of superinfection is greatest when several factors operate together.

The occurrence of fungal infections in compromised hosts generally is reviewed by Young et al (1974) and Williams, Krick and Remington (1976) and there are also accounts of specific diseases such as pulmonary cryptococcosis (Hammermann et al, 1973; Duperval et al, 1977), cryptococcal meningitis (Diamond and Bennett, 1974), phycomycosis (Meyer and Armstrong, 1973), aspergillosis (Young et al, 1970), pulmonary candidiasis (Masur, Rosen and Armstrong, 1977) and generalised candidiasis (Hughes and Remington, 1972; Stone et al, 1974).

There are numerous accounts of the occurrence of opportunistic mycoses among specific groups of patients. Fungal infections in patients with malignancies are well documented (Krick and Remington, 1976; Rosen, 1976; Kaplan, Rosen and Armstrong, 1977; Singer, Kaplan and Armstrong, 1977). Mycoses also develop in patients treated with immunosuppressive agents and steroids related to transplantation surgery. The majority of reports relate to renal transplants (Gallis et al, 1975; Mills, Siegler and Wolfe, 1975) but they have also been reported after heart (Gurwith, Stinson and Remington, 1971) and liver (Schröter et al, 1977) transplantation. Bach et al (1973) found that renal transplant patients treated for rejection of their grafts were most likely to become infected. Fungal infections also occur after cardiac surgery (Evans, 1976a) and commonly take the form of an endocarditis, usually due to candida or aspergillus (Seelig et al, 1974; Kammer and Utz, 1974; Norenberg et al, 1975).

Candida infections have been reported in patients with acute burns (Macmillan, Law and Holder, 1972) and fungaemia, usually due to *Candida albicans*, among general surgery patients (Rodrigues and Wolff, 1974; Ribet et al, 1975). Candida infections can also result from the contamination of intravenous (i.v.) catheters and this is estimated to account for almost a fifth of reported cases of candida sepsis; patients receiving intravenous hyperalimentation appear worst affected (Stone et al, 1974; Rose and Varkey, 1975).

CLINICAL DIAGNOSIS

Clinical criteria can only be used to make a presumptive diagnosis of fungal infection. In the absence of any specific signs or symptoms it is important to consider the possibility of a fungus infection from the outset. At least, a suspected bacterial infection which has failed to respond to seemingly appropriate antibacterial therapy should always be regarded as a possible fungal infection.

There have been few advances in clinical diagnosis but modern techniques for evaluation of patients have been applied to diagnosis of fungal disease.

Pulmonary mycoses have been diagnosed during the evaluation of bronchial brushing (Finley et al, 1974) and lung biopsy techniques (Greenman, Goodall and King, 1975; Bhatt et al, 1977) for diagnosis of opportunistic pulmonary infections in general. The fungal infections they detected included aspergillosis, coccidioidomycosis, candidiasis and phycomycosis.

Scanning techniques have been employed. Thadepalli et al (1977) found that [67]gallium lung scans gave good correlation with conventional methods for diagnosis of pulmonary infections. Four patients with mycoses were included in the study (two *Cryptococcus neoformans* infections, one *C. immitis* and one *H. capsulatum*); those with *Cr. neoformans* and *C. immitis* infections showed an increased uptake of [67]gallium. The diagnostic value of strontium-87m lung scans has been assessed in 10 patients with proven pulmonary aspergillosis (Rohatgi et al, 1977) but the results did not always correlate with radiological findings and false positive results were obtained in control patients with other lung disorders. Bone scanning has been used to assess the extent of skeletal involvement in disseminated coccidioidomycosis (Armbuster et al, 1977). This technique was more sensitive than radiography for detection of early skeletal disease but the two techniques were found to be complementary.

Echocardiography has been used successfully to demonstrate fungal vegetations on heart valves in candida endocarditis of the aortic valve (Gottlieb et al, 1974; Arvan et al, 1976; Gomes et al, 1976) and in aspergillus endocarditis of a Starr-Edwards mitral prosthesis (Schelbert and Muller, 1972). It has been suggested that this procedure should be used routinely, early in the clinical evaluation of drug addicts with suspected endocarditis, particularly when blood cultures are negative and there are systemic emboli (Gottlieb et al, 1974).

The observation that endophthalmitis is a common complication in patients with systemic forms of candidiasis, especially those with candidaemia, has provided the clinician with a most useful diagnostic sign (Griffin et al, 1973; Edwards et al, 1974). The specificity of this sign has been shown in one series of 76 patients with candida endophthalmitis in which 78 per cent of the 37 patients who subsequently died showed evidence of systemic candidiasis at autopsy (Edwards et al, 1974). Yeast endophthalmitis can readily be induced experimentally in rabbits by intravenous (i.v.) inoculation of *C. albicans* but other *Candida* spp. were found to give less consistent results (Edwards et al, 1977). However, in man, several species of *Candida* have been found to cause endophthalmitis.

Endogenous aspergillus endophthalmitis can also occur in patients with invasive aspergillosis (Naidoff and Green, 1975).

LABORATORY DIAGNOSIS

Laboratory procedures often confirm a presumptive clinical diagnosis of fungal infection. In some cases, particularly with some of the opportunistic infections, they only provide further subjective evidence to be considered along with the clinical findings. It is essential that there should be close collaboration between clinician and laboratory worker.

Culture

Recent efforts have in the main been directed towards increasing the sensitivity and selectivity of cultural procedures and finding quicker and more convenient methods for the identification of fungal isolates.

Processing of specimens

A method for enumeration of yeasts in sputum which involves trypsin digestion, homogenization with glass beads, followed by dilution plating is described by Müller, Langer and Jaeger (1977), and they found that with this method the recovery of C. albicans was twice as good as from untreated sputa. Gervasi and Miller (1975) describe a similar procedure which gave improved isolation of Cr. neoformans from sputum. Here the digested sputum is centrifuged to concentrate the yeasts before plating the sediment onto Niger seed medium.

Blood culture techniques have received much attention recently. Biphasic medium has been found to be markedly superior to broth for detection of fungaemia (Roberts and Washington, 1975). Furthermore, it is clear that anaerobic atmospheres in culture bottles are unsuitable for satisfactory growth of fungi. Vacuum blood culture bottles have been shown to inhibit the growth of yeasts and venting the bottles considerably enhances the recovery of these organisms (Gantz et al, 1974; Blazevic, Stemper and Matsen, 1975). The value of hypertonic medium for the isolation of fungi from blood cultures has been assessed by Roberts, Horstmeier and Ilstrup (1976). They compared biphasic medium with and without 15 per cent sucrose in vented bottles and found a higher recovery rate in the medium without sucrose.

A vented, biphasic culture system appears to be best for the recovery of fungi from blood.

Isolation and identification procedures

Procedures for the identification of yeasts have received most attention and although identification of these organisms is still based primarily on their fermentation and assimilation reactions, there have been significant improvements to the standard methodology. Land et al (1975) suggested the incorporation of bromocresol purple dye into the medium for the pour-plate auxanographic technique—the colour change makes positive carbohydrate assimilation results considerably easier to read and visible earlier. Furthermore, this group has devised a rapid method for determining nitrate assimilation in yeasts, based on the detection of nitrate-reductase activity in the cells, which gives results within 10 minutes (Hopkins and Land, 1977). A series of rapid tests for the identification of yeasts based on carbohydrate and nitrate assimilation, fermentation and urease production is described by Huppert et al (1975) and the value of this scheme is endorsed by Segal and Ajello (1976) who found that it correctly identified 94 per cent of isolates within three days.

The rapid identification of C. albicans is based on the production of germ tubes, usually in serum, or of chlamydospores on corn meal or Czapek-Dox and Tween 80 agar. Three solid media have recently been described which allow the sequential development of germ tubes (within 3 h) and chlamydospores (after 24–48 h) by *C. albicans*. One consists of 0.1 per cent glucose agar (Joshi et al, 1975), the second contains rice extract, oxgall and Tween 80 (Beheshti, Smith and Krause, 1975) and a third is a combination of chitosan, trypticase and Tween 80 with antibiotics added to enable the direct isolation and identification of *C. albicans* from clinical specimens (Gunasekaran and Hughes, 1977). Beheshti et al (1975) found, however, that their medium was unable to distinguish satisfactorily between *C. albicans* and *C. stellatoidea*, and indeed this limitation may well apply to all the available methods for the rapid identification of *C. albicans*. *C. stellatoidea* is a relatively infrequent isolate but its inability to assimilate sucrose would appear to be the only satisfactory criterion for readily distinguishing it from *C. albicans*.

Improved methods for identification and isolation of *Cr. neoformans* are also now available. A rapid method for determining urease production by cryptococci is described by Paliwal and Randhawa (1977) and it gives results, based on a colour reaction, within 50 minutes. Many of the media used for the identification of *Cr. neoformans* contain substrates for a phenol oxidase enzyme present in this yeast—the enzyme reaction produces a pigment which turns the colonies brown. Niger seed (*Guizotia abyssinica*) was the original substrate but more recently a medium containing caffeic acid and ferric citrate as substrate has been described by Hopfer and Blank (1975). Moreover, caffeic acid and ferric citrate-impregnated paper discs have been used for the rapid identification of *Cr. neoformans*, giving brown pigmentation within 6 h (Hopfer and Gröschel, 1975) and the general reliability of this rapid method has been confirmed by Wang, Zeimis and Roberts (1977). Caffeic acid has been combined with inositol and urea in a medium intended for the selective isolation and identification of *Cr. neoformans* from clinical specimens (Healy, Dillavou and Taylor, 1977) and with this medium the organism could be detected within 36 h.

Fleming, Hopkins and Land (1977) combine the features of earlier media to formulate a useful dual purpose medium containing oxgall, Tween 80 and caffeic acid which enables rapid presumptive identification of *C. albicans* and *Cr. neoformans*. Results are usually obtained within 3–12 h and in not more than 24 h.

Commercial kits for the identification of medically important yeasts are now available and generally they appear to give satisfactory results, with up to 99 per cent accuracy compared with conventional methods (Bowman and Ahearn, 1976).

Immunological methods for identification of fungi. An immunological method for the rapid and specific identification of *Histoplasma* and *C. immitis* cultures is described by Standard and Kaufman (1976; 1977). The test culture is incubated in broth for three days and the concentrated culture supernatant is tested by immunodiffusion for the presence of antigens homologous to those found in histoplasmin or coccidioidin. The method was sensitive and specific and permitted identification within five days. This approach is interesting and could well be extended to the identification of other fungi.

Significance of culture findings

The significance of a fungal isolate from clinical material depends on its source and identity. The isolation of well established pathogens such as *H. capsulatum* or *C. immitis* from any specimen is generally regarded as evidence of infection with these fungi. However, with the opportunistic pathogens such as candida and aspergillus the situation is not as clear cut; care should be taken in interpretation of culture results and some attention paid to the quantity of fungus isolated. It is important to remember that almost any species of fungus is capable of causing disease in severely compromised patients. The isolation of fungi from blood cultures or cerebrospinal fluid (CSF) provides more reliable evidence of systemic infection than isolations from other clinical material.

Probably the greatest difficulties in interpretation arise with the commensal *Candida* species. Recovery of these organisms from material such as urine, faeces, sputum or bronchial secretions is of relatively little significance as the numbers isolated may be considerable in the absence of infection, particularly among hospitalised patients. The significance of yeasts in urine is discussed by Speller (1975), and it has been said that patients with negative urine cultures are unlikely to have systemic yeast infection (Stone et al, 1974).

Isolation of *Cr. neoformans* from CSF is taken as firm evidence of CNS infection but its isolation from sputum requires further investigation. The yeast has been recovered from the sputum of patients with no evidence of pulmonary cryptococcosis (Hammermann et al, 1973; Randhawa and Pal, 1977) and it has been suggested that *Cr. neoformans* may be a commensal of the respiratory tract, especially among patients with predisposing respiratory disorders.

The recovery of fungi from blood cultures is a more reliable indicator of systemic infection. However, these cultures are frequently negative, particularly in patients with fungal endocarditis, and a series of cultures may be necessary. In one study, cultures of arterial rather than venous blood were found to be more reliable for recovery of candida from the bloodstream (Stone et al, 1974). Unfortunately, isolation of a yeast from a blood culture is not absolute proof of systemic infection as reports of transient candidaemias of no clinical significance have been frequent; these are often related to intravenous catheterization and usually disappear after removal of the catheter. Repeated demonstration of candida in the bloodstream distinguishes between transient candidaemia and true infection. In invasive aspergillosis however, and in other systemic mycoses where the agent is filamentous, blood cultures usually remain negative.

It should be remembered when assessing the results of blood culture that fungi are slower growing than bacteria. Paisley, Todd and Roe (1977) found that subcultures taken from paediatric blood cultures after 4–16 h incubation detected over 60 per cent of the positive bacterial cultures, whereas the four isolates of candida they obtained were seen only in two-day subcultures. As Kobza et al (1976) point out, the concomitant presence of bacteria and candida in blood cultures may be a source of error in diagnosis of candidiasis.

All fungi isolated from blood cultures should be identified fully and regarded as significant until proved otherwise.

Direct microscopy

Direct microscopy of body fluids can be useful for diagnosis of systemic fungal infections and a few recent developments are worthy of mention.

Diagnosis of cryptococcal meningitis by examination of Indian ink preparations of CSF is not always successful. As an alternative, Jameson and Wells (1972) recommend the use of CSF cell preparations made on a cytocentrifuge—the procedure concentrates the cells which can then be stained by Giemsa and PAS methods.

Rapid diagnosis of pulmonary blastomycosis by recognition of *B. dermatitidis* in Papanicolau stained preparations of sputum and bronchial washings is described by Sutliff and Cruthirds (1973) and Sanders et al (1977). Moreover, there have been recent reports of the detection of fungal septicaemia by microscopic examination of blood. Kobza and Steenblock (1977) observed blastospores and pseudohyphae in blood smears from a man with candidaemia and Girard et al (1977) were able to diagnose disseminated histoplasmosis from a peripheral blood film. Block and Young (1977) also describe the early diagnosis of opportunistic infections using microscopic examination of peripheral blood and a membrane filter blood culture technique which gave results within 16–24 h.

Histopathology

Histological examination of biopsy specimens is very useful for diagnosis of systemic fungal infections and in many cases a diagnosis is only made retrospectively on the appearance of the fungus in autopsy material.

Available histological stains, used in combination, can help distinguish between different types of fungi but there is a need for more specific differentiation. In this respect the work of Rolph and Austwick (1973) where they could, for example, differentiate between the hyphae of phycomycetes and those of other fungi using Puchtler and Sweat cresyl fast violet stain for acid mucopolysaccharide, is an encouraging development.

Immunohistology, using fluorescent antibody methods, has been employed for identification of fungi in tissue and this work is briefly reviewed by Kaufman (1976). Improved reagents are needed to increase specificity but the preparation of sufficient quantities of highly specific reagents would remain a problem and it is likely that only a small number of specialist laboratories could carry out such work.

Serology

Serological tests are of proven value in supporting the diagnosis of systemic fungal infections and they may also be used to assess prognosis and response to therapy. The tests used for the diagnosis of some diseases such as histoplasmosis and cryptococcosis give reliable results but for others the tests provide only presumptive evidence of infection and there is a need to improve sensitivity and specificity. In some cases antibodies may be present in the absence of infection and, conversely, some infected patients have little or no detectable antibody response because of their underlying disease condition, chemotherapy or because their infection is at an early stage. Cross reactions are also encountered between some pathogenic fungi and these reflect the crude nature of fungal antigenic extracts. Clearly, the results of serological tests must be interpreted with care but, generally, a high or rapidly rising antibody titre is indicative of infection and a series of tests is more helpful than a single investigation.

The recent literature on fungal serology is voluminous and here it is only possible to summarise some of the main findings and quote selected references. There have been improvements, but perhaps the greatest advance has been the growing realisation of the need to standardise test procedures and reagents. Practical guides to methodology and interpretation of results, such as those by Evans (1976b), Kaufman (1976) and Palmer et al (1977), make it increasingly possible for more laboratories to carry out serological tests and they also result indirectly in standardisation. Commercially produced serodiagnostic kits are also emerging with similar effects.

Techniques for antibody detection

A significant development has been the almost universal acceptance of counter-immunoelectrophoresis (CIE) as a more rapid and sensitive method than immunodiffusion (ID) for detection of precipitins to fungi (Mackenzie and Philpot, 1975). CIE also provides a convenient and rapid method for the estimation of antibody titre (Evans, 1976b). However, ID is still widely used and recently Kaben and Westphal (1977) showed that its sensitivity could be increased by the addition of 2 per cent polyethylene glycol 6000 to the agar as a diffusion agent, and with this modification candida precipitins were detected in 40 per cent more sera.

More sensitive methods for antibody detection such as enzyme immunoassay (ELISA) and radioimmunoassay (RIA) are now being introduced into mycology and are likely to become more widely used. For example, the diagnostic application of ELISA for the detection of antibody to aspergillus and candida has been assessed by Hommel, Kien Truong and Bidwell (1976) and Reiss et al (1977b) have used solid-phase competitive RIA for the detection of antibody to the M antigen of histoplasmin.

Standardisation

The need to find the most satisfactory reagents and methods for carrying out tests is underlined by two inter-laboratory studies on candida serology, which showed that markedly different results are obtained when the same sera are tested in different laboratories with different methods and reagents (Faux et al, 1975; Merz et al, 1977).

Antigenic extracts from fungi are crude mixtures, and purification, with selection of the components most relevant to diagnosis, will ultimately improve specificity. This is made increasingly possible by the availability of better techniques for antigen separation and analysis. In this respect, the application of quantitative crossed immunoelectrophoresis (Laurell) to the study of *C. albicans* antigens, which led to the discovery of 78 different components (Axelsen, 1973), was an important development. Subsequent studies with this technique and its modifications have permitted more precise monitoring of the precipitin response in patients with candida infection and these developments are summarised by Axelsen (1976). These techniques have also been used to study other fungi, for example, *Aspergillus* spp. (Drouhet et al, 1973) and *H. capsulatum* (Mok, Buckley and Campbell, 1977).

A combination of antigenic and chemical analyses as employed by Bradley et al (1974) in a study of the H and M antigens of histoplasmin and by Reiss et al (1977a) for their study of *H. capsulatum* yeast cell walls, shows the approach ultimately necessary with all pathogenic fungi.

Value of tests in diagnosis of infection

Detailed accounts of the serological and skin tests currently used in diagnosis, together with notes on their value and on interpretation of results, are given by Longbottom and Pepys (1975) and Kaufman (1976), and only recent developments are discussed here.

Histoplasmosis

There are recent reports of factors that may interfere with the tests for histoplasmosis. Rheumatoid factor and cold agglutinins were found to block the complement-fixation (CF) reaction to the yeast antigens of *H. capsulatum* but not to histoplasmin antigen (Johnson and Roberts, 1976). A high titre of rheumatoid factor also interferes with the histoplasmin latex agglutination (LA) test and titres of ≥1:32 were seen in patients with no evidence of acute histoplasmosis (Oxenhandler, Adelstein and Rogers, 1977). Furthermore, Di Salvo and Corbett (1976) report apparent false positive LA reactions at titres of ≥1:16 in patients with tuberculosis.

The work of Pine et al (1977) could lead to an increased specificity of tests employing histoplasmin as antigen. They found that purification of the H and M antigens of histoplasmin gave products which were highly reactive and specific when used in a variety of serological tests. These purified reagents did not cross-react with the sera of patients with other fungal infections.

Coccidioidomycosis

Interest has recently focussed on the relative values of coccidioidin and spherulin antigens in serological and skin tests for coccidioidomycosis. Scalarone et al (1974) compared both antigens in the CF test and found spherulin to be more reactive. However, Huppert et al (1977) found no difference in their reactivity with sera submitted for routine *C. immitis* serology, but found that spherulin was considerably less specific than coccidioidin when tested against selected sera from patients with other mycoses.

Spherulin has been found, however, to be more reactive than coccidioidin for skin testing (Stevens et al, 1975). Of the 53 patients with *C. immitis* infection tested, 16 gave positive results with spherulin but negative results with coccidioidin and only in one patient did the opposite occur. Skin tests with spherulin, like those with coccidioidin, do not elicit a humoral antibody response and can be used clinically without affecting the results of serological tests (Deresinski et al, 1977).

The LA test for coccidioidomycosis is highly sensitive but is known to give approximately 6–10 per cent false positive reactions and to be less specific than the tube-precipitin test. In a recent evaluation of LA, Pappagianis, Krasnow and Beall (1976) stress its unreliability for use with CSF samples and also found that caution is needed when it is used with diluted serum.

Paracoccidioidomycosis

Restrepo and Moncada (1974) showed that the sera of patients with para-coccidioidomycosis may contain from one to three precipitins. At diagnosis, 52 per cent of the 54 patients studied had all three precipitin lines, and a strong precipitin response correlated with a high CF titre. On remission of the disease precipitin lines disappeared slowly and in a definite sequence. Cross-reactions with histo-plasmin were observed in eight patients. Cross-reactivity between the antigens of *P. brasiliensis* and *H. capsulatum* is confirmed by Negroni, Iovannitti de Flores and Robles (1976) but it was most evident in CF tests and ID gave almost totally specific results.

Recently Yarzabal et al (1977) isolated a single antigen from a crude metabolic extract of the mycelial phase of *P. brasiliensis* which reacted in ID tests with all 14 sera from patients with paracoccidioidomycosis. It did not react with the sera of two patients with histoplasmosis which had given positive results with crude extracts of *P. brasiliensis*. The reactivity and specificity of this purified antigen is encouraging and it warrants further clinical evaluation.

Blastomycosis

Rippon et al (1977) found the ID test for blastomycosis to be highly sensitive and totally specific when fresh sera were tested with a cell sap extract of *B. dermatitidis*, as opposed to a filtrate antigen obtained by ethanol precipitation. The mating type (+ or −) of the *Ajellomyces dermatitidis* (the sexual stage of *B. dermatitidis*) isolate used to prepare the extract appeared to be important, as an increased number of precipitin lines were observed with the sera of patients in-fected with the same mating type as was used for preparation of the antigenic extract. It is suggested that a polyvalent extract from several strains of the two mating types would be most sensitive.

Attempts have been made to improve the skin test for blastomycosis by purify-ing the antigens. Recently Lancaster and Sprouse (1976) fractionated an alkaline-water soluble extract of the cell wall of *B. dermatitidis* yeast phase and isolated a single component which was highly reactive and specific when used in skin tests to differentiate between guinea-pigs infected with *B. dermatitidis* and *H. capsulatum*. Further evaluation of this fraction is needed in humans, and it may turn out to be an important diagnostic tool.

Cryptococcosis

The LA test for cryptococcal capsular polysaccharide antigen remains one of the best serodiagnostic tests available, but a high rheumatoid factor titre can give non-specific reactions and it is necessary to use appropriate controls to test for this factor. However, this difficulty can be overcome by pre-treatment of samples with 0.003M dithiothreitol (Gordon and Lapa, 1974); the IgM responsible for the non-specific clumping is inactivated while the capsular antigen is unaffected.

Maccani (1977) has found that CIE is also a suitable technique for the detection of cryptococcal capsular polysaccharide in body fluids.

Phycomycosis

There is insufficient information available to assess the diagnostic value of serology in phycomycosis. Antibodies to cellular antigens of phycomycetes have been detected by ID in some patients with rhinocerebral phycomycosis but not in others. However, the appearance of precipitins seemed to correlate with the severity of the disease (Gordon, 1974).

Aspergillosis

Immunodiffusion and CIE for the detection of precipitins are the most widely used tests for the diagnosis of the various forms of aspergillosis.

The use of a highly sensitive radioimmunoassay method enabled Bardana (1974) to show that almost everyone has some level of circulating antibody that reacts with aspergillus antigen. However, these levels are clearly too low to interfere with the ID and CIE tests as the presence of precipitins usually correlates well with disease and non-specific reactions (apart from those due to C-reactive protein) are few. A proportion of patients with bronchial asthma and patients with cystic fibrosis have been found to have precipitating antibodies to *Aspergillus* spp. (Galant et al, 1976) but these are thought to be related either to allergy to or colonisation by the fungus.

It is well known that patients with disseminated invasive aspergillosis may give negative serological results but Bardana et al (1975) found that this lack of antibody applied mainly to patients with acute invasive disease rather than to those with chronic invasion. Nevertheless, regular monitoring of patients by ID was found useful for the early detection of aspergillosis in leukaemic patients (Schaefer, Yu and Armstrong, 1976); six of the 10 patients who developed aspergillosis converted from a negative to positive precipitin reaction and in another patient the reaction intensified.

Other antibody detection techniques have been evaluated in the diagnosis of pulmonary aspergillosis. Early work suggested that the indirect fluorescent-antibody (IFA) test was more sensitive but less specific than tests for the demonstration of precipitins, although false positive reactions were generally at lower titres than those encountered in infection. A recent comparison by Negroni, Iovannitti de Flores and Robles (1977) confirmed the IFA test's lack of specificity and, furthermore, they did not find it to be more sensitive than the other techniques tested (CF, ID, CIE). However, Gordon, Lapa and Kane (1977) report that the use of aspergillus germlings, rather than mature hyphae, as antigen for the IFA test eliminated non-specific diffuse fluorescence and increased the test's specificity.

Passive haemagglutination (PHA) has been found to be sensitive and specific for detecting antibodies to aspergillus and results correlate well with the presence of precipitins. Tönder and Rödsaether (1974) found close agreement between high PHA titres and the presence of aspergillosis, and titres of $\geqslant 1:128$ were highly indicative of disease.

The type of aspergillus extract used is important. Duriez et al (1976) studied the biological activity of extracts prepared from human, animal and saprophytic isolates of *A. fumigatus* and found that their enzyme composition varied. Analysis of antigens by immunoelectrophoresis showed that stronger reactions occurred between the sera of patients with aspergillosis and the isolates obtained from disease processes. Accordingly they suggest that antigenic extracts used in precipitin tests should be prepared from 'pathogenic' strains of *A. fumigatus*. The method of preparation of *A. fumigatus* extracts has also been found to affect their reactivity (Philpot and Mackenzie, 1976).

Candidiasis

Serology is a useful aid to the diagnosis of systemic forms of candidiasis. The most frequently used tests are whole cell agglutination and ID or CIE for the detection of precipitins to somatic extracts of *Candida* spp. These tests are not totally sensitive or specific and results must be interpreted with care (Gordon, 1974; Evans, 1976b).

Earlier findings with the serological diagnosis of candida infections are comprehensively summarised by Taschdjian, Seelig and Kozinn (1973). This group has found the precipitin test to be both sensitive and specific and in one of their most recent studies of 'high risk' patients they found the test to have a sensitivity of 94 per cent, a specificity of 85 per cent and the predictive value of a positive test for the diagnosis of systemic candidiasis was 90 per cent (Kozinn et al, 1976). These findings have been upheld by other investigators but latterly it has become clear from numerous reports, that agglutinins and precipitins to candida are widespread in the absence of overt candidiasis, and often at titres previously regarded as indicative of invasive disease. Holder, Kozinn and Law (1977) concluded that these tests would be of little diagnostic value in burn patients because of the large number of false positives encountered, and similarly, Filice, Yu and Armstrong (1977) found that they were not reliable indicators of invasive candida infection in patients with malignancies because of large numbers of false positive and false negative reactions.

The conflicting findings of different groups are difficult to explain but they are certainly due in large part to differences in reagents, methodology and interpretation of results. The false positive and false negative reactions noted with these tests are to be expected. Evans and Forster (1976) found that in heart surgery patients the appearance of candida antibodies was related to high levels of commensal yeasts in the mouth and gut, and in view of the widespread occurrence of commensal yeasts particularly among hospital patients, it is not surprising that antibodies to these organisms should be equally prevalent. Systemic candida infections develop in severely compromised patients and so it is not surprising either that a significant proportion of these patients should be incapable of mounting a detectable antibody response. Despite their shortcomings, serological tests remain a valuable aid to diagnosis of systemic candidiasis but there is a need for standardisation (Merz et al, 1977). Furthermore, the tests are likely to be most useful when performed regularly over a period of time (Glew et al, 1975); a high or rapidly rising antibody titre suggests infection and, conversely, a reduction in antibody titre is associated with recovery from infection.

Efforts are now being directed towards improving the specificity of available serological tests. Some workers consider that the cell wall mannan, inevitably found in somatic extracts of *Candida* spp. (Syverson and Buckley, 1977), is the component responsible for the majority of positive precipitin reactions in uninfected individuals (false positives), whereas those with a candida infection show, in addition, a reaction to the protein components of the extract. Precipitin lines due to mannan are fuzzy and can usually be distinguished visually from the sharper protein/

glycoprotein lines. However, mannan can be removed from somatic extracts by affinity chromatography with concanavalin A sepharose (Longbottom et al, 1976), and the use of mannan-free somatic extract alongside the original somatic extract enables reactions to the cell wall components to be differentiated from those due to true somatic components. Syverson, Buckley and Gibian (1978) describe a method that enables a similar differentiation to be made. The reaction of candida somatic extract with test serum in crossed immunoelectrophoresis is compared with an adjacent reaction obtained after the extract has been run through an intermediate gel containing concanavalin A to remove mannan. Removal of the cell wall antigens by this method decreased the number of false positive reactions without decreasing sensitivity. The predictive value of the precipitin test for systemic infection was increased from 31 per cent to 71 per cent when used with an 'at risk' patient population. The significance of reactions to the cell wall components of candida has recently been discussed by Frisk (1977).

Analysis of a patient's precipitin response with crossed immunoelectrophoresis has been suggested as a means for differentiating between patients with candidiasis and those with false positive ID reactions. The patient's response is evaluated in relation to a standard antigen-antibody reference system and given a 'precipitin score' which takes account of the number of precipitin lines and the titre. This approach culminated in the study of Axelsen et al (1975) where it was found that the 'precipitin score' was the best criterion for distinguishing patients with candidiasis from controls. A score of $6\frac{1}{2}$ had a diagnostic sensitivity of 88.9 per cent and a specificity of 99.5 per cent. Eleven precipitins were found only in the infected patients' sera but no single line indicated infection and the highest sensitivity for a single precipitin was 33 per cent.

It has been suggested that the specificity of the precipitin test might be increased by the use of antigens specific to the mycelial phase of candida; only patients with candida infection and exposed to the mycelium would have antibodies to these antigens whereas those with antibodies due to commensal blastospores would not react (Evans et al, 1973). Antigenic comparisons of the two growth phases of C. albicans have revealed mycelial specific antigens (Syverson, Buckley and Campbell, 1975; Evans, Richardson and Holland, 1977) but these have yet to be fully evaluated against patients' sera. Antigenic differences between the growth phases were the basis of an IFA test described by Ho et al (1976) where they looked at the differential fluorescence of blastospores and germ tubes of C. albicans in patients with candidiasis and in normal controls. IFA titres were increased in the candidiasis patients but the most marked increase was in the anti-germ tube titre and they suggest that this could be used as a diagnostic test.

Other serological tests have been used for the diagnosis of systemic candidiasis but there is often conflicting evidence as to their value. The LA test has been found to be more sensitive but less specific than ID (Merz et al, 1977). However, it is quantitative, appears to have prognostic value, and has been recommended for use alongside ID (Stickle et al, 1972). Indirect fluorescent antibody and PHA tests have also been evaluated for diagnosis but interpretation of results is difficult unless the class of immunoglobulins to which the antibodies belong is taken into account. Ansorg et al (1977) found that IgG antibodies predominate in the IFA test but that neither IgG nor IgA antibodies could be used to differentiate between

patients with superficial and systemic candidiasis, whereas monitoring IgM antibodies enabled them to do this. High PHA titres, associated with a high proportion
of IgM antibody, were found in the early stages of candida infection, and this is
claimed to make the PHA test particularly suitable for the early diagnosis and
surveillance of 'high risk' patients (Müller and Holtmannspötter, 1975). Moreover,
these investigators found that high IFA titres due to IgG developed in the later
stages of infection making the IHA and IFA tests complementary. However,
Hellwege, Fischer and Bläker (1972) found that in the PHA test IgM antibodies
were the main class of antibodies produced in patients with candida colonisation
and that IgG antibodies were those associated with infection.

Antigen detection
Refinements to antibody detection techniques will be of no value for patients who
for one reason or another produce no antibodies. Tests for the detection of antigen
must, therefore, be used for the diagnosis of infection in these patients. Diagnosis
of cryptococcosis by detection of capsular antigen is well established but tests
are now being developed for the detection of candida and aspergillus antigens
and the results, so far, are encouraging.

The method used by Axelsen et al (1975) to characterise the precipitin response
in patients with candidiasis should also have detected any free candida antigen
present in the patients' serum but none was found. More encouraging results were
obtained by Weiner and Yount (1976) who, using a haemagglutination inhibition
assay, were able to detect circulating mannan in 6 out of 19 patients with invasive
candidiasis, those colonised with yeasts or in patients with other mycotic infections.
was good, and mannan was not detected in the sera of patients with superficial
candidiasis, those colonised with yeasts or in patients with other myotic infections.
More recently, Warren et al (1977) used an enzyme immunoassay (ELISA)
system to demonstrate candida antigen in the sera of rabbits and mice infected
with this yeast, and also in the sera of three patients with systemic candidiasis.

Circulating aspergillus antigen has been detected by CIE in mice with disseminated invasive aspergillosis following i.v. inoculation of the fungus (White et
al, 1977). The antigenaemia became apparent 3–4 days after inoculation but not
all mice gave positive results. Circulating antigen could not be demonstrated in
mice with localised pulmonary infections following inhalation of spores. The importance of using a technique with adequate sensitivity is underlined by the fact
that the antigen detected by CIE could not be demonstrated by ID. Lehman and
Reiss (1978) recently described a novel assay for aspergillus antigen where the
antigen is detected by using an antiserum produced by immunizing one rabbit
with serum from another infected with *A. fumigatus*—the antiserum contains
antibodies to any antigens circulating in the serum of the infected rabbit. This
antiserum, when used in a CIE system, detected a single aspergillus antigen in all
samples of serum and urine from rabbits with experimental aspergillosis and in the
serum of a patient with disseminated aspergillosis. Sera from uninfected control
animals, normal human sera and sera from rabbits infected with candida gave negative results. This looks a particularly promising approach and the authors are now
developing a more sensitive antigen assay system for use with this antiserum. As
they point out, this method can also be applied to other fungal diseases.

In the future, antigen detection is likely to play a significant role in the diagnosis of systemic mycoses.

New approaches to the detection of fungi

Gas liquid chromatography (GLC) has been evaluated for the diagnosis of yeast septicaemia. Miller et al (1974) found that gas chromatograms of sera from patients with candida septicaemia and invasive candidiasis were significantly different from those of normal sera, and that they reverted to normal when infection was eliminated. The additional peaks detected in infected patients were similar to those found in cultures of *C. albicans* grown in serum. Preliminary work by Goullier et al (1976) also showed abnormal GLC peaks in the sera of patients with candida septicaemia.

Electron-capture GLC has been used to examine CSF from patients with crypto-coccosis (Schlossberg, Brooks and Shulman, 1976). Patients with cryptococcal meningitis had similar profiles, which resembled those seen in CSF artificially inoculated with *Cr. neoformans*, but which differed from those of patients with viral meningitis and uninfected controls. Craven et al (1977) also found that this method could distinguish between cryptococcal, tuberculous and viral meningitis.

These chromatographic methods clearly have potential for rapid diagnosis of infection and further evaluation is urgently required.

A *chitin assay* has been used experimentally by Lehman and White (1975) to locate and quantitate aspergillus mycelium in mouse tissues. There is a possibility that this, or some other method based on the same concept of detecting fungal constituents not normally present in animal tissues, could be used to detect fungi in human tissues.

Automation will eventually become commonplace in microbiology. Recently an automated computerised instrument for detection and enumeration of micro-organisms in urine was described and evaluated by Aldridge et al (1977) and Sonnenwirth (1977). The device, which uses selective media and an optical system for quantitation, gave results which showed over 90 per cent agreement with conventional methods when used with urine containing *Candida* spp. and *Torulopsis glabrata*.

REFERENCES

Ajello, L., Chick, E. W. & Furcolow, M. L. eds. (1971) *Histoplasmosis, Proceedings Second National Conference*. Springfield: Charles C. Thomas.

Aldridge, C., Jones, P. W., Gibson, S., Lanham, J., Meyer, M., Vannest, R. & Charles, R. (1977) Automated microbiological detection/identification system. *Journal of Clinical Microbiology*, **6**, 406–413.

Ansorg, R., Gunesch, D., Bandelow, B. & Thomssen, R. (1977) Differenzierung und diagnostische Bedeutung der Immunglobulinklassen humoraler Antikörper gegen Zellwandantigene der Sprosszellen-und Myzelphase von *Candida albicans*. *Mykosen*, **20**, 167–177.

Armbuster, T. G., Goergen, T. G., Resnick, D. & Catanzaro, A. (1977) Utility of bone scanning in disseminated coccidioidomycosis: case report. *Journal of Nuclear Medicine*, **18**, 450–454.

Arvan, S., Cagin, N., Levitt, B. & Kleid, J. J. (1976) Echocardiographic findings in a patient with *Candida* endocarditis of the aortic valve. *Chest*, **70**, 300–302.

Axelsen, N. H. (1973) Quantitative immunoelectrophoretic methods as tools of a polyvalent approach to standardization in the immunochemistry of *Candida albicans*. *Infection and Immunity*, 7, 949–960.

Axelsen, N. H. (1976) Analysis of human *Candida* precipitins by quantitative immunoelectrophoresis. A model for analysis of complex microbial antigen-antibody systems. *Scandinavian Journal of Immunology*, 5, 177–190.

Axelsen, N. H., Buckley, H. R., Drouhet, E., Budtz-Jørgensen, E., Hattel, T. & Andersen, P. L. (1975) Crossed immunoelectrophoretic analysis of precipitins to *Candida albicans* in deep *Candida* infection. Possibilities for standardization in diagnostic *Candida* serology. *Scandinavian Journal of Immunology*, 4, Suppl. 2, 217–230.

Bach, M. C., Adler, J. L., Breman, J., P'eng, F.-K., Sahyouen, A., Schlesinger, R. M., Madras, P. & Monaco, A. P. (1973) Influence of rejection therapy on fungal and nocardial infections in renal-transplant recipients. *Lancet*, 1, 180–184.

Bardana, E. J., Jr. (1974) Measurement of humoral antibodies to aspergilli. *Annals of the New York Academy of Sciences*, 221, 64–75.

Bardana, E. J., Jr., Gerber, J. D., Craig, S. & Cianciulli, F. D. (1975) The general and specific humoral immune response to pulmonary aspergillosis. *American Review of Respiratory Disease*, 112, 799–805.

Beheshti, F., Smith, A. G. & Krause, G. W. (1975) Germ tube and chlamydospore formation by *Candida albicans* on a new medium. *Journal of Clinical Microbiology*, 2, 345–348.

Bhatt, O. N., Miller, R., Riche, J. Le & King, E. G. (1977) Aspiration biopsy in pulmonary opportunistic infections. *Acta Cytologica*, 21, 206–209.

Blazevic, D. J., Stemper, J. E. & Matsen, J. M. (1975) Effect of aerobic and anaerobic atmospheres on isolation of organisms from blood cultures. *Journal of Clinical Microbiology*, 1, 154–156.

Block, C. S. & Young, C. N. (1977) Early diagnosis of opportunistic systemic fungal and nocardial infections. *South African Medical Journal*, 52, 1056–1060.

Bowman, P. I. & Ahearn, D. G. (1976) Evaluation of commercial systems for the identification of clinical yeast isolates. *Journal of Clinical Microbiology*, 4, 49–53.

Bradley, G., Pine, L., Reeves, M. W. & Moss, C. W. (1974) Purification, composition and serological characterization of histoplasmin—H and M antigens. *Infection and Immunity*, 9, 870–880.

Chick, E. W., Balows, A. & Furcolow, M. L. eds. (1975) *Opportunistic fungal infections. Proceedings of the Second International Conference*. Springfield: Charles C. Thomas.

Conant, N. F., Smith, D. T., Baker, R. D. & Callaway, J. L. (1971) *Manual of Clinical Mycology*, 3rd edition. Philadelphia: Saunders.

Craven, R. B., Brooks, J. B., Edman, D. C., Converse, J. D., Greenlee, J., Schlossberg, D., Furlow, T., Gwaltney, J. M., Jr. & Miner, W. F. (1977) Rapid diagnosis of lymphocytic meningitis by frequency-pulsed electron capture gas-liquid chromatography: differentiation of tuberculous, cryptococcal and viral meningitis. *Journal of Clinical Microbiology*, 6, 27–32.

Deresinski, S. C., Levine, H. B., Kelly, P. C., Creasman, R. J. & Stevens, D. A. (1977) Spherulin skin testing and histoplasmal and coccidioidal serology: lack of effect. *American Review of Respiratory Disease*, 116, 1116–1118.

Diamond, R. D. & Bennett, J. E. (1974) Prognostic factors in cryptococcal meningitis. A study in 111 cases. *Annals of Internal Medicine*, 80, 176–181.

Di Salvo, A. F. & Corbett, D. S. (1976) Apparent false positive histoplasmin latex agglutination tests in patients with tuberculosis. *Journal of Clinical Microbiology*, 3, 306–308.

Drouhet, E., Tabet-Derraz, O., Sanchez-Sousa, A. & Viviani, M. A. (1973) Application de l'électrophorèse bidimensionnelle au diagnostic des aspergilloses et à la standardisation des antigènes aspergillaires. Note préliminaire. *Bulletin de la Société Française de Mycologie Médicale*, 2, 7–10.

Duperval, R., Hermans, P. E., Brewer, N. S. & Roberts, G. D. (1977) Cryptococcosis, with emphasis on the significance of isolation of *Cryptococcus neoformans* from the respiratory tract. *Chest*, 72, 13–19.

Duriez, T., Walbaum, S., Tailliez, R. & Biguet, J. (1976) Étude enzymologique comparée de souches de *Aspergillus fumigatus* et de *A. fischeri* d'origine saprophytique ou isolées de lesions humaines ou animales. Repercussions pratique d'ordre diagnostique. *Mycopathologia*, 59, 81–90.

Edwards, J. E., Jr., Foos, R. Y., Montgomerie, J. Z. & Guze, L. B. (1974) Ocular manifestations of *Candida* septicemia: review of seventy-six cases of hematogenous *Candida* endophthalmitis. *Medicine*, 53, 47–75.

Edwards, J. E., Jr., Montgomerie, J. Z., Ishida, K., Morrison, J. O. & Guze, L. B. (1977) Experimental hematogenous endophthalmitis due to *Candida*: species variation in ocular pathogenicity. *Journal of Infectious Diseases*, 135, 294–297.

Emmons, C. W., Binford, C. H., Utz, J. P. & Kwon-Chung, K. J. (1977) *Medical Mycology*, 3rd edition. Philadelphia: Lea and Febiger.

Evans, E. G. V. (1976a) Mycological aspects of open-heart surgery. In *Current Techniques in Extra-corporeal Circulation*, eds. Ionescu, M. I. & Wooler, G. H., pp. 397–406. London: Butterworths.

Evans, E. G. V. (1976b) Ed. Serology of fungal infection and farmer's lung disease. A laboratory manual. British Society for Mycopathology Working Party. Leeds: British Society for Mycopathology.

Evans, E. G. V. & Forster, R. A. (1976) Antibodies to *Candida* after operations on the heart. *Journal of Medical Microbiology*, **9**, 303–308.

Evans, E. G. V., Richardson, M. D., Odds, F. C. & Holland, K. T. (1973) Relevance of antigenicity of *Candida albicans* growth phases to diagnosis of systemic candidiasis. *British Medical Journal*, **4**, 86–87.

Evans, E. G. V., Richardson, M. D. & Holland, K. T. (1977) Demonstration of specific mycelial growth phase antigens of *Candida albicans*. In *Abstracts Second International Mycological Congress*, eds. Bigelow, H. E. & Simmons, E. G., Vol. 1, p. 182. Tampa, Florida.

Faux, J. A., Stanley, V. C., Buckley, H. R. & Partridge, B. M. (1975) A comparison of different extracts of *Candida albicans* in agar gel double diffusion techniques. *Journal of Immunological Methods*, **6**, 235–247.

Filice, G., Yu, B. & Armstrong, D. (1977) Immunodiffusion and agglutination tests for *Candida* in patients with neoplastic disease: inconsistent correlation of results with invasive infections. *Journal of Infectious Diseases*, **135**, 349–357.

Finley, R., Kieff, E., Thomsen, S., Fennessy, J., Beem, M., Lerner, S. & Morello, J. (1974) Bronchial brushing in the diagnosis of pulmonary disease in patients at risk for opportunistic infection. *American Review of Respiratory Disease*, **109**, 379–387.

Fleming, W. H., III, Hopkins, J. M. & Land, G. A. (1977) New culture medium for the presumptive identification of *Candida albicans* and *Cryptococcus neoformans*. *Journal of Clinical Microbiology*, **5**, 236–243.

Frisk, Å. (1977) Serological aspects of candidosis. *Current Therapeutic Research*, **22**, 46–50.

Galant, S. P., Rucker, R. W., Groncy, C. E., Wells, I. D. & Novey, H. S. (1976) Incidence of serum antibodies to several *Aspergillus* species and to *Candida albicans* in cystic fibrosis. *American Review of Respiratory Disease*, **114**, 325–331.

Gallis, H. A., Berman, R. A., Cate, T. R., Hamilton, J. D., Gunnells, J. C. & Stickel, D. L. (1975) Fungal infection following renal transplantation. *Archives of Internal Medicine*, **135**, 1163–1172.

Gantz, N. M., Medeiros, A. A., Swain, J. L. & O'Brien, J. F. (1974) Vacuum blood-culture bottles inhibiting growth of *Candida* and fostering growth of *Bacteroides*. *Lancet*, **2**, 1174–1176.

Gervasi, J. P. & Miller, N. G. (1975) Recovery of *Cryptococcus neoformans* from sputum using new technics for the isolation of fungi from sputum. *American Journal of Clinical Pathology*, **63**, 916–920.

Giraldo, R., Restrepo, A., Cutiérrez, F., Robledo, M., Londoño, F., Hernández, H., Sierra, F. & Calle, G. (1976) Pathogenesis of paracoccidioidomycosis: a model based on the study of 46 patients. *Mycopathologia*, **58**, 63–70.

Girard, D. E., Fred, H. L., Bradshaw, W., Blakely, R. W. & Ettlinger, R. (1977) Disseminated histoplasmosis diagnosed from peripheral blood film. *Southern Medical Journal*, **70**, 65–66.

Glew, R. H., Buckley, H. R., Rosen, H. M., Moellering, R. C., Jr. & Fischer, J. E. (1975) Value of prospective *Candida* precipitins in fungemia in patients with hyperalimentation. *Surgical Forum*, **26**, 113–115.

Gomes, J. A. C., Calderon, J., Lajans, F., Sakurai, H., Friedman, H. S. & Tatz, J. S. (1976) Echocardiographic detection of fungal vegetations in *Candida parapsilosis* endocarditis. *American Journal of Medicine*, **61**, 273–276.

Gordon, M. A. (1974) Serodiagnosis of opportunistic mycoses. In *Opportunistic Pathogens*, eds. Prier, J. E. & Friedman, H., pp. 147–162. London: Macmillan.

Gordon, M. A. & Lapa, E. W. (1974) Elimination of rheumatoid factor in the latex test for cryptococcosis. *American Journal of Clinical Pathology*, **61**, 488–494.

Gordon, M. A., Lapa, E. W. & Kane, J. (1977) Modified indirect fluorescent-antibody test for aspergillosis. *Journal of Clinical Microbiology*, **6**, 161–165.

Gottlieb, S., Khuddus, S. A., Balooki, H., Dominguez, A. E. & Myerburg, R. J. (1974) Echocardiographic diagnosis of aortic valve vegetations in *Candida* endocarditis. *Circulation*, **50**, 826–830.

Goullier, A., Ganansia, Y., Decoux, G., Favier, A., Biguet, J. & Ambroise-Thomas, P. (1976) Apports de la chromatographie en phase gazeuse au diagnostic précoce des septicémies à *Candida*. Essais préliminaires. *Bulletin de la Société Française de Mycologie Médicale*, **5**, 103–107.

Greenman, R. L., Goodall, P. T. & King, D. (1975) Lung biopsy in immunocompromised hosts. *American Journal of Medicine*, **59**, 488–496.

Griffin, J. R., Pettit, T. H., Fishman, L. S. & Foos, R. Y. (1973) Blood-borne *Candida* endophthalmitis. A clinical and pathologic study of 21 cases. *Archives of Ophthalmology*, **89**, 450–456.

Gunasekaran, M. & Hughes, W. F. (1977) A simple medium for isolation and identification of *Candida albicans* directly from clinical specimens. *Mycopathologia*, **61**, 151–157.

Gurwith, M. J., Stinson, E. B. & Remington, J. S. (1971) *Aspergillus* infection complicating cardiac transplantation. *Archives of Internal Medicine*, **128**, 541–545.

Hammerman, K. J., Powell, K. E., Christianson, C. S., Huggin, P. M., Larsh, H. W., Vivas, J. R. & Tosh, F. E. (1973) Pulmonary cryptococcosis: clinical forms and treatment. A Center for Disease Control co-operative mycoses study. *American Review of Respiratory Disease*, **108**, 1116–1123.

Healy, M. E., Dillavou, C. L. & Taylor, G. E. (1977) Diagnostic medium containing inositol, urea and caffeic acid for selective growth of *Cryptococcus neoformans*. *Journal of Clinical Microbiology*, **6**, 387–391.

Hellwege, H. H., Fischer, K. & Bläker, F. (1972) Diagnostic value of *Candida* precipitins. *Lancet*, **2**, 386.

Ho, Y. M., Ng, M. H., Teoh-Chan, C. H., Yue, P. C. K. & Huang, C. T. (1976) Indirect immuno-fluorescence assay for antibody to germ tube of *Candida albicans*—a new dignostic test. *Journal of Clinical Pathology*, **29**, 1007–1010.

Holder, I. A., Kozinn, P. J. & Law, E. J. (1977) Evaluation of *Candida* precipitin and agglutinin tests for the diagnosis of systemic candidiasis in burn patients. *Journal of Clinical Microbiology*, **6**, 219–223.

Hommel, M., Kien Truong, T. & Bidwell, D. E. (1976) Technique immuno-enzymatique (E.L.I.S.A.) appliquée au diagnostic sérologique des candidoses et aspergilloses humaines. Résultats préliminaires. *Nouvelle Presse Médicale*, **5**, 2789–2791.

Hopfer, R. L. & Blank, F. (1975) Caffeic acid-containing medium for identification of *Cryptococcus neoformans*. *Journal of Clinical Microbiology*, **2**, 115–120.

Hopfer, R. L. & Gröschel, D. (1975) Six-hour pigmentation test for the identification of *Cryptococcus neoformans*. *Journal of Clinical Microbiology*, **2**, 96–98.

Hopkins, J. M. & Land, G. A. (1977) Rapid method for determining nitrate utilization by yeasts. *Journal of Clinical Microbiology*, **5**, 497–500.

Hughes, J. M. & Remington, J. S. (1972) Systemic candidiasis, a diagnostic challenge. *California Medicine*, **116**, 8–17.

Huppert, M., Harper, G., Sun, S. H. & Delanerolle, V. (1975) Rapid methods for identification of yeasts. *Journal of Clinical Microbiology*, **2**, 21–34.

Huppert, M., Krasnow, I., Vukovich, K. R., Sun, S. H., Rice, E. H. & Kutner, L. J. (1977) Comparison of coccidioidin and spherulin in complement fixation tests for coccidioidomycosis. *Journal of Clinical Microbiology*, **6**, 33–41.

Jameson, B. & Wells, D. G. (1972) Cytologic diagnosis of cryptococcal meningitis. *New England Journal of Medicine*, **286**, 1267.

Johnson, J. E. & Roberts, G. D. (1976) Blocking effect of rheumatoid factor and cold agglutinins on complement fixation tests for histoplasmosis. *Journal of Clinical Microbiology*, **3**, 157–160.

Joshi, K. R., Bremner, D. A., Parr, D. N. & Gavin, J. B. (1975) The morphological identification of pathogenic yeasts using carbohydrate media. *Journal of Clinical Pathology*, **28**, 18–24.

Kaben, U. & Westphal, H.-J. (1977) Der Nachweis präzipitierender Antikörper bei *Candida*-Infcktionen unter Verwendung eines polyäthylen-glykol-haltigen Agars als Diffusionsmedium. *Mykosen*, **20**, 178–182.

Kammer, R. B. & Utz, J. P. (1974) *Aspergillus* species endocarditis. The new face of a not so rare disease. *American Journal of Medicine*, **56**, 506–521.

Kaplan, M. H., Rosen, P. P. & Armstrong, D. (1977) Cryptococcosis in a cancer hospital: clinical and pathological correlates in forty-six patients. *Cancer*, **39**, 2265–2274.

Kaufman, L. (1976) Serodiagnosis of fungal diseases. In *Manual of Clinical Immunology*, eds. Rose, N. R. & Friedman, H., pp. 363–381. Washington, DC: American Society for Microbiology.

Kobza, K. & Steenblock, U. (1977) Demonstration of *Candida* in blood smears. *British Medical Journal*, **1**, 1640–1641.

Kobza, K., Perruchoud, A., Mihatsch, J. M. & Herzog, H. (1976) Candidaemia and bacterial infections in patients with lung disease. *Lancet*, **2**, 1084.

Kozinn, P. J., Galen, R. S., Taschdjian, C. L., Goldberg, P. L., Protzman, W. & Kozinn, M. A. (1976) The precipitin test in systemic candidiasis. *Journal of the American Medical Association*, **235**, 628–629.

Krick, J. A. & Remington, J. S. (1976) Opportunistic invasive fungal infections in patients with leukaemia and lymphoma. *Clinics in Haematology*, **5**, 249–310.

Lancaster, M. V. & Sprouse, R. F. (1976) Isolation of a purified skin test antigen from *Blastomyces dermatitidis* yeast-phase cell wall. *Infection and Immunity*, **14**, 623–625.

Land, G. A., Vinton, E. C., Adcock, G. B. & Hopkins, J. M. (1975) Improved auxanographic method for yeast assimilations: a comparison with other approaches. *Journal of Clinical Microbiology*, **2**, 206–217.

Lehmann, P. F. & Reiss, E. (1978) Invasive aspergillosis: antiserum for circulating antigen produced after immunization with serum from infected rabbits. *Infection and Immunity*, **20**, 570–572.

Lehmann, P. F. & White, L. O. (1975) Chitin assay used to demonstrate renal localization and cortisone-enhanced growth of *Aspergillus fumigatus* mycelium in mice. *Infection and Immunity*, **12**, 987–992.

Longbottom, J. L. & Pepys, J. (1975) Diagnosis of fungal diseases. In *Clinical Aspects of Immunology*, eds. Gell, P. G. H., Coombs, R. R. A. & Lachmann, P. J., pp. 99–128. Oxford: Blackwell.

Longbottom, J. L., Brighton, W. D., Edge, G. & Pepys, J. (1976) Antibodies mediating type I skin test reactions to polysaccharide and protein antigens of *Candida albicans*. *Clinical Allergy*, **6**, 41–49.

Louria, D. B. (1974) Superinfection: a partial overview. In *Opportunistic Pathogens*, eds. Prier, J. E. & Friedman, H., pp. 1–18. London: Macmillan.

Maccani, J. E. (1977) Detection of cryptococcal polysaccharide using counterimmunoelectrophoresis. *American Journal of Clinical Pathology*, **68**, 39–44.

Mackenzie, D. W. R. & Philpot, C. M. (1975) Counterimmunoelectrophoresis as a routine mycoserological procedure. *Mycopathologia*, **57**, 1–7.

MacMillan, B. G., Law, E. J. & Holder, I. A. (1972) Experience with *Candida* infections in the burn patient. *Archives of Surgery*, **104**, 509–514.

Masur, H., Rosen, P. P. & Armstrong, D. (1977) Pulmonary disease caused by *Candida* species. *American Journal of Medicine*, **63**, 914–925.

Merz, W. G., Evans, G. L., Shadomy, S., Anderson, S., Kaufman, L., Kozinn, P. J., Mackenzie, D. W. R., Protzman, W. P. & Remington, J. S. (1977) Laboratory evaluation of serological tests for systemic candidiasis: a co-operative study. *Journal of Clinical Microbiology*, **5**, 596–603.

Meyer, R. D. & Armstrong, D. (1973) Mucormycosis—changing status. *CRC Critical Reviews in Clinical Laboratory Sciences*, **4**, 421–451.

Miller, G. G., Witwer, M. W., Braude, A. I. & Davis, C. E. (1974) Rapid identification of *Candida albicans* septicemia in man by gas-liquid chromatography. *Journal of Clinical Investigation*, **54**, 1235–1240.

Mills, S. A., Seigler, H. F. & Wolfe, W. G. (1975) The incidence and management of pulmonary mycosis in renal allograft patients. *Annals of Surgery*, **182**, 617–626.

Mok, W. Y., Buckley, H. R. & Campbell, C. C. (1977) Characterization of antigens from type A and B yeast cells of *Histoplasma capsulatum*. *Infection and Immunity*, **16**, 461–466.

Müller, H.-L. & Holtmannspötter, H. (1975) Vergleichende Titerbestimmungen mit dem *Candida*—Hämagglutinationstest und dem *Candida*—Immunfluoreszenztest. *Mykosen*, **18**, 91–96.

Müller, J., Langer, E. & Jaeger, R. (1977) Die Bestimmung der Sprosspilzkonzentration im Sputum. *Mykosen*, **20**, 283–291.

Naidoff, M. A. & Green, W. R. (1975) Endogenous *Aspergillus* endophthalmitis occurring after kidney transplant. *American Journal of Ophthalmology*, **79**, 502–509.

Negroni, R., Iovannitti de Flores, C. & Robles, A. M. (1976) Estudio de las reacciones serologicos cruzadas entre antigenos de *Paracoccidioides brasiliensis* e *Histoplasma capsulatum*. *Revista de la Asociación Argentina de Microbiologia*, **8**, 68–73.

Negroni, R., Iovannitti de Flores, C. & Robles, A. M. (1977) Estudio sobre el valor diagnóstico de la inmunofluorescencia indirecta en la aspergillosis pulmonar. *Sabouraudia*, **15**, 195–200.

Norenberg, R. G., Sethi, G. K., Scott, S. M. & Takaro, T. (1975) Opportunistic endocarditis following open-heart surgery. *Annals of Thoracic Surgery*, **19**, 592–604.

Oxenhandler, R. W., Adelstein, E. H. & Rogers, W. A. (1977) Rheumatoid factor: a cause of false positive histoplasmin latex agglutination. *Journal of Clinical Microbiology*, **5**, 31–33.

Paisley, J. W., Todd, J. K. & Roe, M. H. (1977) Early detection and preliminary susceptibility testing of positive blood cultures with the steers replicator. *Journal of Clinical Microbiology*, **6**, 367–372.

Paliwal, D. K. & Randhawa, H. S. (1977) Rapid method for detection of urea hydrolysis by yeasts. *Applied and Environmental Microbiology*, **33**, 219–220.

Palmer, D. F., Kaufman, L., Kaplan, W. & Cavallaro, J. S. (1977) *Serodiagnosis of mycotic diseases*. Springfield: Charles C. Thomas.

Pan American Health Organisation (1972) *Paracoccidioidomycosis, Proceedings First Pan American Symposium, Medellin, Columbia*. Washington: Pan American Health Organisation.

Pappagianis, D., Krasnow, I. & Beall, S. (1976) False-positive reactions of cerebrospinal fluid and diluted sera with the coccidioidal latex-agglutination test. *American Journal of Clinical Pathology*, **66**, 916–921.

Philpot, C. M. & Mackenzie, D. W. R. (1976) Detection of antibodies to *Aspergillus fumigatus* in agar gel with different antigens and immunodiffusion patterns. *Journal of Biological Standardization*, **4**, 73–79.

Pine, L., Gross, H., Bradley Malcolm, G., George, J. R., Gray, S. B. & Moss, C. W. (1977) Procedures for the production and separation of H and M antigens in histoplasmin: chemical and serological properties of isolated products. *Mycopathologia*, **61**, 131–141.

Randhawa, H. S. & Pal, M. (1977) Occurrence and significance of *Cryptococcus neoformans* in the respiratory tract of patients with bronchopulmonary disorders. *Journal of Clinical Microbiology*, **5**, 5–8.

Reiss, E., Miller, S. E., Kaplan, W. & Kaufman, L. (1977a) Antigenic, chemical and structural properties of cell walls of *Histoplasma capsulatum* yeast-form chemotypes 1 and 2 after serial enzymatic hydrolysis. *Infection and Immunity*, **16**, 690–700.

Reiss, E., Hutchinson, H., Pine, L., Ziegler, D. W. & Kaufman, L. (1977b) Solid-phase competitive-binding radioimmunoassay for detecting antibody to the M antigen of histoplasmin. *Journal of Clinical Microbiology*, **6**, 598–604.

Restrepo, A. & Moncada, L. H. (1974) Characterization of the precipitin bands detected in the immunodiffusion test for paracoccidioidomycosis. *Applied Microbiology*, **28**, 138–144.

Ribet, M., Callafe, R., Delaby, J.-P., Liber, F. & Hassoun, A. (1975) Septicémies à *Candida* dans un service de chirurgie générale. *Chirurgie*, **101**, 441–446.

Rippon, J. W. (1974) *Medical Mycology. The Pathogenic Fungi and the Pathogenic Actinomycetes*. Philadelphia: Saunders.

Rippon, J. W., Anderson, D. N., Jacobsohn, S., Soo Hoo, M. & Garber, E. D. (1977) Blastomycosis: specificity of antigens reflecting the mating types of *Ajellomyces dermatitidis*. *Mycopathologia*, **60**, 65–72.

Roberts, G. D. & Washington, J. A. II (1975) Detection of fungi in blood cultures. *Journal of Clinical Microbiology*, **1**, 309–310.

Roberts, G. D., Horstmeier, C. D. & Ilstrup, D. M. (1976) Evaluation of a hypertonic sucrose medium for the detection of fungi in blood cultures. *Journal of Clinical Microbiology*, **4**, 110–111.

Rodrigues, R. J. & Wolff, W. I. (1974) Fungal septicaemia in surgical patients. *Annals of Surgery*, **180**, 741–746.

Rohatgi, P. K., Simon, D. B., Goldstein, R. A. & Reba, R. C. (1977) Strontium-87m lung scans in pulmonary aspergillosis. *American Journal of Roentgenology*, **129**, 879–882.

Rolph, L. & Austwick, P. K. C. (1973) Differential staining of fungi in tissues. *Journal of Science Technology*, **17**, 22–26.

Rose, H. D. & Varkey, B. (1975) Deep mycotic infection in the hospitalized adult: a study of 123 patients. *Medicine*, **54**, 499–507.

Rosen, P. P. (1976) Opportunistic fungal infections in patients with neoplastic diseases. *Pathology Annual*, **11**, 255–315.

Sanders, J. S., Sarosi, G. A., Nollet, D. J. & Thompson, J. I. (1977) Exfoliative cytology in the rapid diagnosis of pulmonary blastomycosis. *Chest*, **72**, 193–196.

Scalarone, G. M., Levine, H. B., Pappagianis, D. & Chaparas, S. D. (1974) Spherulin as a complement-fixing antigen in human coccidioidomycosis. *American Review of Respiratory Disease*, **110**, 324–328.

Schaefer, J. C., Yu, B. & Armstrong, D. (1976) An *Aspergillus* immunodiffusion test in the early diagnosis of aspergillosis in adult leukemia patients. *American Review of Respiratory Disease*, **113**, 325–329.

Schelbert, H. R. & Muller, O. F. (1972) Detection of fungal vegetations involving a Starr-Edwards mitral prosthesis by means of ultrasound. *Vascular Surgery*, **6**, 20–25.

Schlossberg, D., Brooks, J. B. & Shulman, J. A. (1976) Possibility of diagnosing meningitis by gas chromatography: cryptococcal meningitis. *Journal of Clinical Microbiology*, **3**, 239–245.

Schroter, G. P. J., Hoelscher, M., Putnam, C. W., Porter, K. A. & Starzl, T. E. (1977) Fungus infections after liver transplantation. *Annals of Surgery*, **186**, 115–122.

Seelig, M. S., Speth, C. P., Kozinn, P. J., Taschdjian, C. L., Toni, E. F. & Goldberg, P. (1974) Patterns of *Candida* endocarditis following cardiac surgery: importance of early diagnosis and therapy (an analysis of 91 cases). *Progress in Cardiovascular Diseases*, **17**, 125–160.

Segal, E. & Ajello, L. (1976) Evaluation of a new system for the rapid identification of clinically important yeasts. *Journal of Clinical Microbiology*, **4**, 157–159.

Singer, C., Kaplan, M. H. & Armstrong, D. (1977) Bacteremia and fungemia complicating neoplastic disease. A study of 364 cases. *American Journal of Medicine*, **62**, 731–742.

Sonnenwirth, A. C. (1977) Preprototype of an automated microbial detection and identification system: a developmental investigation. *Journal of Clinical Microbiology*, **6**, 400–405.

Speller, D. C. (1975) Yeasts in urine. *Journal of Antimicrobial Chemotherapy*, **1**, 253–254.

Standard, P. G. & Kaufman, L. (1976) Specific immunological test for the rapid identification of members of the genus *Histoplasma*. *Journal of Clinical Microbiology*, **3**, 191–199.

Standard, P. G. & Kaufman, L. (1977) Immunological procedure for the rapid and specific identification of *Coccidioides immitis* cultures. *Journal of Clinical Microbiology*, **5**, 149–153.

Stevens, D. A., Levine, H. B., Deresinski, S. C. & Blaine, L. J. (1975) Spherulin in clinical coccidioidomycosis. Comparison with coccidioidin. *Chest*, **68**, 697–702.

Stickle, D., Kaufman, L., Blumer, S. O. & McLaughlin, D. W. (1972) Comparison of a newly developed latex agglutination test and an immunodiffusion test in the diagnosis of systemic candidiasis *Applied Microbiology*, **23**, 490–499.

Stone, H. H., Kolb, L. D., Currie, C. A., Geheber, C. E. & Cuzzell, J. Z. (1974) Candida sepsis: pathogenesis and principles of treatment. *Annals of Surgery*, **179**, 697–711.

Sutliff, W. D. & Cruthirds, T. P. (1973) *Blastomyces dermatitidis* in cytologic preparations. *American Review of Respiratory Disease*, **108**, 149–151.

Syverson, R. E. & Buckley, H. R. (1977) Cell wall antigens in soluble cytoplasmic extracts of *Candida albicans* as demonstrated by crossed immuno-affinoelectrophoresis with concanavalin A. *Journal of Immunological Methods*, **18**, 149–156.

Syverson, R. E., Buckley, H. R. & Campbell, C. C. (1975) Cytoplasmic antigens unique to the mycelial or yeast phase of *Candida albicans*. *Infection and Immunity*, **12**, 1184–1188.

Syverson, R. E., Buckley, H. R. & Gibian, J. R. (1978) Increasing the predictive value positive of the precipitin test for the diagnosis of deep-seated candidiasis. *American Journal of Clinical Pathology*. (In press).

Taschdjian, C. L., Seelig, M. S. & Kozinn, P. J. (1973) Serological diagnosis of candidal infections. *CRC Critical Reviews in Clinical Laboratory Sciences*, **4**, 19–59.

Thadepalli, H., Rambhatla, K., Mishkin, F. S., Khurana, M. M. & Niden, A. H. (1977) Correlation of microbiologic findings and [67]gallium scans in patients with pulmonary infections. *Chest*, **72**, 442–448.

Tönder, O. & Rödsaether, M. (1974) Indirect haemagglutination for demonstration of antibodies to *Aspergillus fumigatus*. *Acta Pathologica et Microbiologica Scandinavica*, B, **82**, 871–878.

Vanbreuseghem, R. (1976) Étude clinique, mycologique et histopathologique de l'histoplasmose africaine. *Bruxelles-Médical*, **56**, 85–95.

Wang, H. S., Zeimis, R. T. & Roberts, G. D. (1977) Evaluation of a caffeic acid—ferric citrate test for rapid identification of *Cryptococcus neoformans*. *Journal of Clinical Microbiology*, **6**, 445–449.

Warren, R. C., Bartlett, A., Bidwell, D. E., Richardson, M. D., Voller, A. & White, L. O. (1977) Diagnosis of invasive candidosis by enzyme immunoassay of serum antigen. *British Medical Journal*, **1**, 1183–1185.

Weiner, M. H. & Yount, W. J. (1976) Mannan antigenemia in the diagnosis of invasive *Candida* infections. *Journal of Clinical Investigation*, **58**, 1045–1053.

White, L. O., Richardson, M. D., Newham, H. C., Gibb, E. & Warren, R. C. (1977) Circulating antigen of *Aspergillus fumigatus* in cortisone-treated mice challenged with conidia: detection by counterimmunoelectrophoresis. *FEMS Microbiology Letters*, **2**, 153–156.

Williams, D. M., Krick, J. A. & Remington, J. S. (1976) Pulmonary infection in the compromised host. Part I. *American Review of Respiratory Disease*, **114**, 359–394.

Yarzabal, L. A., Bout, D., Naquira, F., Fruit, J. & Andrieu, S. (1977) Identification and purification of the specific antigen of *Paracoccidioides brasiliensis* responsible for immunoelectrophoretic band E. *Sabouraudia*, **15**, 79–85.

Young, R. C., Bennett, J. E., Vogel, C. L., Carbone, P. P. & De Vita, V. T. (1970) Aspergillosis: the spectrum of the disease in 98 patients. *Medicine*, **49**, 148–173.

Young, R. C., Bennett, J. E., Geelhoed, G. W. & Levine, A. S. (1974) Fungemia with compromised host resistance. A study of 70 cases. *Annals of Internal Medicine*, **80**, 605–612.

5. Meningococcal diseases; pathogenesis and prevention

R. J. Fallon

In recent years considerable advances have been made in the understanding of how meningococci cause disease. Furthermore it is now possible to prevent disease specifically by immunisation rather than by non-specific measures calculated to decrease the chance of spread of the organism from carrier to susceptible subjects.

Although extensive studies have been carried out on recruit populations, particularly in the U.S.A., they have not added greatly to our knowledge of the epidemiology of infection over and above what was well shown by earlier studies (Medical Research Council, 1920) but they have yielded useful information about the antibody response to, carriage of and infection with meningococci and also about the response to and effectiveness of vaccination. Nevertheless in the population at large, meningococcal disease still remains uncontrolled and unpredictable, disease rates fluctuate and epidemics occur without, in most instances, any clear reason. In this review therefore, the new information to be discussed is concerned with the mechanisms by which meningococci cause disease and immunity and with chemoprophylaxis and vaccines in the prevention of disease. Aspects of epidemiology are well discussed by other authors (for example, Christie, 1974).

THE PATHOGENESIS OF MENINGOCOCCAL DISEASE

The meningococcus can give rise to clinical disease ranging from fatal fulminating infection (typically the Waterhouse-Friderichsen syndrome), causing death sometimes even before the typical purpuric rash has time to develop, to chronic meningococcal septicaemia. The common manifestation of disease is meningitis in which the rash may be marked or virtually absent. In addition, meningococci can give rise to disease manifested by blood spread to a single focus, for example a joint or the pericardium as well as to disease spread either by blood or directly to other sites such as the lung or Fallopian tube. The organism is carried in the upper respiratory tract especially the nasopharynx by a proportion of the population which varies with age group and living circumstances and more than one serogroup may be carried at one time. More recently, it has been recognised that meningococci may spread from this site as a result of sexual practices, to the rectum and genital tract.

As in any disease situation the clinical picture is due to the interaction between parasite and host and consideration will be given to the various components of the parasite which may be, or definitely are, involved in the production of disease. The various relevant structures and components of the meningococcus are the pili, or fimbriae, projecting from the surface of the organism, the capsular polysaccharide, the protein antigens and the cell wall, which contains endotoxin.

Pili

For an organism to cause disease by invading the host rather than merely causing an intoxication as seen in tetanus, it must be able to penetrate the layer of secretions which overlie all epithelial surfaces and reach and adhere to the cells beneath. Virulent gonococci of Kellogg's types 1 and 2 are pilated, whereas avirulent strains are not. It has been suggested (Swanson, Kraus and Gotschlich, 1971) that these pili which aid the gonococci to adhere to cells are important components in the production of disease. Virulent gonococci are able to adhere to cells although it is not always certain that pili are responsible for this. Although the association may be fortuitous, a pilated strain of gonococcus resisted ingestion by phagocytes better than a non-pilated strain (Witt, Veale and Smith, 1976). *N. meningitidis* also has pili although these structures are soon lost on subculture. It is tempting to suggest that these pili may enable the meningococcus to adhere to cells of the nasopharynx before penetrating the epithelium and giving rise to systemic disease. Nevertheless, it is worth noting that non-pathogenic neisseria— *N. catarrhalis, N. perflava* and *N. subflava* may also be pilated so that the mere possession of pili is no indication of pathogenicity.

There is no indication as to how meningococci penetrate the mucous secretions of the upper respiratory tract and adhere to the respiratory mucosa, although early studies (Medical Research Council, 1916) indicate that nasal mucus may actually favour the growth of meningococci on artificial culture media. Nevertheless meningococci not only penetrate the layer of mucus but the organisms or their components penetrate the respiratory epithelium in healthy carriers to come into contact with antibody forming cells as evidenced by the production of antibody. Nasopharyngeal carriage is common especially in crowded communities and may last for months.

Antigenic components of the meningococcus

Antibodies are formed both to polysaccharide as well as to protein antigens, the former being better characterised and understood than the latter.

Polysaccharide antigen

It has long been recognised that meningococci can be differentiated into serogroups by agglutination tests, the current classification being established by Branham (1958) with the addition of other serogroups by Slaterus (1961), Slaterus, Ruys and Sieberg (1963) and Evans, Artenstein and Hunter (1968). The classification of meningococci into serogroups depends on their capsular polysaccharide. The chemical composition of the meningococcal group-specific polysaccharides characterised so far is shown in Table 5.1. It is uncommon for meningococci isolated from blood or CSF to be non-groupable, whereas such strains, frequently auto-agglutinable and presumably non-capsulated, are often isolated from the nasopharynx of healthy carriers. Hence possession of a capsular polysaccharide is important in the production of disease and it has been shown, as a result of the development of vaccines from the polysaccharides of group A and C meningococci, that immunity to the capsular polysaccharide protects against disease due to the homologous serogroup.

Although there is a correlation between capsulation and pathogenicity and

Table 5.1 Chemical composition of meningococcal group-specific polysaccharides

Group	Composition
A	N-acetyl-3-0-acetyl mannosamine phosphate (α1–6)
B	N-acetyl neuraminic acid (α2–8)
C	N-acetyl and O-acetyl neuraminic acid (α2–9)
X	N-acetyl glucosamine phosphate (α1–4)
Y	N-acetyl neuraminic acid: glucose*
Z[1]	3-deoxy-D manno-octulosonic acid
W135	N-acetyl neuraminic acid: galactose*

*Y polysaccharide is partially O-acetylated. W135 is not.
Group D and Z polysaccharides have not yet been defined.

between the possession of antibody to the capsular polysaccharide and immunity, the part the polysaccharide plays in the pathogenicity of the organism is not known.

Protein antigen(s)
That the capsular polysaccharide of the meningococcus is not the only antigen able to give rise to protective immunity is evident from the fact that although group B meningococcal polysaccharide is a poor antigen, immunity to group B as well as to other serogroups develops in children as they grow up. This usually correlates well with the decreasing prevalence of infection in older children compared with those in the first few years of life and can be demonstrated in vitro by the presence of bactericidal antibodies (Goldschneider, Gotschlich and Artenstein, 1969a). Hence as children become meningococcal carriers they develop immunity but this is not only to the strain which they carry but to a wide range of serogroups and may occur with carriage of groupable or non-groupable meningococci. This process is not, of course, confined to children but occurs in all age groups studied (Goldschneider, Gotschlich and Artenstein, 1969b; Reller, MacGregor and Beaty, 1973). Hence cross-protective immunity occurs and is not due to polysaccharide antigens. Various workers have shown the presence of cross-reactive antigens in meningococci which are cross-protective, protein in nature (Jennings et al, 1972; Wyle and Kasper, 1971) and stimulate the production of bactericidal antibodies (Kasper et al, 1973a). Frasch and Chapman (1973) studied the protein antigens of group B meningococci in detail and showed that there were over 12 distinct serotypes. The role of the serotype antigens in immunity was further studied by Frasch et al (1976) in the chick embryo. Embryos were inoculated intravenously with a mixture of meningococci and hyperimmune antiserum. Normally chick embryos develop meningitis, sinusitis or pulmonary lesions following inoculation with meningococci. However, in the presence of antiserum to group B polysaccharide there was protection of the embryos, whereas antiserum to the protein, type-specific antigens was poorly protective even though this serum was actively bactericidal in vitro. As the chick has no complement system it was argued that the antibodies produced to group B type-specific protein antigens are complement dependant and poorly opsonic whereas antibodies to the group B polysaccharide which are known to be poorly bactericidal are opsonic.

Group A antibody was more effective than group B in protecting against homologous challenge but group A antibody is both strongly bactericidal and effectively opsonic. The demonstration of type-specific protein antigens in group C similar to those in group B (Munford, Patton and Gorman, 1975) and also in groups W 135 (Jones, 1976) and Y provides a firm laboratory foundation for the epidemiological studies. An interesting and important observation is that group B strains isolated from clinical disease are most commonly of serotype 2 or of complexes related to serotype 2 (Frasch and Chapman, 1973; Jones and Tobin, 1976). As with the group specific polysaccharide, the reason for the association of the type 2 protein antigen with organisms predominantly isolated from disease, as opposed to carriers, is unknown.

Hence, there are two major antigenic components of the meningococcus, the group specific polysaccharide conferring group-specific immunity and the type-specific protein conferring a broader immunity shared between a number of serogroups. Doubtless the situation is more complex than this in that cross protective antibodies are stimulated by less well defined components of the meningococcus and also possibly of other organisms. In this latter connection it has been shown that group B meningococcal polysaccharide is identical with the K1 antigen of *Escherichia coli* (Kasper et al, 1973b; Fallon and McIllmurray, 1976) and there may be other similar relationships (Robbins et al, 1972).

Disease-producing components of the meningococcus

One fraction from meningococci that has been studied by a number of workers is the lipopolysaccharide but its importance as an antigen is not yet known. Nevertheless, when it comes to the production of disease as opposed to the stimulation of an immune response the endotoxin of the meningococcus is of prime importance. In common with other Gram-negative bacteria *N. meningitidis* produces an endotoxin which is associated with the protein-lipopolysaccharide complex of the cell wall. In culture meningococci show blebs on the cell wall and these blebs, which are released into the medium, contain endotoxin. DeVoe and Gilchrist (1973) showed, using keto-deoxyoctonic acid (KDO) assay, that 18 per cent of the bacterial endotoxin was in these released blebs. Hence, it may not be necessary for the meningococci to be lysed for them to release endotoxin. Furthermore although phagocytosed meningococci are rapidly destroyed by polymorphonuclear leucocytes, the residual material egested by the phagocytes contains meningococcal 'ghosts' with the cytoplasmic membrane and outer wall membrane relatively intact (DeVoe, Gilchrist and Storm, 1973; DeVoe, 1976). This egested material sensitises animals to endotoxin, although it appears that endotoxin is modified by polymorphonuclear leucocytes (in terms of measurement of KDO). In contrast to the results obtained in rabbits given purified lipopolysaccharide subcutaneously then intravenously which resulted in the development of the localised Shwartzman reaction alone, 12 of 32 rabbits given egested material subcutaneously followed by intravenous lipopolysaccharide or cell wall blebs developed disseminated intravascular coagulation (DIC) (DeVoe and Gilka, 1976).

Meningococcal endotoxin may differ from endotoxin derived from enterobacteriaceae in its ability to give rise to skin lesions. Hence, Davis and Arnold (1974) found that purified lipopolysaccharides from enterobacteria and meningococci of groups A, B and C were equally potent for the production of the generalised Shwartzman reaction and for mouse lethality but that the meningococcal lipopolysaccharide was 5–10 times more potent in inducing the dermal Shwartzman reaction. These authors believe that this explains the prominence of purpura in meningococcal septicaemia—these lesions being indistinguishable from the dermal Shwartzman reaction. Meningococcal endotoxin, therefore, has properties similar to other endotoxins but may also have enhanced dermotropic properties and, in possibly synergistic combination with egested meningococcal products following phagocytosis, can give rise to DIC. The similarity of meningococcal endotoxin to other endotoxins has been emphasised recently by Davis, Ziegler and Arnold (1978). They found that antibodies to *E. coli* neutralised meningocoaccal endotoxaemia in rabbits from all three major meningococcal capsular serogroups using the dermal necrosis of the local Schwartzman phenomenon and the renal cortical necrosis of this phenomenon as assays. Although antisera raised against endotoxin from meningococci of groups A, B and C provided good protection against endotoxaemia from homologous capsular groups, the *E. coli* endotoxin protected against endotoxaemia from all groups. The authors interpret their findings as indicating that the endotoxin core is the toxic moiety of meningococcal lipopolysaccharide and that this core is immunologically similar to enteric lipopolysaccharide. They suggest the antigenically variable side chains of meningococcal lipopolysaccharide interfere with the production of antibody protective against the common core. The practical application which they suggest is that antibodies prepared against the *E. coli* strain (J5) with which they worked, could interrupt the course of meningococcal endotoxaemia in patients, regardless of the capsular serogroup of the infecting strain.

Pathology of meningococcal infection
There has been no recent advance in the understanding of how the meningococcus passes from the nasopharynx into the blood or nervous system. The current state of knowledge is summarised by Christie (1974). Epidemiological and experimental studies show that acute meningococcal infection occurs in subjects without antibody. Whether circulating antibody will protect against direct invasion of the nervous system as against blood stream invasion is uncertain, particularly in view of the report of Griffiss et al (1974) of a child with bactericidal antibodies who developed a recurrence of infection with the same strain of meningococcus as that causing the initial infection. However, it may well be that the vital protective factor is secretory IgA in the nasopharynx.

The gross pathology of meningococcal infection is well described in standard textbooks. However, recent studies on what may well be the essential lesion in meningococcal septicaemia are of importance. A consistent feature noted in several studies of large series of fatal cases of meningococcal infection has been the vascular lesions. Hence, Ferguson and Chapman (1948) noted the presence of widely spread thrombi in patients dying of the Waterhouse-Friderichsen syndrome and Hardman and Earle (1967) in a review of 200 fatal cases noted acute vasculitis to be present. Intravascular coagulation was seen more commonly in patients dying at a time when group B infection was prevalent as opposed to cases dying when group A predominated. Dalldorf and Jennette (1977) studied seven fatal cases of meningococcal septicaemia and observed the presence of widespread pulmonary micro-vascular thrombosis, the thrombi consisting of platelets and leucocytes, and also of DIC with the formation of fibrin thrombi. Six of the cases died in shock and all these showed pulmonary capillary thrombosis. All seven patients had bilateral haemorrhagic infarction of the adrenal glands with extensive fibrin thrombi in the adrenal cortical capillaries and four patients also had similar thrombi in the renal glomeruli. The pulmonary lesions paralleled those produced experimentally in rabbits which were inoculated intraperitoneally with meningococci and mucin (Gaskins and Dalldorf, 1976). It is of interest that fatal pulmonary oedema was reported by Frankel, Bennett and Borland (1976) in two cases of meningococcal meningitis. No mention was made in the postmortem findings of intravascular coagulation, but they noted that mention of pulmonary oedema in meningococcal meningitis had only been made in two other clinical reports.

In a study of the cutaneous lesions in acute meningococcal septicaemia Sotto et al (1976) noted endothelial necrosis, thrombosis and necrosis of muscle cells and pericytes in the vascular wall. These features resemble those of the local Shwartzman reaction but in addition immunoglobulins and complement were present in the vascular wall of most patients. This would correlate with the demonstration of circulating immune complexes found in some patients with meningococcal disease. Fibrin thrombi in renal and adrenal cortical capillaries are seen in the generalised Shwartzman reaction which is endotoxin-induced and it may well be that meningococcal endotoxin, as noted by Davis and Arnold (1974) can act both generally and also at a local level in skin. An important point made by Dalldorf and Jennette (1977) is that whereas the micro-thrombi which form as a result of endotoxin action may be prevented by heparin therapy, the toxic thrombi in the lungs would not be because the precipitating factor is increased cell adhesion which is not affected by heparin although it may be influenced by aspirin.

Another aspect of meningococcal infection which has received attention recently is the formation of immune complexes and the part this plays in the final picture of disease. An immunological investigation of four patients with meningococcal meningitis who developed arthritis or cutaneous lesions (Greenwood, Whittle and Bryceson, 1973) suggested that immune complex formation may have occurred in two or possibly three of the patients, C_3 levels in serum falling on the sixth day of illness. They also showed, in one case, evidence of the presence of immunoglobulin, meningococcal antigen and C_3 deposition in and around blood vessel walls as noted also by Sotto et al (1976). Greenwood et al (1973) also found immunoglobulin, meningococcal antigen and C_3 in the synovial fluid cells of both patients investigated for this. These workers were unable to demonstrate the presence of circulating immune complexes but Davis et al (1976) demonstrated such complexes both in serum and synovial fluid of a woman infected with a group C meningococcus who developed sterile bilateral knee effusions on the 15th day of illness. Larson et al (1977) demonstrated immune complexes in cells and fluid from the knees of a boy who developed arthritis of wrists and knees the day after treatment commenced for meningococcal meningitis. The complexes were complement-fixing and the authors assumed that the local reaction was a complement-mediated sterile inflammatory reaction which caused much of his later general illness, fever and most of his joint disease. In a study of 211 patients with meningo-coccal disease, Greenwood, Onyewotu and Whittle (1976) showed that 13 patients with meningococcal septicaemia without meningitis had low serum C_3 levels and suggested that complement activation may have contributed to the peripheral circulatory collapse that was responsible for the deaths of nine of these cases. In line with their earlier findings (Greenwood et al, 1973) they found a transient fall in serum C_3 levels in 13 patients positive for serum antigen who subsequently developed arthritis or intravenous vasculitis. It is interesting to note that all 13 cases with meningococcaemia were infected with group C meningococci, as was the case of Davis et al (1976), in view of the observation that in the same population, group A meningococci caused meningitis but no cases of septicaemia (Evans-Jones et al, 1977). This accords with studies in the U.S.A. (Hardman, 1968) that group C infection appeared more commonly than group A to be associated with adrenal haemorrhage.

Man's interaction with the meningococcus seems, then, to depend on what happens at the moment of first contact as carriage before disease, certainly with group C meningococci, appears to be short (Edwards et al, 1977). A patient either becomes a carrier or much less commonly, a case. In either situation the host pro-duces antibody to both group and type antigens of the meningococcus resulting in both group specific and cross-protective immunity. In any antigenic challenge the quality as well as quantity and speed of antibody response is important. It has been suggested that in some cases of meningoccal septicaemia IgM deficiency may be present but this finding has yet to be confirmed. Also Whittle et al (1976) have presented evidence to suggest that patients with meningococcal meningitis may have a familial immune defect resulting in a decreased ability to respond to polysaccharide antigens.

In infection the blood stream is invaded, with the meninges usually being secondarily affected. The septicaemia gives rise to endotoxaemia and dissemination of meningococci into capillaries giving rise to local lesions and also to DIC. Com-plement activation may well occur due to the action of endotoxin and immune complexes may form later, contributing to skin manifestations and vasculitis as well to the arthritis, iritis and neuropathy seen in some cases. Complement activa-tion may be important in the unfavourable outcome of septicaemic illness and DIC may give rise to pulmonary oedema.

Although a complex but composite picture is emerging in acute disease, less progress has been made in the understanding of the uncommon condition of chronic meningococcal septicaemia. Niklasson and Svanbom (1973) studied four cases but, apart from showing the presence of complement-fixing antibodies to meningococci in two cases and vasculitis in skin biopsy from one case, no immuno-logical or other investigations were performed which might explain the basis of the condition. The presence of vasculitis, skin lesions and joint involvement suggests that immune complexes are formed and play a part in the picture of disease but there is no indication as to the difference in the host-parasite relationship here and in acute infection.

As might be expected in a septicaemic illness, meningococci have been isolated from many sites with involvement of many organs. This aspect of meningococcal disease as well as a discussion on the pathogenesis of the Waterhouse-Friderichsen syndrome is considered in a useful review by Bell and Silber (1971). Meningo-cocci have been isolated from cases of pneumonia on many occasions and the relevant literature has been reviewed by Putsch, Hamilton and Wolinsky (1970). Whether the organism has been the primary pathogen is difficult to establish, not only because meningococci may be found in the pharynx without causing disease, but also because routine laboratory investigations for evidence of viral, rickettsial and mycoplasmal infection have only become widely available relatively recently. Jacobs and Norden (1974) reported the isolation of meningococci from both blood and sputum of a patient with pneumonia who had no evidence of influenza, adeno-virus, coxsackievirus or mycoplasmal pneumonia; Irwin, Woelk and Coudon (1975) reported the isolation of meningococci from transtracheal aspirates from three cases of pneumonia. Interestingly their cases and that of Jacobs and Norden (1974) were of group Y infection and two had evidence of recent viral infection. In the discussion of their results, Irwin et al (1975) raise the question of the relation-ship of preceding virus infection to meningococcal disease. However, Artenstein et al (1967) in a survey of army recruits found that their results suggested that viral respiratory disease is not a significant factor either in the spread of meningo-cocci in recruits nor in invasion of the host following nasopharyngeal colonisation.

Recently reports have appeared of meningococci being isolated from genital sites and also from the rectum. In some instances these may be chance infections (Fallon and Robinson, 1974), whereas others may be the result of sexual activity (Wilmott, 1976; Beck, Fluker and Platt, 1974; Givan and Keyl, 1974).

THE PREVENTION OF MENINGOCOCCAL DISEASE

Disease due to microbial agents can be prevented by (1) elimination of the agent from the environment; (2) reduction in the chance of a carrier or case trans-mitting the agent to susceptibles, either by isolating and treating the case or by reducing the closeness of physical contact by avoiding overcrowding which, as experience in recruit camps shows, is a most important factor in meningococcal disease; (3) preventing the organism from multiplying in the patient once it has reached him, as by chemoprophylaxis; (4) immunisation.

Of these possibilities only the last two are specific and relevant.

Chemoprophylaxis
Until the recognition of disease due to sulphonamide-resistant meningococci in 1963 chemoprophylaxis with sulphonamides was the accepted method of attempt-ing to prevent acquisition of meningococci, and disease due to them. Since that time there has been world wide recognition of the existence of fully resistant strains as well as of strains of partial resistance which were unlikely to be eradicated from the nasopharynx of carriers by sulphonamide therapy. Most antibiotics are inefficient in eradicating meningococcal carriage. However, in 1969 Deal and Sanders first reported the effect of rifampicin on meningococcal carriage and since that time studies have been made both in service and civilian populations. Devine et al (1971a) studied the effectiveness of minocycline in eradicating meningococci from the nasopharynx of carriers. Both agents are effective, although not all

carriers are cleared. Hence with rifampicin Devine et al (1971b) found that 89 of 93 servicemen were cleared of nasopharyngeal meningococci after two days treatment with 600 mg of rifampicin given twice daily. The four remaining carriers, although yielding rifampicin sensitive strains initially, carried resistant strains after the course of treatment. In their study on minocycline Devine et al (1971a) found a reduction of 67.6 per cent in meningococcal carriers following a two-day course. No resistant strains were isolated in a further study using both drugs sequentially (Devine et al, 1973) and only seven of 1258 carriers continued to carry organisms after treatment, one of the seven strains being rifampicin resistant. Unfortunately, minocycline has unpleasant side effects and also is unsuitable for use in children, so that rifampicin is the favoured drug of the two despite the fact that resistant organisms may appear after treatment. Chemoprophylaxis was employed in a civilian population in the epidemic of group C infection in Brazil (Munford et al, 1974). The carriage rate two weeks after sulphadiazine treatment was 49 per cent, 17 per cent after minocycline, 9 per cent after rifampicin and 0 per cent after a combination of the latter two drugs. However, 33 per cent of those taking minocycline and rifampicin experienced side effects.

Chemoprophylaxis of meningococcal infection has to be considered whenever a case occurs because more than 50 per cent of secondary cases occur less than five days after the index case and so vaccination, even if available, would be ineffective. There are two situations where action may be thought to be warranted: (1) in the family of the patient, (2) in the contacts where a case occurs in a situation where there may be a number of susceptibles—e.g. a boarding school or a recruit camp. In the first situation, although second cases in a family are rare, there is an enhanced risk of infection occurring compared with the general population. This appears to be as much as 1000 fold according to a recent survey (Meningococcal Disease Surveillance Group, 1974) and is much higher than in non family contacts. Also consideration has to be given to the age of family contacts. Hence, children and young adults are more susceptible to infection than adults. Kaiser et al (1974) found that the secondary attack rate in all close household contacts was 5.9 per cent but was 11.8 per cent in contacts aged 1–4 years.

Where the organism is known to be sulphonamide sensitive, sulphadiazine can be given (for children 1–12 years old, 500 mg 12 hourly for two days, adults 1 g 12 hourly for two days). If the sensitivity is unknown but sulphonamide-resistant strains are uncommon, sulphadiazine could be given pending the results of culture. Where sulphonamide resistance is present (in the U.K. about 15 per cent of all serogroups are fully resistant, the rate varying from group to group) rifampicin should be used, as the problem of the emergence of resistant strains of meningococci or other organism is not likely to be of significance if the antibiotic is only used infrequently and in special circumstances. Rifampicin is given twice daily for two days in the following oral dosage: adults 600 mg, children 1–12 years 10 mg/kg, under 1 year 5 mg/kg. A simple algorithm for prophylaxis has been published by Jacobson and Fraser (1976).

Vaccination
The group-specific polysaccharides of groups A and C meningococci are potent antigens giving rise to the production of group-specific protective antibodies.

Highly purified polysaccharides have been produced and can be used as vaccines. The background to this development has been described by Gotschlich (1975). More recently the specifications for meningococcal polysaccharide vaccines (WHO Technical Report Series No. 594, 1976) and a summary of their efficacy (WHO Technical Report Series No. 588, 1976) have been published. The dosage and efficacy of vaccination have been studied in adults, children and pregnant women and their babies. Studies have been made of the prevention of infection in high risk situations such as recruit camps as well as in the face of epidemics and there is now much information available on dosage, serological response, side effects and efficacy. The salient features of the various studies are that, firstly, there should be enough disease due to a particular serogroup to warrant the production of a vaccine. This applies to group A which gives rise to epidemics in Africa and has recently given rise to epidemics in Brazil and Finland, and to group C which has given rise to epidemics in Brazil, in the U.S. armed forces and which appears to be of importance now in Africa. It also applies to group B. Secondly, the polysaccharide should be a good antigen. This applies to groups A and C especially if the polysaccharide is of high molecular weight. However, group B polysaccharide is a poor antigen (Wyle et al, 1972) and here one must look to the possibility of producing a vaccine dependant on the cross protective protein antigens—especially of type 2 and related types in view of the greater association of these with disease.

Thirdly, the vaccine should give a good and durable response in all age groups, without unacceptable side effects.

Although vaccines are needed for the prevention of disease due to groups A, B and C they are only available for group A and C.

Group A vaccine is intrinsically unstable but if stabilised by lactose can be stored, as can the more stable group C vaccine, at or below 5°C. The vaccines are usually given separately but a combined A and C vaccine has been used in Brazil. The dosage depends on the characteristics of a particular batch but is usually 50 μg. In Finland in 1974–75 the dose of group A vaccine used was equivalent to 30 μg polysaccharide (50 μg gave many side reactions) except for children 3–5 months old who received 20 μg (Peltola et al, 1976). The response to vaccination differs with age. Group A and C vaccines give rise to immunity in subjects over the age of 6 years but there is less certainty yet about the response in younger children and infants. Hence, with group C vaccine no protection was seen in infants aged 6–23 months but protection was seen in children aged 2–3 years (Taunay et al, 1974). A poor response is seen in children given group C vaccine in infancy and given a second dose 4–10 months later, although a booster effect has been reported in older children by Monto, Brandt and Artenstein (1973) who also noted a better response in children given 100 μg rather than 50 μg of vaccine. Käyhty and Mäkelä (1977) found the mean antibody response to primary group A vaccination was lower in children under 1 year old than in older children but after a booster dose rose to a level of over 1 μg/ml (the mean adult level) in 60 per cent of children aged 3–5 months and in 90 per cent of those aged 6–11 months. Nearly 100 per cent of children aged 1 year reached this level after primary vaccination. In a study carried out in Brazil (Carvalho et al, 1977) 21 pregnant women and 29 infants were examined for response to a combined group A and C vaccine. Most of the women sero-converted or showed a rise in antibody titre. Seven of the infants born to the 21 women were found to have passively transferred antibody to group A and 14 to group C. The immunity lasted for 2–5 months. Vaccination in the 29 infants only resulted in one sero-conversion, despite the fact that in all but two the mothers had been vaccinated one year previously. Both vaccines may produce a fall in the rate of new acquisitions of the respective serogroup of meningococci but do not affect those carrying the organisms at the time of vaccination. The efficacy of the vaccines has been shown in that the incidence of group C disease in servicemen has been reduced to very low levels following vaccination, and similar results have been obtained in the face of epidemics. Hence, in Finland in a double blind trial, no case of group A disease occurred in 49 295 vaccinated children, whereas nine cases occurred in 31 906 unvaccinated children. The vaccines do not produce serious side effects and in most studies in adults and infants, no side effects have been reported. However in Finnish children aged three months to five years vaccinated with 50 μg of group A polysaccharide, 71 per cent had local symptoms, 37 per cent mild systemic reactions and 1.8 per cent fever over 38.5°C. The dose was subsequently reduced to 25 μg. The duration of immunity as shown by the possession of antibody following vaccination is uncertain. The longest period so far reported is three years with group A vaccine (WHO Technical Report Series No. 588, 1976) and five years with group C (Brandt and Artenstein, 1975).

A novel use of vaccination against group A meningococcal infection has recently been described by Greenwood, Hassan-King and Whittle (1978). They vaccinated 523 contacts with tetanus toxoid and 520 contacts with meningococcal vaccine. Five of those who received tetanus toxoid developed meningococcal meningitis and another four probably had meningococcal disease but only one possible case of meningococcal infection occurred amongst the contacts vaccinated with group A vaccine. However, in view of the fact that secondary cases of meningococcal infection may often occur very shortly after the index case in a family, it would seem wise to combine chemoprophylaxis with vaccination of contacts.

Although group B meningococci do not usually produce outbreaks they have done so in recent times and are the commonest serogroup isolated in many countries including the United Kingdom. Immunisation in infancy with a good group B vaccine would eradicate much of meningococcal disease in many countries. For example, in Scotland 202 of 314 cases of meningococcal disease occurring between 1972 and 1976 were due to group B and 82 per cent of these occurred in children under the age of five years. Serogroups other than A, B and C are of little numerical importance as yet so that the use of a polysaccharide vaccine would not be warranted. Nevertheless, if a broadly cross-protective vaccine could be developed this could reduce the prevalence of meningococcal infection, particularly if it was effective in infants who are so greatly at risk. Anyone who has seen how deadly and rapidly lethal the meningococcus can be will realise that eradication of disease due to this organism is a worthwhile objective.

REFERENCES

Artenstein, M. S., Rust, J. H., Jr., Hunter, D. H., Lawson, T. H. & Buescher, E. L. (1967) Acute respiratory disease and meningococcal infection in army recruits. *Journal of the American Medical Association*, **201**, 1004–1008.

Beck, A., Fluker, J. L. & Platt, D. J. (1974) *Neisseria meningitidis* in urogenital infection. *British Journal of Venereal Diseases*, **50**, 367–369.

Bell, W. E. & Silber, D. L. (1971) Meningococcal meningitis: past and present concepts. *Military Medicine*, **136**, 601–611.

Brandt, B. L. & Artenstein, M. S. (1975) Duration of antibody responses after vaccination with group C *Neisseria meningitidis* polysaccharide. *Journal of Infectious Diseases*, **131**, supplement, S69–S72.

Branham, S. E. (1958) Reference strains for the serologic groups of meningococcus (*Neisseria meningitidis*). *International Bulletin of Bacteriological Nomenclature and Taxonomy*, **8**, 1–15.

Carvalho, A. de A., Giampaglia, C. M. S., Kimura, H., Pereira, O. A. de C., Farhat, C. K., Neves, J. C., Prandini, R., Carvalho, E. da S. & Zarvos, A. M. (1977) Maternal and infant antibody response to meningococcal vaccination in pregnancy. *Lancet*, **2**, 809–811.

Christie, A. B. (1974) *Infectious Diseases. Epidemiology and Clinical Practice*, 2nd edition. Edinburgh: Churchill Livingstone.

Dalldorf, F. G. & Jennette, J. C. (1977) Fatal meningococcal septicemia. *Archives of Pathology and Laboratory Medicine*, **101**, 6–9.

Davis, C. E. & Arnold, K. (1974) Role of meningococcal endotoxin in meningococcal purpura. *Journal of Experimental Medicine*, **140**, 159–171.

Davis, C. E., Ziegler, E. J. & Arnold, K. S. (1978) Neutralisation of meningococcal endotoxin by antibody to core glycolipid. *Journal of Experimental Medicine*, **147**, 1007–1017.

Davis, J. A. S., Peters, N., Mohammed, I., Major, G. A. C. & Holborow, E. J. (1976) Circulating immune complexes in a patient with meningococcal disease. *British Medical Journal*, **1**, 1445–1446.

Deal, W. B. & Sanders, E. (1969) Efficacy of rifampin in treatment of meningococcal carriers. *New England Journal of Medicine*, **281**, 641–645.

Devine, L. F., Johnson, D. P., Hagerman, C. R., Pierce, W. E., Rhode, S. L. III & Pekinpaugh, R. O. (1971a) The effect of minocycline on meningococcal nasopharyngeal carrier state in naval personnel. *American Journal of Epidemiology*, **93**, 337–345.

Devine, L. F., Johnson, D. P., Rhode, S. L. III, Hagerman, C. R., Pierce, W. E. & Pekingpaugh, R. O. (1971b) Rifampicin: effect of two-day treatment on the meningococcal carrier state and the relationship to the levels of drug in sera and saliva. *American Journal of Medical Sciences*, **261**, 79–83.

Devine, L. F., Pollard, R. B., Krumpe, P. E., Hoy, E. S., Mammen, R. E., Miller, C. H. & Peckinpaugh, R. O. (1973) Field trial of the efficacy of a previously proposed regimen using minocycline and rifampin sequentially for the elimination of meningococci for healthy carriers. *American Journal of Epidemiology*, **97**, 394–401.

DeVoe, I. W. (1976) Egestion of degraded meningococci by polymorphonuclear leukocytes. *Journal of Bacteriology*, **125**, 258–266.

DeVoe, I. W. & Gilchrist, J. E. (1973) Release of endotoxin in the form of cell wall blebs during the in vitro growth of *Neisseria meningitidis*. *Journal of Experimental Medicine*, **138**, 1156–1167.

DeVoe, I. W., Gilchrist, J. E. & Storm, D. W. (1973) Ultrastructural studies on the fate of Group B meningococci in human peripheral blood leukocytes. *Canadian Journal of Microbiology*, **19**, 1355–1359.

DeVoe, I. W. & Gilka, F. (1976) Disseminated intravascular coagulation in rabbits: synergistic activity of meningococcal endotoxin and materials egested from leucocytes containing meningococci. *Journal of Medical Microbiology*, **9**, 451–458.

Edwards, E. A., Devine, L. F., Sengbusch, C. H. & Ward, H. W. (1977) Immunological investigation of meningococcal disease. III. Brevity of Group C acquisition prior to disease occurrence. *Scandinavian Journal of Infectious Diseases*, **9**, 105–110.

Evans, J. R., Artenstein, M. S. & Hunter, D. S. (1968) Prevalence of meningococcal serogroups and description of three new groups. *American Journal of Epidemiology*, **87**, 643–646.

Evans-Jones, L. G., Whittle, H. C., Onyewotu, I. I., Egler, L. J. & Greenwood, B. M. (1977) Comparative study of group A and group C meningococcal infection. *Archives of Disease in Childhood*, **52**, 320–323.

Fallon, R. J. & McIllmurray, M. B. (1976) *Escherichia coli* K1. *Lancet*, **1**, 201.

Fallon, R. J. & Robinson, E. T. (1974) Meningococcal vulvovaginitis. *Scandinavian Journal of Infectious Diseases*, **6**, 295–296.

Ferguson, J. H. & Chapman, O. D. (1948) Fulminating meningococcic infections and the so-called Waterhouse-Friderichsen syndrome. *American Journal of Pathology*, **24**, 763–796.

Frankel, R. J., Bennett, E. D. & Borland, C. D. (1976) Pulmonary oedema in meningococcal meningitis. *Postgraduate Medical Journal*, **52**, 529–531.

Frasch, C. E. & Chapman, S. S. (1973) Classification of *Neisseria meningitidis* Group B into distinct serotypes. III. Application of a new bactericidal inhibition technique to distribution of serotypes among cases and carriers. *Journal of Infectious Diseases*, **127**, 149–154.

Frasch, C. E., Parkes, L., McNelis, R. M. & Gotschlich, E. C. (1976) Protection against group B meningococcal disease. I. Comparison of group-specific and type-specific protection in the chick embryo model. *Journal of Experimental Medicine*, 144, 319–329.

Gaskins, R. A., Jr. & Dalldorf, F. G. (1976) Experimental meningococcal septicemia: effect of heparin therapy. *Archives of Pathology and Laboratory Medicine*, 100, 318–324.

Givan, K. F. & Keyl, A. (1974) The isolation of *Neisseria* species from unusual sites. *Canadian Medical Association Journal*, 111, 1077–1079.

Goldschneider, I., Gotschlich, E. C. & Artenstein, M. S. (1969a) Human immunity to the meningococcus. I. The role of humoral antibodies. *Journal of Experimental Medicine*, 129, 1307–1326.

Goldschneider, I., Gotschlich, E. C. & Artenstein, M. S. (1969b) Human immunity to the meningococcus. II. Development of natural immunity. *Journal of Experimental Medicine*, 129, 1327–1348.

Gotschlich, E. (1975) Development of polysaccharide vaccines for the prevention of meningococcal disease. *Monographs in Allergy*, 9, 245–258.

Greenwood, B. M., Hassan-King, M. & Whittle, H. C. (1978) Prevention of secondary cases of meningococcal disease in household contacts by vaccination. *British Medical Journal*, 1, 1317–1319.

Greenwood, B. M., Onyewotu, I. I. & Whittle, H. C. (1976) Complement and meningococcal infection. *British Medical Journal*, 1, 797–799.

Greenwood, B. M., Whittle, H. C. & Bryceson, A. D. M. (1973) Allergic complications of meningococcal disease. II—immunological investigations. *British Medical Journal*, 1, 737–740.

Griffiss, J. M., Bannatyne, R. M., Artenstein, M. S. & Anglin, C. S. (1974) Recurrent meningococcal infection with an antigenically identical strain. *Journal of the American Medical Association*, 229, 68–70.

Hardman, J. M. (1968) Fatal meningococcal infections: the changing pathologic picture in the '60s. *Military Medicine*, 133, 951–964.

Hardman, J. M. & Earle, K. M. (1967) Meningococcal infection. A review of 200 fatal cases. *Journal of Neuropathology*, 26, 119.

Irwin, R. S., Woelk, W. K. & Coudon, W. L. III (1975) Primary meningococcal pneumonia. *Annals of Internal Medicine*, 82, 493–498.

Jacobs, S. A. & Norden, C. W. (1974) Pneumonia caused by *Neisseria meningitidis*. *Journal of the American Medical Association*, 227, 67–68.

Jacobson, J. A. & Fraser, D. W. (1976) A simplified approach to meningococcal disease prophylaxis. *Journal of the American Medical Association*, 236, 1053–1054.

Jennings, H. J., Martin, A., Kenny, C. P. & Diena, B. B. (1972) Cross-protective antigens of *Neisseria meningitidis* obtained from Slaterus group Y. *Infection and Immunity*, 5, 547–551.

Jones, D. M. (1976) Serotypes of meningococci. *Journal of Clinical Pathology*, 29, 1045.

Jones, D. M. & Tobin, B. M. (1976) Serotypes of group B meningococci. *Journal of Clinical Pathology*, 29, 746–748.

Kaiser, A. B., Hennekens, C. H., Saslaw, M. S., Hayes, P. S. & Bennett, J. V. (1974) Seroepidemiology and chemoprophylaxis of disease due to sulfonamide-resistant *Neisseria meningitidis* in a civilian population. *Journal of Infectious Diseases*, 130, 217–224.

Kasper, D. L., Winkelhake, J. L., Brandt, B. L. & Artenstein, M. S. (1973a) Antigenic specificity of bactericidal antibodies in antisera to *Neisseria meningitidis*. *Journal of Infectious Diseases*, 127, 378–387.

Kasper, D. L., Winkelhake, J. I., Zollinger, W. D., Brandt, B. L. & Artenstein, M. S. (1973b) Immunochemical similarity between polysaccharide antigens of *Escherichia coli* 07 :K1(L) :NM and group B *Neisseria meningitidis*. *Journal of Immunology*, 110, 262–268.

Käyhty, H. & Mäkelä, P. H. (1977) Extent and duration of serum antibody response to the group A meningococcal polysaccharide vaccine. Paper presented at the Scottish-Scandinavian Conference on Infectious Diseases, Uppsala.

Larson, H. E., Nicholson, K. G., Loewi, G., Tyrrell, D. A. J. & Posner, J. (1977) Arthritis after meningococcal meningitis. *British Medical Journal*, 1, 618.

Medical Research Council, 1916. Report of the Special Advisory Committee upon bacteriological studies of cerebrospinal fever during the epidemic of 1915. *Special Report series* No. 2. H.M. Stationery Office, London.

Medical Research Council, 1920. Cerebrospinal fever. Studies in the bacteriology, prevention, control and specific treatment of cerebrospinal fever among the military forces, 1915–19. *Special Report series* No. 50. H.M. Stationery Office, London.

Meningococcal Disease Surveillance Group (1974) Meningococcal disease. Secondary attack rate and chemoprophylaxis in the United States, 1974. *Journal of American Medical Association*, 235, 261–265.

Monto, A. S., Brandt, B. L. & Artenstein, M. S. (1973) Response of children to *Neisseria meningitidis* polysaccharide vaccines. *Journal of Infectious Diseases*, 127, 394–400.

Munford, R. S., de Vasconcelos, Z. J. S., Phillips, C. J., Gelli, D. S., Gorman, G. W., Risi, J. B. &

Feldman, R. A. (1974) Eradication of carriage of *Neisseria meningitidis* in families: a study of Brazil. *Journal of Infectious Diseases*, **129**, 644–649.

Munford, R. S., Patton, C. M. & Gorman, G. W. (1975) Epidemiologic studies of serotype antigens common to groups B and C *Neisseria meningitidis*. *Journal of Infectious Diseases*, **131**, 286–290.

Niklasson, P.-M. & Svanbom, M. (1973) Prolonged meningococcal septicemia. A report of four cases and a comparison with benign gonococcal septicemia. *Scandinavian Journal of Infectious Diseases*, **5**, 29–33.

Peltola, H., Mäkelä, P. H., Elo, O., Pettay, O., Renkonen, O.-V. & Sivonen, A. (1976) Vaccination against meningococcal Group A disease in Finland, 1974–75. *Scandinavian Journal of Infectious Diseases*, **8**, 169–174.

Putsch, R. W., Hamilton, J. D. & Wolinsky, E. (1970) *Neisseria meningitidis*, a respiratory pathogen? *Journal of Infectious diseases*, **121**, 48–54.

Reller, L. B., MacGregor, R. R. & Beaty, H. N. (1973) Bactericidal antibody after colonization with *Neisseria meningitidis*. *Journal of Infectious Diseases*, **127**, 56–62.

Robbins, J. B., Myerowitz, R. L., Whisnant, J. K., Argaman, M., Schneerson, R., Handzel, Z. T. & Gotschlich, E. C. (1972) Enteric bacteria cross-reactive with *Neisseria meningitidis* groups A and C and *Diplococcus pneumoniae* types I and III. *Infection and Immunity*, **6**, 651–656.

Slaterus, K. W. (1961) Serological typing of meningococci by means of micro-precipitation. *Antonie von Leeuwenhoek*, **27**, 305–315.

Slaterus, K. W., Ruys, A. C. & Sieberg, I. G. (1963) Types of meningococci isolated from carriers and patients in a non-epidemic period in the Netherlands. *Antonie von Leeuwenhoek*, **29**, 265–271.

Sotto, M. N., Langer, B., Hoshino-Shimizu, S. & de Brito, T. (1976) Pathogenesis of cutaneous lesions in acute meningococcemia in humans: light, immunofluorescent, and electron microscopic studies of skin biopsy specimens. *Journal of Infectious Diseases*, **133**, 506–514.

Swanson, J., Kraus, S. J. & Gotschlich, E. C. (1971) Studies on gonococcus infection. I. Pili and zones of adhesion: their relation to gonococcal growth patterns. *Journal of Experimental Medicine*, **134**, 886–906.

Taunay, A. de E., Galvao, P. A., de Morais, J. S., Gotschlich, E. C. & Feldman, R. E. (1974) Disease prevention by meningococcal serogroup C polysaccharide vaccine in pre-school children: results after eleven months in Sao Paulo, Brazil. *Pediatric Research*, **8**, 429.

Whittle, H. C., Oduloju, A., Evans-Jones, G. & Greenwood, B. M. (1976) Evidence for familial immune defect in meningococcal meningitis. *British Medical Journal*, **1**, 1247–1250.

WHO Technical Report Series No. 588 (1976) World Health Organization, Geneva.

WHO Technical Report Series No. 594 (1976) World Health Organization, Geneva.

Willmot, F. E. (1976) Meningococcal salpingitis. *British Journal of Venereal Diseases*, **52**, 182–183.

Witt, K., Veale, D. R., Smith, H. (1976) Resistance of *Neisseria gonorrhoeae* to ingestion and digestion by phagocytes of human buffy coat. *Journal of Medical Microbiology*, **9**, 1–12.

Wyle, F. A. & Kasper, D. L. (1971) Immunochemical studies on serotype antigens of *Neisseria meningitidis*. Bacteriological Proceedings, 99.

Wyle, F. A., Artenstein, M. S., Brandt, B. L., Tramont, E. C., Kasper, D. L., Alticri, P. L., Berman, S. L. & Lowenthal, J. P. (1972) Immunologic response of man to group B meningococcal polysaccharide vaccines. *Journal of Infectious Diseases*, **126**, 514–522.

6. The rapid detection of bacterial antigens

D. M. Jones

Traditionally, pathogenic organisms causing infection are cultured from pathological material on appropriate media and, when growth has taken place, identification by further tests follows. These methods are inherently as slow as the rate of growth of bacteria. Recently attention has turned to methods that will demonstrate the presence of bacterial antigens or other products directly in the pathological material. Given techniques of sufficient sensitivity and specificity, identification of the infecting microorganism may be possible without waiting for the organisms to grow on artificial media. With the need for sensitivity tests and other information about the organisms such methods cannot usually supplant culture but may be applicable as additional techniques. This review will cover some immunological methods for the detection of bacterial antigens in body fluids and also some non-immunological methods for detection of bacterial components and metabolites.

COUNTERCURRENT IMMUNOELECTROPHORESIS (CIE)

Cell-free bacterial antigens have been recognised since early in this century, but it was in the 1930s that it was shown, for example by Maegraith (1935), that some cases of meningococcal meningitis could be diagnosed quickly by a precipitin method. He observed that in cases due to meningococci from Group I-III (now group A) precipitin lines were easily obtained but that with Group II cases (group B) this was not usually so. This was a difficulty that we shall see remains with more modern techniques. The precipitin method was not widely adopted although some workers continued to report on its usefulness (Alexander, 1937). More recently the sensitivity of the precipitin reaction has been increased by the use of countercurrent immunoelectrophoresis (CIE; synonym immunoelectroosmophoresis = IEOP, or l'électrosynérèse as it was termed by the originator, Bussard, 1959). The inherent sensitivity and specificity of this technique was clear from a forensic application to the identification of blood stains, semen and saliva (Culliford, 1964). It was the discovery of Australia antigen and its association with serum hepatitis in 1965, coupled with the early shortage of suitable reagents, that resulted in the widespread use of CIE in laboratories. This has, however, lately been superseded by more sensitive methods for the detection of hepatitis B surface antigen. With the technique more widely available in laboratories other applications were developed such as the detection of bacterial antigens. Cerebrospinal fluid (CSF), serum, urine and other body fluids are suitable for testing by CIE. Antibodies may also be detectable by CIE but the method is usually much less sensitive when used in this mode.

The technique

Small wells to hold the antigen and antibody are made a few mm apart in an agar gel and an electric current is then passed through the gel. Antibody is forced to move towards the cathode by an electroosmotic flow while the antigen moves eletrophoretically to the anode. In the absence of an excess of either reactant a precipitin line is formed in a short time. Because the flows of antigen and antibody are generally in the direction of each other, rather than radial, there is an increase in both rate of reaction and in sensitivity over ordinary diffusion methods. However, the optimal conditions for reaction depend on a complex compromise of both physical and chemical conditions which can vary with different antigen/ antibody systems and there is no simple formula which meets every case. There have often been pleas for the standardisation of CIE techniques but it is very doubtful if this is possible. It may be helpful to deal with some of the variables.

Buffer has a dual role; it maintains both the ionic strength and the pH in the support system and in the electrode compartments. Barbital buffer 0.05–0.1M producing a slightly alkaline pH is popular for bacterial antigen systems. With higher ionic strengths most of the current is carried by the buffer and therefore other molecules will move more slowly. A variation is to use buffer in the electrode compartment that has a lower or higher ionic strength than that of the support gel ('discontinuous buffer'). The principle is that the zone of discontinuity travels through the gel and compacts the antigen-antibody precipitate into a finer, denser line, rendering it more visible and thus giving a gain in sensitivity. This desired effect is not always observed.

Antigen in the fluid under examination should be soluble and this may be critically affected by pH. Fluids may be concentrated before examination and this is a worthwhile procedure if the examination of the undiluted body fluid has given negative results. A polyacrylamide gel such as Lyphogel (Gelman) will give a 4- or 5-fold concentration of quite small volumes. An ultrafiltration cell will give greater increases in concentration quickly but in practice the volume of the specimen provided, if it is cerebrospinal fluid (CSF), is often too small for this method to be used.

In the support medium, under the influence of the electric field, water molecules and antibodies stream to the cathode while antigens migrate to the anode. The streaming of γ-globulin is the reverse of the expected because the electroosmotic flow overcomes the weak electrophoretic tendency, carrying the antibody to the cathode on a 'tide'. The degree of electroosmophoresis can be varied by using different agar/agarose mixtures, and this may be necessary in some systems to achieve a precipitin line nicely placed between the wells. For example polysaccharide antigens may be detected much more effectively in agarose because of this increased endosmotic flow towards the cathode. An alternative support system is cellulose acetate which may have certain advantages. It is a ready-to-use material and can be indented, when wet, into shallow wells, as described by Kohn and Kahan (1976). The resulting precipitates are readily stained with nigrosin to give permanent preparations.

The electric field is produced at either constant voltage or, more commonly, at a constant current. Passage of a too powerful current in an attempt to shorten the reacting time may result in overheating of the gel and inactivation of antibody.

The possibility of electrocution from the equipment should not be forgotten (Spencer, Ingram and Levinthal, 1966).

Sera should be specific and have high precipitin titres: some commercial sera raised for agglutination or other techniques may not be satisfactory. Reactions of identity may be obtained by CIE using a triple well array (Kohn, 1970) but care is needed to avoid prozone effects and it is necessary to have reference and test material present in approximately equivalent concentrations.

In summary, CIE can be a rapid and specific test for the presence of various soluble bacterial antigens in body fluids. The conditions of the test have to be chosen carefully and a good deal of trial and error may be necessary before maximum sensitivity is obtained for a particular antigen/antibody system. Countercurrent immunoelectrophoresis has been applied to the rapid detection of antigens in clinical bacteriology, notably in pyogenic meningitis, pneumonia, bacteraemia and arthritis.

Meningitis

Early observations of Edwards (1971) and Greenwood, Whittle and Dominic-Rajkovic (1971), on the usefulness and sensitivity of the method for detecting group C and group A meningococcal polysaccharides respectively in CSF have been amply confirmed by many others. The list of antigens has been extended to include the polyribosephosphate antigen from *Haemophilus influenzae* type b and the capsular polysaccharides from the many types of *Streptococcus pneumoniae* (Coonrod and Rytel, 1972; Fossieck, Craig and Paterson, 1973). The method has been found to be a useful adjunct to conventional diagnostic methods for pyogenic meningitis in many parts of the world (Myhre, 1974; Higashi et al, 1974). CIE has been particularly useful in northern Nigeria where large epidemics of group A meningococcal meningitis occur and produce an overwhelming load on hospital and laboratory facilities. Under these conditions rapid aetiological diagnosis and prompt appropriate treatment are essential because of the large number of cases that occur at the height of an epidemic. CSF may be dried on filter paper under field conditions and posted to the laboratory to be tested by CIE with only slight loss of sensitivity. In this way information of epidemiological value may be collected. For the evaluation of CIE in purely diagnostic terms, a comparison of Gram film, culture and CIE with the whole spectrum of pyogenic meningitis is helpful. Denis, Abibou and Chiron (1977), reporting from Dakar, found CIE more sensitive than culture in 55 cases of pneumococcal meningitis, 14 cases of *H. influenzae* meningitis and 6 meningococcal infections. Colding and Lind (1977) made the comparison in a selection of 283 specimens of CSF from cases of pyogenic meningitis. The appropriate pathogen was detected in 85 per cent by culture, 77 per cent by microscopy and in only 55 per cent by CIE. By combining microscopy and CIE, a rapid etiological diagnosis was achieved in as many cases as those eventually obtained by culture alone. In 12 per cent of cases in this series CIE was positive when culture was negative.

Edwards (1971) showed that the presence of group C meningococcal antigen in the serum of patients with meningitis was associated with a poor prognosis. It was also shown that when antigen was detectable in the serum these patients were slow to produce antibody (Hoffman and Edwards, 1972). Careful studies of group

A meningococcal meningitis in Nigeria by Whittle and co-workers (1975) revealed how antigen may persist in CSF despite treatment before admission to hospital and that high levels of antigen with slow clearance were associated with neurological damage. They also related antigenaemia to a poor prognosis and to increased frequency of complications.

In another study Greenwood and Whittle (1974) showed that the absence of detectable antigen in CSF in patients proven to have meningococcal meningitis was associated with a very favourable prognosis. Feldman (1977), who studied mainly cases of *H. influenzae* meningitis, suggested that with this infection it was the numbers of organisms in the CSF that was a more prognostic observation than the amount of antigen detectable. According to Fosseick et al (1973) persisting pneumococcal antigen in serum and urine after clearance from the CSF may also be associated with a persistent focus of infection in the lungs or elsewhere. Although clinical signs such as shock and coma are of prognostic value in meningitis, accompanying antigenaemia and the persistence of bacterial antigen in the CSF have been found to be additional indications of a poor prognosis. Antigen usually disappears from CSF within 24–48 hours after treatment has begun and any longer persistence is a bad sign. Apart from association with the more severe infections antigen persistence may occasionally be an indication of inadequate therapy. When arthritis occurs as part of the infection syndrome, bacterial antigen may be demonstrated by CIE in the synovial fluid (Feldman and DuClos, 1973).

The most successful diagnostic applications of CIE have been in areas where the group B meningococcus is not a major cause of meningitis. Commercial sera raised against *H. influenzae* type b, the pneumococcus types and the clinically important meningococcal groups A, C, W135 and Y are usually satisfactory for CIE. Suitable antiserum to the group B meningococcal polysaccharide is much more difficult to prepare and commercially available sera have been unsatisfactory. Even with adequate serum the sensitivity of CIE for the detection of group B polysaccharide may be lower than for the other organisms (Tobin and Jones, 1972). The situation has improved with the demonstration that *Escherichia coli* K1 antigen is similar to, or identical with, the group B meningococcal polysaccharide. An anti-K1 serum was reported to be effective for detecting the antigen of the group B meningococcus by Fallon and McIllmurray (1976), who also showed that reduction of the ionic strength of the buffer in the support gel was necessary for this antigen/antibody system. Robbins (1977) has also reported how a potent precipitating antiserum to the group B meningococcus may be prepared. With any system for antigen detection cross-reactions with other organisms having similar antigens remains a possibility. *Bacillus* sp. exist that cross-react with type III *Strep. pneumoniae*, *H. influenzae* b, and *Neisseria meningitidis* group A, but these are unlikely to be found in clinical material (Myerowitz, Gordon and Robbins, 1973). The normal bacterial flora may also occasionally contain cross-reactive bacteria and some pneumococcal types cross-react with *H. influenzae* type b (Bradshaw et al, 1971); these cross-reactions do not seem to cause confusion in practice. An important cross-reaction is that already noted between the antigens of *E. coli* K1 and group B meningococci because strains of *E. coli* that cause neonatal meningitis may carry the K1 antigen (Robbins et al, 1974; Cheasty,

Cross and Rowe, 1977). Thus a precipitin line with CSF from a neonate with meningitis and group B meningococcal antiserum may occasionally signify *E. coli* infection.

Pneumococcal infections

Systemic pneumococcal infection may be associated with demonstrable pneumo-coccal antigen in the serum. Dorff, Coonrod and Rytel (1971) reported antigen detected by CIE in 3 of 17 patients who had positive blood cultures. They used 'Omniserum', a polyvalent antiserum, against a large number of pneumococcal capsule types (Statens Seruminstitut, Copenhagen) and this serum has been widely used since. These findings have been extended by other workers, and in a later study Coonrod and Rytel (1973) were able to detect antigen in serum or urine from nearly half of the cases of pneumococcal pneumonia that they studied. The observation that partially degraded pneumococcal antigen was detectable in urine for some days after the start of therapy was a useful diagnostic finding. Tugwell and Greenwood (1974) examined sputum by CIE in addition to serum and urine from patients admitted with lobar pneumonia. Pneumococcal capsular antigen was found in 79 per cent of purulent sputa, 54 per cent of urine samples and 27 per cent of serum samples. They suggested that pneumococcal capsular poly-saccharide was detectable in sputum only in the presence of significant infection and also pointed out that the results were unaffected by antibiotics given just prior to admission. Although pneumococcal antigen can usually be detected by CIE in sputum when culture is also positive, it is undoubtedly useful when therapy has begun and cultural methods are likely to be unsuccessful. Occasionally in severe pneumococcal pneumonia response to penicillin therapy is slow and the tempta-tion to change therapy can be resisted if pneumococcal antigen can be shown still to be present in the sputum. The individual capsule type of infecting pneumo-coccus can also readily be identified by CIE using type-specific antisera. Capsule types 7 and 14 have been more difficult to detect because of the basic nature of these antigens and modification of the gel buffer to one containing sulphonated phenylboronic acid was used to overcome this by Anhalt and Yu (1975). El-Refaie and Dulake (1975), in a careful and comprehensive study, found that a gel at pH 6.6 instead of the more usual pH 8.6 was superior for detection of pneumococcal antigens in sputum. These workers detected antigen in 44 per cent of unselected chest infections but were able to culture pneumococci from only 15 per cent of their patients. They stressed the value of the speed with which a diagnosis could be made by CIE and how this could make a valuable contribution to the establishment of the correct antibiotic therapy in chest infection. Perlino and Shulman (1976) also considered CIE of sputum to be a rapid, sensitive and specific method for diagnosing pneumococcal infection and superior to con-ventional culture methods. In an interesting study of post-mortem material El-Refaie et al (1976) demonstrated pneumococcal capsular antigen in 55 per cent of lungs showing evidence of acute pneumonia at necropsy. Pneumococci were not cultured from any of these cases, probably due to antibiotic therapy ante-mortem and the overgrowth of contaminating bacteria. Cross-reacting bacteria were care-fully sought but only one *E. coli* strain was encountered that cross-reacted with a specific pneumococcal antiserum. This investigation has clearly shown that terminal pneumococcal chest infection is much commoner than one would suppose from conventional cultural studies.

Haemophilus influenzae infections

In addition to meningitis, CIE has been applied to the diagnosis of other infections due to *H. influenzae* type b. In three cases of epiglottitis Duncan and Hansman (1977) reported failure to detect antigenaemia, but Smith and Ingram (1975) found antigen in the serum of three of eight cases. These latter workers also demonstrated antigen in pericardial fluid and serum in three cases of pericarditis. It would seem that in those cases where there is a bacteraemia the rapidity with which CIE results are available may mean a useful contribution to the early choice of appropriate therapy in the severe childhood infections with *H. influenzae*. High antigen levels in serum and CSF have been found to indicate a poor prognosis (Shackelford, Campbell and Feigin, 1974).

The examination of sputum by CIE using specific sera against *H. influenzae* types a–f has yielded some interesting results. Although uncapsulated strains of *H. influenzae* are commonly isolated from the respiratory tract, a study by McIntyre (1978) has shown that capsulate strains may be quite common. As with pneumococcal infection, the bacterial antigens were found in sputum more frequently than *H. influenzae* was grown and the results were available much sooner.

Assorted infections

The following are examples of the application of CIE to the diagnosis of various infections and show some of the possibilities. In a hospital epidemic of cross-infection by *Klebsiella aerogenes* type K2, CIE was used by Simpson and Speller (1977) for the rapid and accurate diagnosis of both septicaemia and urinary tract infection. Riter, Menge and Hill (1975) noted that Group D streptococcal antigen was readily demonstrable in urine, 2-hour broth cultures and 12-hour blood cultures as an aid to rapid identification. In severe *Pseudomonas aeruginosa* infections, specific bacterial antigens were detected by Bartram et al (1974) using a polyvalent serum active against 13 serotypes. The diagnosis of a single case of neonatal meningitis due to Group B streptococcus was reported by Henning and Tenstam (1973) using commercial streptococcal grouping sera.

LATEX AGGLUTINATION TEST (LAT)

Latex particles can readily be sensitised with a globulin solution prepared by salt precipitation of an antiserum. The resulting reagent may then be used in a conventional slide agglutination test with CSF or serum. The reagent is reasonably stable and sensitised latex particles retain their sensitivity for at least 4–6 months if kept at 4°C. A possible source of false positive reactions is rheumatoid factor although this reacts with human rather than animal immunoglobulin.

Meningitis

The LAT was used for the diagnosis of *H. influenzae* meningitis by Newman, Stevens and Gaafar (1970) and the test was positive in 28 of 30 cases examined. Severin (1972) investigated the method for the diagnosis of meningococcal meningitis and concluded that for groups A and C meningococci it was slightly more sensitive than CIE and much simpler to perform. Group B polysaccharide could not be detected in CSF or even in culture supernates by either the LAT or CIE presumably due to the use of an inadequate antiserum. The LAT was used for examining CSF from meningococcal, pneumococcal and *H. influenzae* meningitis by Whittle et al (1974). In their hands the LAT was as sensitive as CIE for detecting meningococcal antigens (Group A only) and *H. influenzae*, but less sensitive for pneumococcal antigens. They commented that the LAT was simple, inexpensive and perhaps ideally suited to laboratories without sophisticated equipment. These workers also made the interesting observation that the group A meningococcal antigen detected by the LAT was not the same as that reacting in CIE. The antigen detected by the LAT was not entirely heat resistant and probably had a protein component in addition to polysaccharide. In a further evaluation of the LAT for the detection of pneumococcal antigens in CSF or serum, Coonrod and Rylko-Bauer (1976) found the LAT to be much inferior to CIE. Both groups of workers used Omniserum to sensitise the latex (supplemented with type 3 antiserum by Whittle et al) and it may be that variation in the sensitising ability of the polyvalent serum accounted for some difference in the results, but there was agreement that the LAT was in some degree less sensitive than CIE for detecting pneumococcal antigens. The LAT was successfully used for demonstrating meningococcal (groups A and C) and *H. influenzae* type b antigens in CSF by Leinonen and Herva (1977). They failed to get agglutination with meningococcal group B antigen using a commercial antiserum but were more successful with the high titre serum supplied by Dr J. B. Robbins. It is our experience that the LAT can be used satisfactorily for the detection of group B meningococcal antigen but we have not been able to increase the sensitivity of the test above that of CIE.

Latex agglutination has been useful for the detection of certain bacterial antigens and with these it is a sensitive, cheap and reliable technique, having the advantage over CIE of simplicity. Deficiencies in performance with group B meningococcal antigen and pneumococcal antigens may limit the general usefulness of the test, but if these were overcome it may well be the rapid method of choice in the diagnosis of meningitis.

COAGGLUTINATION

Strains of *Staphylococcus aureus* that have protein A on their outer surface bind immunoglobulin G. The protein A binds with the Fc portion of the IgG molecule and leaves the Fab part free to combine with antigen. The staphylococci are first stabilised by treatment with formaldehyde and heating to $80°C$, washed and then allowed to react with antiserum. The staphylococci may be treated with three or four different antisera without loss of specificity and suspensions usually retain reactivity for about one month if kept at $4°C$, although this may be variable. It seems that IgG slowly leaches away from the protein A and sensitivity may sometimes be restored to a suspension by rewashing. In the test antigen and suspension are mixed together on a slide and rapid coagglutination occurs. It has been found that some patients' sera react with unsensitised staphylococci and may therefore give a false positive result; this activity can often be removed by absorption. The method was described by Kronvall (1973) as a method for typing pneumococci and since then it has been used for serological identification with several bacterial genera; for example Salmonella, shigella, gonococci and the grouping of streptococci. Coagglutination has been used directly with CSF, serum and urine for detecting the presence of bacterial antigens.

Meningitis

In 1975 Olcen, Danielsson and Kjellander reported some preliminary results using polyvalent suspensions to detect meningococcal antigen in CSF. They found that protein present in some CSF samples gave rise to false positive agglutination but that this could be abolished by preliminary treatment of the CSF with protein A. They used staphylococci sensitised with pooled meningococcal antisera but their results seemed to lack some specificity. Using staphylococci sensitised with commercial *H. influenzae* type-specific sera, Suksansong and Dajani (1977) found coagglutination to be superior to CIE for detection of *H. influenzae* type b antigen in CSF, serum and urine. They found the test to be type-specific and with CSF was more sensitive than CIE, giving more positive results after the commencement of therapy when culture had become negative. When testing serum they used a control suspension of unsensitised staphylococci and if there was agglutination with this they were able to remove this activity successfully by absorption with staphylococci. Coagglutination with undiluted urine detected haemophilus antigen in 64 per cent of samples whereas only 17 per cent were positive by CIE. Although these workers experienced false positives only with serum, these also occur with CSF samples that contain large amounts of protein. It is therefore both a prudent and simple procedure to pretreat each CSF with unsensitised staphylococci for five minutes before proceeding to slide coagglutination. Coagglutination has been found to be more sensitive than CIE for detecting group A and C meningococcal antigen in CSF and of equal sensitivity for demonstration of group B antigen (Eldridge et al, 1978). Experience is still limited with the method for detecting pneumococcal and haemophilus antigens but it may again be slightly more sensitive than CIE. More experience of coagglutination with serum is also needed to assess the frequency of false positive reactions and the reliability of absorption to remove these.

LIMULUS LYSATE TEST FOR ENDOTOXIN

Levin and Bang (1964) demonstrated that blood from the primitive horse-shoe crab (*Limulus polyphemus*) clotted in the presence of small amounts of endotoxin derived from Gram-negative bacteria. It was found that the endotoxin sensitivity resides in the only type of blood cell present in this crab, the amoebocyte. These cells may be extracted from the blood, lysed with distilled water and the resulting supernatant contains the active principle. A dilution of this preparation will form a coagulum in the presence of as little as 0.1 ng endotoxin and it is essential that fluids to be tested and all reagents are handled in endotoxin-free glassware or plastic. Glassware may be freed of endotoxin contamination by heat, for example, by autoclaving for one hour followed by dry heat at 200°C for two hours. The Limulus Lysate Test (LLT) compares favourably with other methods for endotoxin detection (Rojas-Corona et al, 1969). It has therefore been used as a test for pyrogens in pharmaceutical preparations, being cheaper and simpler than the rabbit test, although its use for this purpose is not yet officially recognised. A recent modification of the test has been claimed to give even more sensitivity by substituting protein precipitation for the observation of gelation (Nandan and Brown, 1977). With the potential for large scale application in the pharmaceutical field the materials necessary for the performance of the LLT are becoming commercially available.

Endotoxaemia

The test has been applied directly to the detection of endotoxin in plasma and other body fluids. Reinhold and Fine (1971) demonstrated the specificity of the test for endotoxin and found endotoxin in plasma from patients with Gram-negative sepsis. They further demonstrated that the test could be used for the quantitative measurement of circulating endotoxin. Undiluted plasma was found to have an endotoxin-binding capacity which may reduce the sensitivity of the test, although if the plasma is diluted further than 1:32 this effect was abolished. Others have shown that this inhibitor may also be extracted with chloroform. Levin et al (1970), in a study on patients with suspected infections, obtained a good correlation between a positive limulus test and bacteraemia with Gram-negative organisms. They further obtained some positive endotoxin tests in patients with localised Gram-negative infections without a demonstrated bacteraemia, and negative limulus tests in bacteraemia due to Gram-positive cocci. Caridis et al (1972) were also able to detect circulating endotoxin with the limulus test in a series of patients with a confirmed Gram-negative bacteraemia. These workers also obtained positive results in a number of patients who did not have obvious sources of infection, particularly those with haemorrhage, circulatory collapse or hepatic injury. They accounted for these results with the postulation that endotoxin normally absorbed from the gut is not inactivated by the reticulo-endothelial system in patients with severe haemorrhage or trauma. This controversial aspect does not concern us here; suffice it to say that the limulus test has been found by many workers to be positive in association with demonstrated Gram-negative bacteraemia or sepsis (Levin et al, 1972; Fossard and Kakkar, 1974). However, the clinical usefulness of the limulus test has been questioned in the context of Gram-negative bacteraemia. It seems that as 1.5×10^3 Gram-negative bacteria per ml are required to give a positive limulus test, blood culture methods are more sensitive for the demonstration of bacteraemia. Elin and co-workers (1975) have pointed out that as endotoxin is rapidly cleared from the circulation by the liver, the presence of liver impairment may be an important factor that contributes to a positive limulus test. These workers also commented on the differing levels of sensitivity of limulus lysates obtained from various sources. Their experiences of the test led them to the conclusion that it was not clinically useful and that it did not give the early evidence of endotoxaemia that would lead to clinical action. The limulus test was found to be unhelpful in typhoid fever; Magliulo et al (1976) could not relate endotoxaemia to the occurrence of fever or other clinical symptoms and the closest correlation was with positive blood culture. These workers found that with infections with salmonellae other than

Salmonella typhi, a positive test for endotoxin without a demonstrable bacteraemia occurred in nearly half the patients they studied, especially those less than one year old. They also found that the limulus test did not contribute to the diagnosis or to the management of the patient. Goldstein, Reller and Wang (1976) used the limulus test on plasma from neonates to determine if endotoxin could be detected when the gut was first colonised and if the test had any clinical application in the detection of bacteraemia: this study was small and inconclusive. The use of the limulus test for the diagnosis of Gram-negative bacteraemia has not been particularly successful, possibly due to factors such as inhibitory effect of plasma, which may vary from patient to patient, and the occasional presence of endotoxin originating from the gut or from localised infections without bacteraemia. Antibiotics may also affect the limulus test (McCullough and Scolnick, 1976). Endotoxaemia has even been reported from a significant proportion of patients with Gram-positive infections (Stumacher, Kovnat and McCabe, 1973).

Meningitis

Applying the limulus test to CSF from 38 culture-proved cases of meningitis, Nachum, Lipsey and Siegel (1973) obtained a positive result with every one. In 13 the gram film failed to show any organism. Negative limulus tests were given by samples from 74 patients with other forms of meningitis. These results were much more clear-cut than those described above obtained by examining plasma. The Gram-negative organisms in this study were limited to *H. influenzae*, *N. meningitidis*, *Citrobacter freundi* and *Eikenella corrodens*. The result of the limulus test was available soon after lumbar puncture and it was claimed that the test would be useful for distinguishing between Gram-positive or Gram-negative infections in the absence of a positive gram film. In a study of 145 infants with suspected meningitis, Dyson and Cassady (1976) encountered six infants with Gram-negative meningitis and had positive limulus test results available on these infants within 30 minutes. The organisms obtained on culture were *E. coli* and *Serratia marcescens*. Further encouraging results with meningitis were recorded by Ross et al (1975). They obtained a positive limulus test on 37 of 38 cases of meningitis with Gram-negative etiology, the majority of which were due to *H. influenzae*. A presumptive answer on the possibility of infection due to Gram-negative bacteria was rapidly available using the limulus test, so allowing more rational choice of antibiotic therapy. The specificity of the limulus test when applied to CSF was further confirmed by Clumeck, Lauwers and Butzler (1977) who had no false positives in 18 cases of non-Gram-negative meningitis and 23 out of 24 positive test results with Gram-negative meningitis. In only 11 of the cases due to Gram-negative bacteria in this series were organisms seen in the gram film. Positive limulus tests were obtained by Tuazon et al (1977) with CSF and joint fluids from assorted Gram-negative infections which were all culture-positive. It is clear that the test has specificity but sensitivity is more difficult to assess. Reports so far seem to equate positive culture with positive limulus test; there is no evidence of the latter being positive in a significant number of instances when culture is negative, although no doubt more data will become available. It is clear that the technical snags that surround the examination of plasma do not hamper the application of the limulus test to CSF and there is some evidence (Trippodo et al, 1973) that the blood-brain barrier may be impervious to circulating endotoxin.

Urinary tract infection

The limulus test has been applied to the detection of Gram-negative bacteriuria with apparent success (Jorgensen et al, 1973). By simple quantitative comparison these workers found that if the limulus test was positive at urine dilution of 1:100 or 1:1000 this indicated a colony count greater than 100 000 Gram-negative bacteria per ml. The test would of course not detect urinary tract infection with Gram-positive bacteria and seems to be unnecessarily complicated and expensive for enumerating coliforms.

Mastitis

Another body fluid that has been tested with the limulus lysate system is milk. Hartman, Ziv and Saran (1976) were able to detect endotoxin in milk from individual quarters of the udders of cows with mastitis at dilutions ranging from $1:10^4$ to $1:10^9$. Normal milk, as long as it was diluted to $1:10^3$, gave consistently negative results. The limulus test gave good presumptive evidence of Gram-negative mastitis under field conditions.

Local lesions

The rapid presumptive diagnosis of Gram-negative infection in a corneal ulcer caused by what proved to be *Ps. aeruginosa* was achieved by testing corneal scraping with limulus lysate. Poirier and Jorgensen (1977) claimed that the result was available in less time than it took to prepare and examine a gram film thoroughly.

GAS-LIQUID CHROMATOGRAPHY

Although not strictly a method for antigen detection this technique may be used in a variety of ways to detect the presence of microorganisms and is therefore included. Gas-liquid chromatography (GLC) is a long-established analytical method within chemistry but the last 15 years has found increasing application in microbiology. Volatilised microbial cell components or metabolites can be analysed by GLC and the chromatograph used to characterise and identify microorganisms. Decomposition of whole cells by heat (pyrolysis GLC), or of hydrolysed or derivatised cell extracts or the detection of metabolites in media are variations in the application of the technique. The gas chromatograph has a high degree of sensitivity and resolution; it is an easy device to operate and, relative to much of the equipment found in a modern biochemistry department, not particularly expensive. Choice of type and sensitivity of detector system will depend on the application required. GLC has been used to characterise bacteria and fungi sometimes to generic level and sometimes to specific level, and even antigenically different strains of *E. coli* have been distinguishable by their pyrograms. The list of microorganisms to which the method has been applied is now very large indeed and is increasing. Standardisation between laboratories is difficult and this may be a serious flaw in the use of the method, but the application of GLC to microbiology holds a great deal of promise. For a general account the reader is referred to Mitruka (1975).

Clearly GLC has potential for microbial discrimination in vitro and it is a logical extension to apply the method directly to clinical specimens. The concentration of bacterial products in such specimens is likely to be much less than in cultures and therefore the most sensitive detector systems such as electron-capture will probably be appropriate.

Bacteraemia

Mitruka, Jonas and Alexander (1970) produced bacteraemia in mice by intra-peritoneal injection of various *Clostridium* sp., *Staph. aureus*, *E. coli* and *Salmonella typhimurium*. Samples of serum taken at appropriate times were extracted and screened for the presence of microbial metabolites. Peaks were produced that were absent at time of inoculation and in control uninfected mice but appeared in the course of the infection. Some of the peaks were similar to those obtained from in vitro growth of the same organism. Although many peaks were present in the chromatographs there was at least one peak characteristic for each particular type of infection among those studied. This work showed that GLC can be used to detect particular bacterial activity in vivo through the presence of either bacterial metabolites or host response. The finding that each of these bacterial species produced some specific trace is encouraging and the range of infections studied in this way could be extended with benefit. It seems that further study of the specific parts of the chromatograph may yield important information perhaps leading to reliable standard methods for the presumptive identification of infecting organisms at an early stage of the infection.

Application of GLC to mixed cultures (Mitruka et al, 1973) was a necessary further step in the evaluation of the method. These workers demonstrated that characteristic bacterial markers could still be distinguished in mixed cultures of two or three different species. They also examined serum taken from rats infected simultaneously with both *S. typhimurium* and *Ps. aeruginosa*. Several metabolites from rats with mixed infections were identical to those with monospecific infections and in addition some compounds were similar to those detected in both single and mixed in vitro cultures. Thus the presence of mixed infection seems unlikely to confuse the chromatographic method.

Arthritis

Gas-liquid chromatography has been used to analyse synovial fluid from patients with septic arthritis (Brooks et al, 1974). The synovial fluid was extracted and derivatised and an electron capture detector used. The chromatographs were sufficiently distinctive to allow the differentiation between arthritis due to staphylococcal, streptococcal or gonococcal infection. The authors concluded that the volatile metabolites detected were derived from the infecting microorganism or were metabolites of the host modified by the bacterium: if this were so it follows that the chromatographs are likely to be specific. Synovial fluid from traumatic aseptic arthritis showed none of the features associated with infection. The method described by these authors took about three hours to complete. With more knowledge of the specific compounds related to specific infections, interpretation will become simpler and the profile produced by a particular organism may become more readily identifiable at various stages of the course of the infection and ensuing treatment.

Meningitis

Electron capture GLC techniques have been applied to the diagnosis of some forms of meningitis. Schlossberg, Brooks and Shulman (1976) examined CSF taken from patients with cryptococcal meningitis and various forms of virus meningitis. Both infected groups had profiles that differed from the uninfected controls; eight cryptococcal infections all gave similar patterns; the patterns from the various virus infections differed from each other and from the cryptococcal pattern. Brooks et al (1977) identified the presence of a substance, possibly 3-(2'ketohexyl) indoline, in the CSF of patients with tuberculous meningitis. Although the origin of this substance is at present unknown it may represent a marker for tuberculous meningitis and it was not demonstrated in either cryptococcal meningitis or virus meningitis. In addition there are preliminary results that may suggest that the CSF from pyogenic meningitis gives patterns that are different from those of cryptococcal meningitis. If the profiles prove to be characteristic for the various common microbial causes of meningitis, GLC would become an important and valuable method in the diagnosis of meningitis. It seems that already application of GLC could be useful where established methods are inevitably slow e.g. in the diagnosis of tuberculous meningitis.

Anaerobic infections

Bacteroides, clostridia and fusobacteria all produce short chain fatty acids by the metabolism of carbohydrate and proteins, and these end-products are so regularly produced that the chromatographs can be used for identification of some species. GLC has been used to detect these fatty acids in pus or serous fluid. Gorbach et al (1976) compared careful cultural studies with the demonstration of fatty acids in pus from 20 cases, nearly all of which were mixed infections due to aerobic and anaerobic bacteria. The presence of fatty acids correlated extremely well with the presence of anaerobes on culture. In contrast samples of pus that did not contain fatty acids yielded mainly aerobes or anaerobic cocci; *Clostridium welchii* was isolated from one fatty acid-free sample of pus. A few samples of pus that were delayed in transit before being cultured showed fatty acids but no anaerobes were grown. In these instances it was inferred that the metabolic markers had persisted although the organisms had become irrecoverable. Phillips, Tearle and Willis (1976) reported a very similar study on 44 consecutive samples of pus. Mixed growths including anaerobes were obtained from 24 of these and in all volatile fatty acids were detected; in 16 no acids or acetic acid only were found and these had aerobic growths only; 4 samples were sterile with no acids. Again this study demonstrated GLC analysis will rapidly and reliably produce evidence for the presumptive presence of anaerobes in pus. Tissue extracts of appendices removed at operation were also studied by these workers but the chromatographs were unrelated to the clinical state of the appendix or its flora. Such an effective method for demonstrating the presumptive presence of anaerobes in pus will have stimulatory and improving effect on the efficiency of the culture methods which are still necessary for confirmation and for appropriate antibiotic sensitivity tests to be made.

CONCLUSION

Rapid methods for microbial antigen detection should be of clinical value. This may be derived from speed, but only if the result is available in time to affect the management and treatment of the patient from the outset. If this requirement is not met then a result obtained next day by conventional methods may be quite adequate. If culture is unlikely to be successful or time consuming then the balance is in favour of antigen detection. In chest infection antigen detection may be particularly valuable for the common infecting organisms. Nevertheless antigen detection should usually be regarded as an adjunct to culture because of the need for sensitivity testing and perhaps further identification of the organisms. In circumstances where culture methods are too complex or difficult, as in field conditions in developing countries, then simple antigen detection methods may be especially valuable. The prognostic value of antigen detection has been commented on by many authors although there is often little action that can be taken despite possession of the result. If it is decided that a rapid method is applicable then the choice will vary depending on the facilities available: no one method is a universal best choice. In the future, methods of increased sensitivity will continue to be tried. Haemagglutination-inhibition has been shown to be more sensitive than CIE for the detection of meningococcal polysaccharide (Greenwood and Whittle, 1974) but the necessity to prepare the reagents for the test make it quite unsuitable for acute clinical application although good for retrospective studies. Radioimmune techniques are more sensitive than many of the methods described (Käyhty, Mäkelä and Ruoslahti, 1977) but the need for expensive equipment for these methods may restrict their application. Enzyme-linked immunoadsorbent assay (ELISA) has recently been applied to the detection of hepatitis B surface antigen and it is probably equally as sensitive as radioimmunoassay but can be performed without the need for too much expensive hardware. This may be one of the directions of future development for bacterial antigen detection together with further exploitation of the potential of the gas-liquid chromatograph.

REFERENCES

Alexander, H. E. (1937) Prognostic value of the precipitin test in meningococcal meningitis. *Journal of Clinical Investigation*, **16**, 207–211.

Anhalt, J. P. & Yu, P. K. W. (1975) Counterimmunoelectrophoresis of pneumococcal antigens: improved sensitivity for the detection of types VII and XIV. *Journal of Clinical Microbiology*, **2**, 510–515.

Bartram, C. E., Crowder, J. G., Beeler, B. & White, A. (1974) Diagnosis of bacterial diseases by detection of serum antigens by counterimmunoelectrophoresis, sensitivity, and specificity of detecting Pseudomonas and pneumococcal antigens. *Journal of Laboratory and Clinical Medicine*, **83**, 591–598.

Bradshaw, M. W., Schneerson, R., Parke, J. C. & Robbins, J. B. (1971) Bacterial antigens cross-reactive with the capsular polysaccharide of *Haemophilus influenzae* Type b. *Lancet*, **1**, 1095–1097.

Brooks, J. B., Kellog, D. S., Alley, C. C., Short, H. B., Handsfield, H. H. & Huff, B. (1974) Gas chromatography as a potential means of diagnosing arthritis. I. Differentiation between staphylococcal, streptococcal, gonococcal and traumatic arthritis. *Journal of Infectious Diseases*, **129**, 660–668.

Brooks, J. B., Choudhary, G., Craven, R. B., Alley, C. C., Liddle, J. A., Edman, D. C. &

Converse, J. D. (1977) Electron capture gas chromatography detection and mass spectrum identification of 3-(2'-ketohexyl) indoline in spinal fluids of patients with tuberculous meningitis. *Journal of Clinical Microbiology*, **5**, 625–628.

Bussard, A. (1959) Description d'une technique combinant simultanément l'électrophorèse et la précipitation immunologique dans un gel: l'électrosynérèse. *Biochimica et Biophysica Acta*, **34**, 258–260.

Caridis, D. T., Reinhold, R. B., Woodruff, P. W. H. & Fine, J. (1972) Endotoxaemia in man. *Lancet*, **1**, 1381.

Cheasty, T., Gross, R. J. & Rowe, B. (1977) Incidence of K1 antigen in *Escherichia coli* isolated from blood and cerebrospinal fluid of patients in the U.K. *Journal of Clinical Pathology*, **30**, 945–947.

Clumeck, N., Lauwers, S. & Butzler, J. P. (1977) Limulus test and meningitis. *British Medical Journal*, **1**, 777.

Colding, H. & Lind, I. (1977) Counterimmunoelectrophoresis in the diagnosis of bacterial meningitis. *Journal of Clinical Microbiology*, **5**, 405–409.

Coonrod, J. D. & Rylko-Bauer (1976) Latex agglutination in the diagnosis of pneumococcal infection. *Journal of Clinical Microbiology*, **4**, 168–174.

Coonrod, J. D. & Rytel, M. W. (1972) Determination of aetiology of bacterial meningitis by counter-immunoelectrophoresis. *Lancet*, **1**, 1154–1157.

Coonrod, J. D. & Rytel, M. W. (1973) Detection of type-specific pneumococcal antigens by counterimmunoelectrophoresis. II. Etiological diagnosis of pneumococcal pneumonia. *Journal of Laboratory and Clinical Medicine*, **81**, 778–786.

Culliford, B. J. (1964) A new method for precipitin reactions of forensic blood, semen and saliva strains. *Nature*, **201**, 1092–1094.

Denis, F., Abibou, S. & Chiron, J. (1977) Bacterial meningitis diagnosis by counterimmunoelectrophoresis. *Journal of the American Medical Association*, **238**, 1248–1249.

Dorff, G. J., Coonrod, J. D. & Rytel, M. W. (1971) Detection by immunoelectrophoresis of antigen in sera of patients with pneumococcal bacteraemia. *Lancet*, **1**, 578–579.

Duncan, S. & Hansman, D. (1977) Detection of bacterial capsular polysaccharide in the body fluids of patients with haemophilus epiglottitis or meningitis. *Pathology*, **9**, 73–74.

Dyson, D. & Cassady, G. (1976) Use of Limulus lysate for detecting Gram-negative neonatal meningitis. *Pediatrics*, **58**, 105–109.

Edwards, E. A. (1971) Immunologic investigations of meningococcal disease. I. Group-specific *Neisseria meningitidis* antigens present in the serum of patients with fulminant meningococcemia. *Journal of Immunology*, **106**, 314–317.

Eldridge, J., Sutcliffe, E. M., Abbott, J. D. & Jones, D. M. (1978) Serological grouping of meningococci and detection of antigen in cerebrospinal fluid by coagglutination. *Medical Laboratory Sciences*, **35**, 63–66.

Elin, R. J., Robinson, R. A., Levine, A. S. & Wolff, S. M. (1975) Lack of clinical usefulness of the Limulus test in the diagnosis of endotoxaemia. *New England Journal of Medicine*, **293**, 521–524.

El-Refaie, M. & Dulake, C. (1975) Counter-current immunoelectrophoresis for the diagnosis of pneumococcal chest infection. *Journal of Clinical Pathology*, **28**, 801–806.

El-Refaie, M., Tait, R., Dulake, C. & Dische, F. E. (1976) Pneumococcal antigen in pneumonia. A post-mortem study with histological and bacteriological findings. *Postgraduate Medical Journal*, **52**, 497–500.

Fallon, R. J. & McIllmurray, M. B. (1976) *Escherichia coli* K1. *Lancet*, **1**, 201.

Feldman, S. A. & DuClos, T. (1973) Diagnosis of meningococcal arthritis by immunoelectrophoresis of synovial fluid. *Applied Microbiology*, **25**, 1006–1007.

Feldman, W. E. (1977) Relation of concentrations of bacteria and bacterial antigen in cerebrospinal fluid to prognosis in patients with bacterial meningitis. *New England Journal of Medicine*, **296**, 433–435.

Fossard, D. P. & Kakkar, V. V. (1974) The Limulus test in experimental and clinical endotoxaemia. *British Journal of Surgery*, **61**, 798–804.

Fossieck, B., Craig, R. & Paterson, P. Y. (1973) Counterimmunoelectrophoresis for rapid diagnosis of meningitis due to *Diplococcus pneumoniae*. *Journal of Infectious Diseases*, **127**, 106–109.

Goldstein, J. A., Reller, L. B. & Wang, W. L. (1976) Limulus amoebocyte lysate test in neonates. *American Journal of Clinical Pathology*, **66**, 1012–1015.

Gorbach, S. L., Mayhew, J. W., Bartlett, J. G., Thadepalli, H. & Onderdonk, A. B. (1976) Rapid diagnosis of anaerobic infections by direct gas-liquid chromatography of clinical specimens. *Journal of Clinical Investigation*, **57**, 478–484.

Greenwood, B. M. & Whittle, H. C. (1974) Antigen-negative meningitis due to Group A *Neisseria meningitidis*. *Journal of Infectious Diseases*, **129**, 201–204.

Greenwood, B. M., Whittle, H. C. & Dominic-Rajkovic, O. (1971) Counter-current immunoelectrophoresis in the diagnosis of meningococcal infections. *Lancet*, **2**, 519–521.

Hartman, I., Ziv, G. & Saran, A. (1976) Application of the Limulus amoebocyte lysate test to the detection of Gram-negative bacterial endotoxins in normal and mastitic milk. *Research in Veterinary Science*, **20**, 342–343.

Henning, C. & Tenstam, J. (1973) Meningitis in an infant due to Group B streptococcus demonstrated with immunoelectroosmophoresis (IEOP). *Scandinavian Journal of Infectious Diseases*, **5**, 313–315.

Higashi, G. I., Sippel, J. E., Girgis, N. I. & Hassan, A. (1974) Counterimmunoelectrophoresis: an adjunct to bacterial culture in the diagnosis of meningococcal meningitis. *Scandinavian Journal of Infectious Diseases*, **6**, 233–235.

Hoffman, T. A. & Edwards, E. A. (1972) Group-specific polysaccharide antigen and humoral antibody response in disease due to *Neisseria meningitidis*. *Journal of Infectious Diseases*, **126**, 636–644.

Jorgensen, J. H., Carvajal, H. F., Chipps, B. E. & Smith, R. F. (1973) Rapid detection of Gram-negative bacteriuria by use of the Limulus endotoxin assay. *Applied Microbiology*, **26**, 38–42.

Käyhty, H., Mäkelä, P. H. & Ruoslahti, E. (1977) Radioimmunoassay of capsular polysaccharide antigens of groups A and C meningococci and *Haemophilus influenzae* type b in cerebrospinal fluid. *Journal of Clinical Pathology*, **30**, 831–833.

Kohn, J. (1970) Method for the detection and identification of alpha$_1$ fetoprotein in serum. *Journal of Clinical Pathology*, **23**, 733–735.

Kohn, J. & Kahan, M. (1976) Countercurrent immunoelectrophoresis on cellulose acetate. *Journal of Immunological Methods*, **11**, 303–309.

Kronvall, G. (1973) A rapid slide-agglutination method for typing pneumococci by means of specific antibody adsorbed to protein A-containing staphylococci. *Journal of Medical Microbiology*, **6**, 187–190.

Leinonen, M. & Herva, E. (1977) The latex agglutination test for the diagnosis of meningococcal and *Haemophilus influenzae* meningitis. *Scandinavian Journal of Infectious Diseases*, **9**, 187–191.

Levin, J. & Bang, F. B. (1964) The role of endotoxin in the extracellular coagulation of Limulus blood. *Bulletin of the Johns Hopkins Hospital*, **115**, 265–274.

Levin, J., Poore, T. E., Zauber, N. P. & Oser, R. S. (1970) Detection of endotoxin in the blood of patients with sepsis due to Gram-negative bacteria. *New England Journal of Medicine*, **283**, 1313–1316.

Levin, J., Poore, T. E., Young, N. S., Margolis, S., Zauber, N. P., Townes, A. S. & Bell, W. R. (1972) Gram-negative sepsis: detection of endotoxaemia with the Limulus test. *Annals of Internal Medicine*, **76**, 1–7.

Louis, J. (1909) Sur la précipito réaction de Vincent dans la méningite cérébrospinale. *Comptes Rendus des Seances de la Societe de Biologie et de ses Filiales*, **1**, 814.

Maegraith, B. G. (1935) The rapid diagnosis of cerebrospinal fever. *Lancet*, **1**, 545–546.

Magliulo, E., Scevola, D., Fumarola, D., Vaccaro, R., Bertotto, A. & Burberi, S. (1976) Clinical experience in detecting endotoxaemia with the Limulus test in typhoid fever and other salmonella infections. *Infection*, **4**, 21–24.

McCullough, K. Z. & Scolnick, S. A. (1976) Effect of semisynthetic penicillins on the Limulus lysate test. *Antimicrobial Agents and Chemotherapy*, **9**, 856–858.

McIntyre, M. (1978) The detection of capsulated *Haemophilus influenzae* in chest infections by countercurrent immunoelectrophoresis. *Journal of Clinical Pathology*, **31**, 31–34.

Mitruka, B. M. (1975) *Gas Chromatographic Applications in Microbiology and Medicine.* New York: John Wiley & Sons.

Mitruka, B. M., Jonas, A. M. & Alexander, M. (1970) Rapid detection of bacteraemia in mice by gas chromatography. *Infection and Immunity*, **2**, 474–478.

Mitruka, B. M., Jonas, A. M., Alexander, M. & Kundargi, R. S. (1973) Rapid differentiation of certain bacteria in mixed populations by gas-liquid chromatography. *Yale Journal of Biology and Medicine*, **46**, 104–112.

Myerowitz, R. L., Gordon, R. E. & Robbins, J. B. (1973) Polysaccharides of the genus *Bacillus* cross-reactive with the capsular polysaccharides of *Diplococcus pneumoniae* Type III, *Haemophilus influenzae* Type b, and *Neisseria meningitidis* Group A. *Infection and Immunity*, **8**, 896–900.

Myhre, E. B. (1974) Rapid diagnosis of bacterial meningitis. *Scandinavian Journal of Infectious Diseases*, **6**, 237–239.

Nachum, R., Lipsey, A. & Siegel, S. E. (1973) Rapid detection of Gram-negative bacterial meningitis by the Limulus lysate test. *New England Journal of Medicine*, **289**, 931–934.

Nandan, R. & Brown, D. R. (1977) An improved in vitro pyrogen test: to detect picograms of endotoxin contamination in intravenous fluids using Limulus amoebocyte lysate. *Journal of Laboratory and Clinical Medicine*, **89**, 910–918.

Newman, R. B., Stevens, R. W. & Gaafar, H. A. (1970) Latex agglutination test for the diagnosis of *Haemophilus influenzae* meningitis. *Journal of Laboratory and Clinical Medicine*, **76**, 107–113.

Olcen, P., Danielsson, D. & Kjellander, J. (1975) The use of protein A-containing staphylococci sensitised with antimeningococcal antibodies for grouping *Neisseria meningitidis* and demonstration of meningococcal antigen in cerebrospinal fluid. *Acta Pathologica et Microbiologica Scandinavica, Section B*, **83**, 387–396.

Perlino, C. A. & Shulman, J. A. (1976) Detection of pneumococcal polysaccharide in the sputum of patients with pneumococcal pneumonia by counterimmunoelectrophoresis. *Journal of Laboratory and Clinical Medicine*, **87**, 496–502.

Phillips, K. D., Tearle, P. V. & Willis, A. T. (1976) Rapid diagnosis of anaerobic infections by gas-liquid chromatography of clinical material. *Journal of Clinical Pathology*, **29**, 428–432.

Poirier, R. H. & Jorgensen, J. H. (1977) Endotoxin assay for rapid diagnosis of pseudomonas corneal ulcer. *Lancet*, **2**, 85–86.

Reinhold, R. B. & Fine, J. (1971) A technique for quantitative measurement of endotoxin in human plasma. *Proceedings of the Society for Experimental Biology and Medicine*, **137**, 334–340.

Riter, M. A., Menge, S. K. & Hill, H. R. (1975) Identification of group D streptococci by counter-immunoelectrophoresis. *Abstracts of the Annual Meeting of the American Society of Microbiology*, p.36.

Robbins, J. B. (1977) Test antiserum for group B meningococci. *British Medical Journal*, **1**, 1220.

Robbins, J. B., McCracken, G. H., Gotschlich, E. C., Orskov, F., Orskov, I. & Hanson, L. A. (1974) *Escherichia coli* K1 polysaccharide associated with neonatal meningitis. *New England Journal of Medicine*, **290**, 1216–1220.

Rojas-Corona, R. R., Skarnes, R., Tamakuma, S. & Fine, J. (1969) The *Limulus* coagulation test for endotoxin. A comparison with other assay methods. *Proceedings of the Society for Experimental Biology and Medicine*, **132**, 599–601.

Ross, S., Rodriguez, W., Controni, G., Korengold, G., Watson, S. & Khan, W. (1975) Limulus lysate test for Gram-negative bacterial meningitis. *Journal of the American Medical Association*, **233**, 1366–1369.

Schlossberg, D., Brooks, J. B. & Shulman, J. A. (1976) Possibility of diagnosing meningitis by gas chromatography: cryptococcal meningitis. *Journal of Clinical Microbiology*, **3**, 239–245.

Severin, W. P. J. (1972) Latex agglutination in the diagnosis of meningococcal meningitis. *Journal of Clinical Pathology*, **25**, 1079–1082.

Shackelford, P. G., Campbell, J. & Feigin, R. D. (1974) Countercurrent immunoelectrophoresis in the evaluation of childhood infections. *Journal of Pediatrics*, **85**, 478–481.

Simpson, R. A. & Speller, D. E. C. (1977) Detection of bacteraemia by countercurrent immunoelectrophoresis. *Lancet*, **1**, 206.

Smith, E. W. P. & Ingram, D. L. (1975) Counterimmunoelectrophoresis in *Hemophilus influenzae* Type b epiglottitis and pericarditis. *Journal of Pediatrics*, **86**, 571–573.

Spencer, E. W., Ingram, V. M. & Levinthal, C. (1966) Electrophoresis: an accident and some precautions. *Science*, **152**, 1722–1723.

Stumacher, R. J., Kovnat, M. J. & McCabe, W. R. (1973) Limitations of the usefulness of the *Limulus* assay for endotoxin. *New England Journal of Medicine*, **288**, 1261–1264.

Suksansong, M. & Dajani, A. S. (1977) Detection of *Haemophilus influenzae* type b antigens in body fluids, using specific antibody-coated staphylococci. *Journal of Clinical Microbiology*, **5**, 81–85.

Tobin, B. M. & Jones, D. M. (1972) Immunoelectroosmophoresis in the diagnosis of meningococcal infections. *Journal of Clinical Pathology*, **25**, 583–585.

Trippodo, N. C., Jorgensen, J. H., Priano, L. L. & Traber, D. L. (1973) Cerebrospinal fluid levels of endotoxin during endotoxemia. *Proceedings of the Society for Experimental Biology and Medicine*, **143**, 932–937.

Tuazon, C. U., Perez, A. A., Elin, R. J. & Sheagren, N. (1977) Detection of endotoxin in cerebrospinal and joint fluids by limulus assay. *Archives of Internal Medicine*, **137**, 55–56.

Tugwell, P. & Greenwood, B. M. (1974) Bacteriological findings in pneumonia. *Lancet*, **1**, 95.

Whittle, H. C., Egler, L. J., Tugwell, P. & Greenwood, B. M. (1974) Rapid bacteriological diagnosis of pyogenic meningitis by latex agglutination. *Lancet*, **2**, 619–621.

Whittle, H. C., Greenwood, B. M., Davidson, N. M., Tomkins, A., Tugwell, P., Warrell, D. A., Zalin, A., Bryceson, A. D. M., Parry, E. H. O., Brueton, M., Duggan, M., Oomen, J. M. V. & Rajkovic, A. D. (1975) Meningococcal antigen in diagnosis and treatment of Group A meningococcal infections. *American Journal of Medicine*, **58**, 823–828.

7. The pathogenesis of diarrhoea of bacterial origin

H. P. Lambert

Acute diarrhoeal diseases account for much illness at all ages and in all countries. In parts of the world where malnutrition is common and good standards of hygiene hard to achieve, this group of illnesses remains a dominant cause of death in early childhood. The 1970s have witnessed a great increase in knowledge relevant to these illnesses, about normal and disordered physiology, about the microbial populations of the gastro-intestinal tract and their interactions, and about the causes and pathogenesis of gastro-intestinal infections. Many important mechanisms have been delineated, notably the identification of organisms which act by adhering to the small bowel mucosa and there elaborating toxins causing intraluminal fluid accumulation, and others which act mainly by mucosal invasion, of the large and sometimes the small intestine. The distinction between 'toxin' and 'invasive' diarrhoeas makes a useful starting point, but, since so many aspects of the pathogenesis of bacterial diarrhoeas are still obscure, over-rigid classification, more precise than our present understanding can justify, has been eschewed in the following account.

In order to become pathogenic, an infecting organism must first overcome the formidable defences and normal homeostatis of the gastro-intestinal tract. Normal gastric acid is an effective barrier, and the infecting dose of many organisms including cholera and Salmonellas can be much reduced by temporary neutralisation of gastric acidity, while achlorhydria from disease or previous gastrectomy is associated with Salmonella infections of unusual severity. The mechanisms of antimicrobial immunity associated with mucosal surfaces have attracted much recent interest; in addition to the specific cellular and humoral components, the importance of non-specific defence mechanisms is now increasingly recognised. Interaction between the normal gut flora and the host mucosa is seen as as a crucial process which limits and regulates colonisation by exogenous organisms. Short-term, semi-physiological factors may also be important, inhibition of bowel motility, for example, greatly reduces resistance of the bowel to infection.

ENTEROTOXINS IN *ESCHERICHIA COLI* DIARRHOEA

Two lines of research have provided the impetus for recent advances in the study of enterotoxin diarrhoea. First, work on cholera during the last two decades and second, the study of animal diarrhoeas caused by enterotoxigenic strains of *E. coli*. In cholera there is extensive colonisation of the bowel but no systemic invasion by the causal vibrio, and no acute inflammation of the mucosa. All the features of the illness are attributable to losses of water and electrolytes from the small bowel. These changes can be produced by the toxin elaborated by *V. cholerae* which is thought to act by stimulating adenyl cyclase activity in the small bowel mucosa with a resulting increase in isotonic fluid secretion induced by the increased cellular concentration of adenosine 3′, 5′-cyclic monophosphate, or cyclic AMP. The pathogenesis of cholera will not be discussed in detail here and full information can be found in the excellent monograph by Barua and Burrows (1974). A number of model systems have been developed for the study of cholera toxin beginning with the demonstration by De and Chatterjee (1953) that ligated loops of intestine in the anaesthetised rabbit could be used for this purpose. These techniques were also applied to *E. coli* diarrhoeas of calves and pigs and revealed that two forms of toxin could be produced by *E. coli*. The heat labile form (LT) has some similarities to cholera toxin, is antigenic and, like cholera toxin, stimulates the adenyl cyclase system and so induces isotonic fluid secretion. Heat stable enterotoxin (ST) also induces fluid secretion in some of the test systems, but its mode of action is not yet known. It is now evident that enterotoxigenic *E. coli* strains of human origin may also produce either LT and ST together or, less

Table 7.1   Test systems for enterotoxin production in *E. coli*

Rabbit ileal loop
Infant rabbit
Infant mouse
Rabbit skin permeability
Adrenal cells Y1
Chinese hamster ovary (CHO)
Human embryonic intestine

commonly, LT or ST alone. Tests for enterotoxin production are listed in Table 7.1. The tissue culture methods using Chinese hamster ovary (CHO) or Y1 adrenal cells test LT as does the permeability factor test in rabbit skin. The infant mouse test detects mainly ST while the rabbit ileal loop and infant rabbit test probably detect both forms depending on timing and other technical factors (Evans, Evans and Pierce, 1973).

Enterotoxin production in *E. coli* strains of animal origin is governed by a transmissible plasmid, and this mechanism has also been shown to operate in strains of human origin (Smith and Lingood, 1971). Gyles, So and Falkow (1974) found at least one transmissible plasmid in 90 per cent of 96 toxigenic strains but in only 36 per cent of 204 non-toxigenic strains, and they have defined and characterised the plasmids coding for heat-labile and heat-stable enterotoxin production. By contrast, toxin production in *V. cholerae* is chromosomally determined.

Enterotoxigenic *E. coli* diarrhoea in man

The extension to other bacteria of the techniques of enterotoxin assay first used in cholera, and the impetus from the study of toxigenic *E. coli* diarrhoea in animals, has led to intensive study of toxin production by *E. coli* in man. Gorbach et al (1971) examined the microflora of the small and large bowel of 17 patients in Calcutta with acute undifferentiated diarrhoea. All had extensive small bowel colonisation, but in eight of them the most prevalent species was *E. coli* distributed through small and large gut. These strains of *E. coli*, only one of which was a classical enteropathogenic serotype, gave positive results in the rabbit ileal loop test for enterotoxin production. Volunteer studies (Dupont et al, 1971) confirmed the clinical relevance of toxin production. Subjects who swallowed large inocula of several toxigenic *E. coli* strains developed profuse watery diarrhoea without fever and, in three who were intubated, the causal strain of *E. coli* was found in the jejunum in concentrations of 10^5–10^7. From these important studies have stemmed many attempts to estimate the importance of enterotoxin production in *E. coli* in diarrhoeal disease in man, using a variety of tests for heat labile and heat stable forms of *E. coli* enterotoxin.

Travellers' diarrhoea
Strong evidence is now available, especially from prospective studies, suggesting that an appreciable proportion of patients with this universal and troublesome

Table 7.2   Enterotoxic *E. coli* in travellers' diarrhoea

Source	Population	Place	Test system	No. positive/No. tested Diarrhoea	Controls
Shore et al, 1974	Adults	Various	Infant mouse	4/11	0/17
Gorbach et al, 1975	Adults	Mexico	Rabbit skin permeability	26/38	6/41
Merson et al, 1976	Adults	Mexico	CHO, Y1 adrenal Infant mouse Rabbit ileal loop	23/59	6/62
Sack et al, 1977	Adults	Kenya	Y1 adrenal Infant mouse	17/27	1/12

complaint have been infected with enterotoxin-producing strains of *E. coli*. Gorbach and his colleagues (Gorbach et al, 1975), using the rabbit skin permeability assay, found enterotoxic *E. coli* in 26 of 36 (72 per cent) of U.S. students who developed diarrhoea in Mexico but only in 6 of 41 (15 per cent) who remained well. The toxigenic strains usually cleared from the stool within five days. Merson et al (1976) used the adrenal Y1 cell, Chinese hamster ovary and the infant mouse assays, confirming positive tests with the rabbit ileal loop. Fifty-nine of 121 physicians or their families travelling to Mexico developed diarrhoea, of whom 23 acquired enterotoxigenic strains of *E. coli*, some producing LT and ST, some LT only and a few ST only. Toxin producing strains were also isolated from 3 of 13 patients with loose stools not amounting to diarrhoea and from 3 of 49 who remained well. Another prospective study, in American Peace Corps volunteers travelling to Kenya, confirmed that most enterotoxigenic strains found in travellers' diarrhoea are LT or LT/ST producing, while a few produce stable toxin only (Sack et al, 1977). Studies on travellers' diarrhoea are summarised in Table 7.2.

Non-cholera diarrhoea in the tropics
Following the early report from Calcutta (Gorbach et al, 1971) the importance of enterotoxigenic *E. coli* in the tropics has been confirmed in other studies. Nalin

et al (1975) made an extensive study of females over one year old and males aged 1 to 14 years in a village community in Bangladesh. CHO positive *E. coli* strains were found in 19.2 per cent of all cases, but in 33 per cent of the more severely ill in-patients. Since this test detects LT and most human strains elaborate both LT and ST, these authors also tested for ST only strains in a random selection from the isolates negative by the CHO test, finding 7 of 23 tested produced ST only. Ryder et al (1976a), also working in Bangladesh and using the Y1-adrenal cell and infant mouse tests together with antitoxin estimation, found evidence of infection with enterotoxigenic *E. coli* in 11 of 48 patients. Positive results varied with age, however, toxigenic strains being found in 10 of 18 patients over 10 years old, in 1 of 5 children between 2 and 10, but in none of the 25 infants less that two years old.

Diarrhoea of infancy and childhood

In contrast to the situation in travellers' diarrhoea, in which prospective studies and control groups are fairly easily organised, the role of enterotoxigenic strains in childhood diarrhoea has proved hard to evaluate. Results with human strains in the animal laboratory models are less clear cut than with strains of animal origin, and it has only recently become evident that strains producing ST only, as well as those producing LT or LT/ST, may be associated with infant diarrhoea. Gorbach and Khurana (1972), using the infant rabbit assay method and testing 600 strains of *E. coli* from children with diarrhoea in Chicago, found enterotoxin production in strains from 24 of 29 children in the acute stage of their illness. Two or three different serotypes producing enterotoxin were often found in a stool from one patient. Results elsewhere in infant diarrhoea have varied enormously, and the variety of tests used by different investigators makes it difficult to obtain an over-all view. Sack et al (1975) found enterotoxigenic strains in 10 of 64 diarrhoea episodes (16 per cent) in Apache children but it is notable that an enterotoxigenic strain was found in only 1 of 21 small bowel intubations. Guerrant et al (1975), found positive results with the CHO test in 20 of 40 Brazilian infants and children, and in none of 20 controls without diarrhoea. By contrast, Echeverria, Blacklow and Smith (1975) found no LT producing strains in 61 Boston children aged five years or less with diarrhoea, and Gross, Scotland and Rowe (1976) found no evidence of toxin production by Y1-mouse adrenal, CHO, and infant mouse tests in strains from any of six fully studied outbreaks of infantile enteritis caused by classical enteropathogenic serotypes. Studies using the infant mouse test only, which detects ST strains, have also given variable results. Whereas Rudoy and Nelson (1975) obtained positive results in 31 of 36 children with diarrhoea and none of 17 controls, Dean et al (1972) had obtained completely negative results in 37 diarrhoeal children. Although differences in testing techniques may account for some of this variability, it is evident, now that several test systems are often used in parallel, that ST strains may be associated with infant diarrhoea as well as with travellers' diarrhoea in adults. Such an outbreak has been recorded from a special care nursery of a children's hospital in Texas (Ryder et al, 1976b) in which an *E. coli* serotype 078:K80:H12, a strain producing ST and of known association with diarrhoea in Bangladesh and India, was found in 18 of 25 infants with diarrhoea and in 14 of 55 infants without bowel disturbance. Gross et al (1976)

Table 7.3   Enterotoxic *E. coli* in diarrhoea of infancy and childhood

Source	Place	Test system	No. positive/No. tested Diarrhoea	Control
Gorbach & Khurana, 1972	Chicago	Infant rabbit	24/29	
Dean et al, 1972	Honolulu	Infant mouse	0/37	
Sack et al, 1975a	Arizona	Rabbit ileal loop		
		Infant rabbit	10/64	
		Adrenal Y1		
Rudoy & Nelson, 1975	Texas	Infant mouse	31/36	0/17
Guerrant et al, 1975	Brazil	CHO	20/40	
Echeverria et al, 1975	Boston,	Adrenal Y1		
	U.S.A.	Rabbit ileal loop	0/61	
		Serology		
Nalin et al, 1975	Bangladesh	CHO	95/498	
		Dog loop		
Ryder et al, 1976a	Bangladesh	Adrenal Y1	11/18 (> 10 yrs old)	
		Infant mouse	0/12 (< 2 yrs old)	
Ryder et al, 1976b	Texas	Adrenal Y1	18/25	14/55
		Infant mouse		
Gross, Scotland & Rowe, 1976	U.K.	Adrenal Y1		
		CHO	0/6 outbreaks	
		Infant mouse		

have also described outbreaks of infant diarrhoea caused by another ST producing strain 0159:H20. Table 7.3 shows some important studies in summary form.

'Enterotoxigenic' and 'enteropathogenic' serotypes

The most serious dilemma presented by recent work on *E. coli* gastroenteritis is the discrepancy between the two types of evidence obtained from serotyping and from toxin testing. The association of certain specific 'O' serotypes, about 17 in number, with diarrhoea in infancy was based largely on epidemiological evidence, although supported in part by volunteer studies and by occasional episodes of waterborne or food-borne infection in adults. Most enterotoxigenic strains do not belong to classical serotypes, and since both LT and ST are plasmid-determined, it is to be expected that these characteristics are not type-specific, although it does now appear that some otherwise rare serotypes are found frequently to be producers of enterotoxin, even when isolated from very different parts of the world (Ørskov et al, 1976). For most classical enteropathogenic serotypes, evidence of pathogenicity is based on epidemiological grounds and toxin production has not in general been detected in these strains (Gross, Scotland and Rowe, 1976). Gangarosa and Merson (1977), in a thoughtful review of the historical evidence, have shown that the epidemiological association between 'classical' serotypes and infant diarrhoea is now much less strong than in the 1950s when many major outbreaks were recorded, associated particularly with serotypes 0111, 055 and 0127. Experiments at that time suggested that at least some of these strains did produce toxin. Has a change in their pathogenic properties in the community been paralleled by a general loss of toxigenicity in strains stored in the laboratory for many years, or do the classical strains cause diarrhoea by mechanisms not depending on the production of enterotoxin? Neither postulate can easily be invoked to resolve the dilemma. While loss of toxigenic capacity on prolonged storage does occur, many strains can be shown to produce toxin over long periods in laboratory conditions. It may be that infant diarrhoea caused by classical sero-types depends on pathogenic mechanisms in which toxin production plays no part, but this postulate fails to explain the striking resemblances between cholera and severe infantile diarrhoea caused by enteropathogenic *E. coli*. Scott Thomson pointed to this analogy in 1955 when he showed that, in babies with acute gastroenteritis caused by the now classical types 0111, 055 and 026, the causal organism could be found throughout the bowel in numbers usually found only in faeces. So far the pathogenesis of diarrhoea caused by the classical strains re-mains enigmatic.

On the other hand, demonstration of toxin production in the laboratory does not necessarily indicate that this characteristic is expressed in vivo or is significant in pathogenesis; epidemiological and other evidence needs also to be provided and this has been done with particular success in travellers' diarrhoea. Finally, entero-toxin production is not confined to *E. coli* among the Enterobacteriaceae, since a number of other species, especially Klebsiellas, have been shown capable of forming toxin.

COLONISATION AND MUCOSAL ADHERENCE

One of the most important—and obscure—aspects of the pathogenesis of bacterial diarrhoeas is the multiplication of the initial inoculum and its colonisa-tion at a site relevant to its pathogenic potential. The associations of particular bacteria with particular mucosal surfaces has attracted much study in recent years. Mucosal adherence has been established as a necessary precondition for patho-genicity of certain organisms, and bacterial receptor sites on the host mucosa, and specific interactions between host and parasite can be identified. The best established example in gastroenteritis relates to the K88 antigen in entero-pathogenic *E. coli* diarrhoeas of newborn piglets, which enables strains possessing it to adhere to pig intestinal mucosa, and to proliferate in the bowel (Jones and Rutter, 1972). McNeish et al (1975) developed a method measuring the extent of attachment of cultures of *E. coli* to fragments of human foetal intestine. Although a wide experimental variation was noted, two known pathogenic strains (026:K60:H11 and 078:H12) showed a much greater tendency to adhere to the mucosa than did non-pathogenic serotypes. These workers (Williams et al, 1977) have now found that, like the animal mucosal adherence factors, capacity to adhere in one of the human strains is controlled by a transmissible plasmid. Many mucosa-bacterial interactions are highly specific both for bacterial and host species, and for types of mucosa, but others are less specific and positive chemotaxis towards rabbit gut mucosa has been identified in strains of *V. cholerae*, *E. coli* and *S. typhimurium* (Allweiss et al, 1977). Such a mechanism might be important in the earliest stages of infection. A related aspect of colonisation has been studied by Evans et al (1975) who measured the ability of an enterotoxigenic *E. coli* strain of human origin to colonise the infant rabbit gut, and in doing so, to produce a diarrhoeal response. The strain possessed a pilus-like surface structure which was absent from a laboratory derived variant and, although both strains were able to produce enterotoxin as judged by the rabbit ileal loop, the derived strain was unable to multiply in the infant rabbit gut. Moreover, adsorbed serum specific for the surface-associated antigen protected against colonisation by the wild strain. The responsible antigen is plasmid-controlled. By analogy with the K88 antigen, a surface structure of this type could well play a role in mucosal adherence, but other mechanisms might be responsible for the capacity of the strain possessing this antigen to multiply in the bowel in defiance of the regulatory forces tending to maintain a constant bowel flora. The same pilus-associated colonisation factor (Cf) has recently been identified (Evans, Evans and Dupont, 1977) in an ST only strain of *E. coli* (078:H12) isolated from a number of episodes of diarrhoea in a children's hospital in Texas.

DYSENTERIC SYNDROMES

Bacillary dysentery forms a notable contrast with cholera and the enterotoxic *E. coli* diarrhoeas. Shigella infections have their main impact on the colon. The changes of acute inflammation are seen on sigmoidoscopy and biopsy and in the stool which contains blood and mucus. The systemic effects of the infection are fever and neutrophilia, sometimes accompanied by meningism and convulsions in children. Less severe illnesses are hard to distinguish from diarrhoeas of small intestinal origin, but microscopic examination of mucus or stool provides a simple screening test. Faecal leucocytes are seen in dysenteric illnesses and in salmonella infections (which often affect both small and large bowel, q.v.) but not in cholera, enterotoxigenic *E. coli* infections or in viral diarrhoeas (Harris, Dupont and Hornick, 1972). The mucosal invasion characteristically caused by the Shigellae and by other organisms with a similar mode of action can be matched to some extent by laboratory models; such organisms evoke conjunctivitis in guinea-pigs (Serény test), and cytopathic effect on HeLa cells in tissue culture.

The pathogenic mechanisms in shigellosis are still not fully understood. The paralytic effects of the exotoxin of *Sh. dysenteriae* I (Shiga bacillus) in experimental animals led to its description as a neurotoxin, its action apparently irrelevant in human disease. Recently, however, this organism has been shown to induce intestinal fluid secretion apparently by the activation of mucosal adenyl cyclase (Charney et al, 1976). Keusch and Jacewicz (1975) have found that Shiga enterotoxin and neurotoxin are at least closely related if not identical. Shiga extracts also cause an inflammatory response with epithelial damage in intestinal loops, and are cytotoxic to HeLa cells. The cytotoxic effect is produced by a separate fraction, of smaller molecular weight than that associated with neurotoxin and enterotoxin. The relevance of these toxins to the pathogenesis of shigellosis is still in dispute. Attempts made to analyse the effects of bacterial components by the use of deficient mutants indicated that invasiveness and not toxigenicity is the main virulence determinant but an apparently non-toxigenic mutant was able to produce cytotoxin under special conditions and did in fact evoke anti-cytotoxin antibody in infected volunteers (Keusch et al, 1976). It is therefore possible that toxins produced in small amounts might still play an important role at cellular level.

'Dysenteric' *Escherichia coli*

Just as some serotypes of *E. coli* cause diarrhoea by a cholera-like mechanism, a limited number of strains act in a dysentery-like manner. The strains generally share cross-reacting O antigens with Shigella serotypes and were first identified as causing diarrhoea in children and adults in Japan (Ogawa, Nakamura and Sakazaki, 1968). One of them, *E. coli* 0124:B17, caused a large number of episodes of diarrhoea in the U.S.A., traced to imported French cheese. The isolates were shown to cause acute inflammatory changes in the rabbit gut mucosa and they gave positive results in the Serény test (Tulloch et al, 1973). The volunteer studies of Dupont et al (1971) also show clearly that strains of *E. coli* of this type can induce a dysenteric syndrome, with acute colonic inflammation, fever, and systemic illness, but without colonisation of the small bowel. This form of *E. coli* diarrhoea is much less common than the enterotoxic variety and 'dysenteric' *E. coli* strains have rarely been isolated from outbreaks of infant diarrhoea.

SALMONELLA INFECTIONS

The histological changes induced in the bowel by infection with Salmonella species differ in many respects both from the choleraic and dysenteric forms of bowel infection. Typhoid fever, in the main a septicaemic rather than a diarrhoeal illness, shows a mononuclear inflammatory response in the affected tissues. Salmonella gastroenteritis, by contrast, is characterised by acute inflammatory changes and polymorphonuclear infiltration affecting especially the lamina propria. Although in traditional accounts of salmonellosis mucosal changes and colonic involvement are not emphasised, Mandal and Mani (1976) demonstrated colonic inflammation in 21 of 23 hospital patients with Salmonella diarrhoea. Studies in monkeys have shown both colitis and an impaired mucosal transport mechanism in the small bowel, with evidence of activation of adenyl cyclase. Koupal and Deibel (1975) have characterised an enterotoxin produced by a strain of *S. enteritidis*, showing properties in common with both ST and LT of *E. coli*. It seems, therefore, that the pathogenic processes in Salmonella infections have features in common with the enterotoxic and the dysenteric forms of bacterial diarrhoea. The relative importance of small and large bowel involvement may differ with the infecting strain and with other factors yet to be defined.

OTHER ENTEROTOXIC FORMS OF BACTERIAL DIARRHOEA

Clostridial food poisoning

This familiar variety of food poisoning is associated with ingestion of living organisms of certain strains of *Clostridium perfringens* type A. Most outbreaks in Britain are caused by strains with heat-resistant spores, but food poisoning strains are otherwise not easily distinguished by routine methods. An antigenic heat-labile toxin formed during sporulation, and different from the other toxins produced by *Cl. perfringens*, has been extracted which causes accumulation of fluid in ileal loops, apparently by a cytotoxic effect demonstrable in tissue culture (McDonel, 1974). The toxin also causes an erythematous reaction after intradermal injection in guinea-pigs and rabbits.

Staphylococcal food poisoning

The acute illness is caused by ingestion of pre-formed heat-stable staphylococcal enterotoxin, now known to exist in five distinct antigenic types which do not cross-react. Its exact mode of action has been a matter of dispute for many years, work being hampered by the absence of good experimental models. Experiments using primates gave some support to the belief that its primary site of action might not be in the bowel, but in the central nervous system, and that the vomiting, so prominent in this illness, might be of central origin. Recent studies have, however, shown clearly that staphylococcal enterotoxin causes decreased absorption in the small intestine mainly by direct action on the mucosa but also to a lesser extent acting on bowel remote from the site of application (Elias and Shields, 1976).

A different process is seen in staphylococcal enterocolitis, in which intense local damage is associated with proliferation of a toxigenic strain in the affected area of bowel.

LESS COMMON BACTERIAL DIARRHOEAS

Vibrio parahaemolyticus

Some strains of this halophilic marine vibrio are a common cause of food poisoning in Japan, but have been identified also in the U.S.A., Britain and other countries. The clinical syndrome varies a good deal; some outbreaks are characterised by profuse watery stools, while in others the illnesses are dysenteric in type; septicaemia is not found. Evidence from rabbit intestinal loop experiments has given conflicting results. The loops show an inflammatory reaction with bacterial invasion of the epithelium, but supernatant culture fluids and purified haemolysins (the pathogenic strains are characterised by production of a haemolysin) usually fail to elicit fluid accumulation (Barker and Gangarosa, 1974).

Bacillus cereus

Outbreaks of food poisoning associated with ingestion of this organism take one of two forms. In some the incubation period is long and in the other, that associated with boiled or fried rice and a large infecting dose, there is a short incubation period of one to six hours. Little is yet known of pathogenesis, but several strains have been shown to cause fluid accumulation in rabbit ileal loops. Increased rabbit-skin permeability, and a necrotic reaction after intradermal injection in guinea-pig skin have also been described (Portnoy et al, 1976).

Yersinia enterocolitica

Human infections with this organism, recognised especially in Scandinavia, are characterised by septicaemia as well as diarrhoea, fever and an acute terminal ileitis with mesenteric lymphadenitis. Arthritis and erythema nodosum often follow the acute illness. An experimental model has been developed in mice which can be infected by oral or parenteral challenge. The initial infection is located in the Peyer's patches of the distal ileum, followed by caseous necrosis of the mesenteric glands and involvement of distant sites. The mode of spread apparently involves direct bacterial invasion, and toxin has not been found in cultures of *Y. enterocolitica*.

Campylobacter enteritis

Although known for many years as an occasional cause of diarrhoeal illness or septicaemia in man, and a familiar cause of infectious abortion in cattle and ewes, only recently have technical advances permitted a closer study of the role of this organism in human disease. Affected patients experience fever, malaise and other general symptoms as well as profuse diarrhoea and abdominal colic, and the diarrhoea is often macroscopically or microscopically bloody. The organism has been found in the stomach, jejunum and ileum. Haemorrhagic necrosis has been described in the small bowel in fatal cases, and inflammatory oedema of the ileum observed at laparotomy (Skirrow, 1977).

CONCLUSION

A number of separate and important factors in the pathogenesis of bacterial diarrhoeas have been identified and explored in recent years. Most clearly defined are those which enable the initial inoculum to colonise the bowel and to adhere to the intestinal mucosa; enterotoxin production acting to increase intra-luminal fluid in the small bowel; and direct inflammation of the mucosa of the large, and sometimes the small bowel. Between the polar forms of pathogenesis represented by cholera at one extreme and classical bacillary dysentery at the other lie a number of syndromes, and it is likely that more than one pathogenic mechanism operates in many of them. Other important factors certainly remain to be discovered; in particular, future advances will much depend on increased knowledge of the complex and normally remarkably stable microbial-host interactions in the intestine, and how these may be disturbed by pathogenic bacteria.

REFERENCES

Allweiss, B., Dostal, J., Carey, K. E., Edwards, T. F. & Freter, R. (1977) The role of chemotaxis in the ecology of bacterial pathogens of mucosal surfaces. *Nature*, **266**, 488–450.

Barker, W. H. & Gangarosa, E. J. (1974) Food poisoning due to *Vibrio parahaemolyticus*. *Annual Review of Medicine*, **25**, 75–81.

Barua, D. & Burrows, W. Ed. (1974) *Cholera*. Philadelphia: W. B. Saunders.

Charney, A. N., Gots, R. E., Formal, S. B. & Gianella, R. A. (1976) Activation of intestinal mucosal adenylate cyclase by *Shigella dysenteriae* I enterotoxin. *Gastroenterology*, **70**, 1085–1090.

De, S. N. & Chatterjee, D. N. (1953) An experimental study of the mechanism of action of *Vibrio cholerae* on the intestinal mucous membrane. *Journal of Pathology and Bacteriology*, **66**, 559–562.

Dean, A. G., Ching, Y.-C., Williams, R. G. & Harden, L. B. (1972) Test of *Escherichia Coli* enterotoxin using infant mice; application in a study of diarrhoea in children in Honolulu. *The Journal of Infectious Diseases*, **125**, 407–411.

Dupont, H., Formal, S. B., Hornick, R. B., Snyder, M. J., Libonati, J. P., Sheahan, D. G., Labrec, E. H., & Kalas, J. P. (1971) Pathogenesis of *Escherichia coli* diarrhoea. *New England Journal of Medicine*, **285**, 1–9.

Echeverria, P., Blacklow, N. R. & Smith, D. H. (1975) Role of heart-labile toxigenic *Escherichia coli* and Reovirus-like agent in diarrhoea in Boston children. *Lancet*, **ii**, 1113–1116.

Elias, J. & Shields, R. (1976) Influence of staphylococcal enterotoxin on water and electrolyte transport in the small intestine. *Gut*, **17**, 527–535.

Evans, D. G., Evans, D. J. & Pierce, N. F. (1973) Differences in the response of rabbit small intestine to heat-labile and heat-stable enterotoxins of *Escherichia coli*. *Infection and Immunity*, **7**, 873–880.

Evans, D. G., Evans, D. J. & DuPont, H. (1977) Virulence factors of enterotoxigenic *Escherichia coli*. *Journal of Infectious Diseases*, **136**, S118–S123.

Evans, D. G., Silver, R. P., Evans, D. J., Chase, D. G. & Gorbach, S. L. (1975) Plasmid controlled colonization factor associated with virulence in *Escherichia coli* enterotoxigenic for humans. *Infection and Immunology*, **12**, 656–667.

Gangarosa, E. J. & Merson, M. H. (1977) Curent concepts: relevance of enteropathogenic serotypes of *Esch. coli* in diarrhoea. *New England Journal of Medicine*, **296**, 1210–1213.

Gorbach, S. L., Banwell, J. G., Chatterjee, B. D., Jacobs, B. & Sack, R. B. (1971) Acute undifferentiated human diarrhoea in the Tropics. 1. Alterations in intestinal microflora. *Journal of Clinical Investigation*, **50**, 881–889.

Gorbach, S. L., Kean, B. H., Evans, D. G., Evans, D. J. & Bessudo, D. (1975) Travellers diarrhoea and toxigenic *Escherichia coli*. *The New England Journal of Medicine*, **292**, 933–936.

Gorbach, S. L. & Khurana, C. M. (1972) Toxigenic *Escherichia coli*. *New England Journal of Medicine*, **287**, 792–795.

Gross, R. J., Rowe, B., Henderson, A., Byatt, M. E. & MacLaurin, J. C. (1976) A new *Escherichia coli* O-group, 0159 associated with outbreaks of enteritis in infants. *Scandinavian Journal of Infectious Diseases*, **8**, 195–198.

Gross, R. J., Scotland, S. M. & Rowe, B. (1976) Enterotoxin testing of *Escherichia coli* causing epidemic infantile enteritis in the U.K. *Lancet*, **i**, 629–631.

Guerrant, R. L., Moore, R. A., Kirschenfeld, P. M. & Sande, M. A. (1975) Role of toxigenic and invasive bacteria in acute diarrhoea of childhood. *New England Journal of Medicine*, **293**, 567–573.

Gyles, C., So, M. & Falkow, S. (1974) The enterotoxin plasmids of *Escherichia coli*. *The Journal of Infectious Diseases*, **131**, 40–49.

Harris, J. C., Dupont, H. L. & Hornick, R. B. (1972) Fecal leukocytes in diarrhoeal illness. *Annals of Internal Medicine*, **76**, 697–703.

Jones G. W. & Rutter, J. M. (1972) Role of K88 antigen in the pathogenesis of neonatal diarrhoea caused by *Escherichia coli* in piglets. *Infection and Immunity*, **6**, 918–927.

Keusch, G. T. & Jacewicz, M. (1975) The pathogenesis of Shigella diarrhoea. V. Relationship of Shiga enterotoxin, neurotoxin and cytotoxin. *Journal of Infectious Diseases*, **131**, S33–S39.

Keusch, G. T., Jacewicz, M., Levine, M. M., Hornick, R. B. & Kochwa, S. (1976) Pathogenesis of shigella diarrhoea. Serum anticytotoxin antibody response produced by toxigenic and non toxigenic Shigella dysenteriae 1. *Journal of Clinical Investigation*, **57**, 194–202.

Koupal, L. R. & Deibel, R. H. (1975) Assay characterization and localization of an enterotoxin produced by salmonella. *Infection and Immunity*, **11**, 14–22.

McDonel, J. L. (1974) In vivo effects of *Clostridium perfringens* enteropathogenic factors on the rat ileum. *Infection and Immunity*, **10**, 1156–1162.

McNeish, A. S., Turner, P., Fleming, J. & Evans, N. (1975) Mucosal adherence of human enteropathogenic *Escherichia coli*. *Lancet*, **ii**, 946–948.

Mandal, B. K. & Mani, V. (1976) Colonic involvement in salmonellosis. *Lancet*, **i**, 887–888.

Merson, M. H., Morris, G. K., Sack, D. A., Wells, J. G., Feeley, J. C., Sack, R. B., Creech, W. B., Kapikian, A. Z. & Gangarosa, E. J. (1976) Travelers' diarrhoea in Mexico. *The New England Journal of Medicine*, **294**, 1299–1305.

Nalin, D. R., Rahaman, M., McLaughlin, J. C., Yunus, M. & Curlin, G. (1975) Enterotoxigenic *Escherichia coli* and idiopathic diarrhoea in Bangladesh. *Lancet*, **ii**, 1116–1119.

Ogawa, H., Nakamura, A. & Sakazaki, R. (1968) Pathogenic properties of 'enteropathogenic' *Escherichia coli* from diarrhoeal children and adults. *Japanese Journal of Medical Science and Biology*, **21**, 333–349.

Ørskov, F., Ørskov, I., Evans, D. J., Sack, B. R., Sack, D. A. & Wadstrom, T. (1976) Special *Escherichia coli* serotypes among enterotoxigenic strains from diarrhoea in adults and children. *Medical Microbiology and Immunology*, **162**, 73–80.

Portnoy, B. L., Goepfert, J. M. & Harmon, S. M. (1976) An outbreak of *Baccilus cereus* food poisoning resulting from contaminated vegetable sprouts. *American Journal of Epidemiology*, **103**, 589–594.

Rudoy, R. C. & Nelson, J. D. (1975) Enteroinvasive and enterotoxigenic *Escherichia coli*. *American Journal of Diseases of Children*, **129**, 668–672.

Ryder, R. W., Sack, D. A., Kapikian, A. Z., McLaughlin, J. C., Chakraborty, J., Rahman, A. S. M., Merson, M. H. & Wells, J. C. (1976a) Enterotoxigenic *Escherichia coli* and Reovirus-like agent in rural Bangladesh. *Lancet*, **i**, 659–662.

Ryder, R. W., Wachsmuth, I. K., Buxton, A. E., Evans, D. G., DuPont, H. L., Mason, E. & Barrett, F. F. (1976b) Infantile diarrhoea produced by heat-stable enterotoxigenic *Escherichia coli*. *The New England Journal of Medicine*, **295**, 849–853.

Sack, R. B., Hirschhorn, N., Brownlee, I., Cash, R. A., Woodward, W. E. & Sack, D. A. (1975)

Enterotoxigenic *Escherichia coli*—associated diarrheal disease in Apache children. *New England Journal of Medicine*, **292**, 1041–1045.

Sack, D. A., Kaminsky, D. C., Sack, R. B., Warnola, I. A., Ørskov, F., Ørskov, I., Slack, R. C. B., Arthur, R. R. & Kapikian, A. Z. (1977) Enterotoxigenic *E. coli* diarrhoea of travelers: a prospective study of American Peace Corps volunteers. *Johns Hopkins Medical Journal*, **141**, 63–70.

Sack, D. A., Wells, J. G., Merson, M. H., Sack, R. B. & Morris, G. K. (1975) Diarrhoea associated with heat-stable enterotoxin-producing strains of *Escherichia coli*. *Lancet*, **ii**, 239–241.

Shore, E. G., Dean, A. G., Holik, K. J. & Davis, B. R. (1974) Enterotoxin-producing *Escherichia coli* and diarrhoeal disease in adult travelers; a prospective study. *Journal of Infectious Diseases*, **129**, 577–582.

Skirrow, M. B. (1977) Campylobacter enteritis: a 'new' disease. *British Medical Journal*, **2**, 9–11.

Smith, H. W. & Lingood, M. A. (1971) The transmissible nature of neterotoxin production in a human enteropathogenic strain of *Escherichia coli*. *The Journal of Medical Microbiology*, **4**, 301–305.

Thomson, S. (1955) The role of certain varieties of *Bacterium coli* in gastro-enteritis of babies. *Journal of Hygiene*, **53**, 357–367.

Tulloch, E. F., Ryan, K. J., Formal, S. B. & Franklin, F. A. (1973) Invasive enteropathic *Escherichia coli* dysentery. *Annals of Internal Medicine*, **79**, 13–17.

Williams, P. H., Evans, N., Turner, P. & George, R. H. (1977) Plasmid mediating mucosal adherence in human enteropathogenic *Escherichia coli*. *Lancet*, **i**, 1151.

8. Aminoglycoside pharmacology

G. E. Mawer

Antibiotic pharmacology embraces several disciplines. The microbiologist measures *antibacterial activity* and compares this with host toxicity. If a new agent proves selectively toxic to pathogens it is then relevant to study its *pharmaco-kinetics* and to discover how it is handled in the body. Equipped with this basic information the clinician then tries to identify patients likely to benefit from the drug and to define the dosage schedule for a satisfactory *clinical response.*

ANTIBACTERIAL ACTIVITY

Although they differ in activity against specific bacteria there are strong pharma-cological similarities between the different aminoglycoside antibiotics developed since the original introduction of streptomycin in 1944. They are each active against Gram-negative bacilli and the tubercle bacillus but not against anaerobes or streptococci. Their antibacterial activity is greatest at alkaline pH. When dosage is inappropriately high they can each permanently damage the organs of hearing and balance and can produce reversible acute renal failure and potentiate the effect of neuromuscular blocking drugs.

The antibacterial actions of the aminoglycosides are due to inhibition of protein synthesis. The drugs bind to ribosomes and interfere with amino acid poly-merisation (Weinstein, 1975). Nothing is known however of the biochemical basis for the toxic effects on the vulnerable hair cells of the cochlea and vestibule.

The in vitro antibacterial activity of the aminoglycosides is illustrated by Figure 8.1 taken from the early work of Klein, Eickhoff and Finland (1964) on

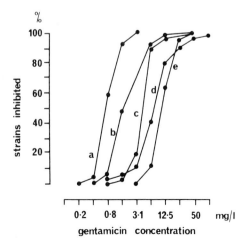

Fig. 8.1 Antibacterial activity of gentamicin against (a) *Staphylococcus aureus,* (b) *Klebsiella pneumoniae/Aerobacter aerogenes,* (c) *Escherichia coli,* (d) *Pseudomonas aeruginosa* and (e) *Proteus species.* The vertical scale indicates the proportion of studied strains which were inhibited by a given concentration of antibiotic in agar. The use of undiluted cultures gave higher inhibitory concentrations than often reported (Klein, Eickhoff and Finland, 1964).

gentamicin. Most strains of *E. coli* and *Klebsiella pneumoniae* for example were in-hibited by antibiotic concentrations up to 6 mg/l of agar. Concentrations of this order are attained in plasma during the first hour after the administration of recommended doses. On the other hand several strains of *Proteus* species and *Pseudomonas aeruginosa* were only inhibited by concentrations above 12 mg/l. Plasma concentrations of this level are avoided because of the risk of toxicity.

Three features of the aminoglycosides have acted as a continuing stimulus to the development of new drugs; resistance can be acquired by bacteria which previously were sensitive; certain Gram-negative bacteria are naturally resistant; there is only a small difference between the therapeutic dose and the toxic dose.

Acquired resistance
These antibiotics all consist of amino-substituted sugars and alicyclic alcohols linked through glycosidic bonds. Thus they carry many polar and reactive —OH and —NH_2 groupings. The resulting low lipid solubility is responsible for failure to penetrate cell membranes and tissue barriers; absorption from the gut and penetration into brain and CSF are poor. Penetration into bacteria would be equally poor were it not for the presence of carrier mediated transport mechanisms specific for the reactive groupings. Bacteria become resistant when they acquire conjugating enzymes which mask these groups by acetylation, adenylation or phosphorylation (Davies and Courvalin, 1977). Such resistance quickly became obvious with streptomycin and reduced the effective antibacterial spectrum of kanamycin when it was widely used. Acquired resistance to gentamicin is still very uncommon amongst Gram-negative isolates from infected hospital patients in the United Kingdom. In North America however it is common enough for the publication of studies on series of such patients. In one major hospital for example the incidence of gentamicin-resistant isolates rose from 0.8 per cent in 1971 to 8 per cent in 1975 (Guerrant et al, 1977).

In an attempt to keep ahead of bacterial innovation semi-synthetic amino-glycoside derivatives are being developed. Amikacin is an L-amino-α-hydroxybutyric acid derivative of kanamycin A (Fig. 8.2a) which is effective against many kanamycin- and gentamicin-resistant strains (Davies and Courvalin, 1977). Similarly netilmicin is an ethyl derivative of a dehydrogenated C_{1a} gentamicin (Fig. 8.2b) which is active against gentamicin-resistant strains of *Esch. coli* and *Klebsiella pneumoniae* (Rahal et al, 1976). These derivatives are relatively stable in the presence of many aminoglycoside-inactivating bacterial enzymes (see also Ch. 11); the steric effect of the synthetic side chain appears to discourage further masking of reactive groupings without preventing uptake by the bacterial cell. There must however be limited scope for useful structural modification. We must conserve existing aminoglycosides by careful and planned use rather than relying on the continuous development of new agents (Neu, 1976a). There are strong microbiological if not commercial arguments for discouraging oral and topical use of aminoglycosides and for reserving newer agents for the treatment of infections where there is a high likelihood of gentamicin-resistance (Editorial, 1977).

Anti-pseudomonal activity

After its introduction in 1963 gentamicin was shown to be more active than streptomycin or kanamycin particularly against *Klebsiella pneumoniae, Proteus species* and *Pseudomonas aeruginosa*. Nevertheless several pseudomonas strains are inhibited only by concentrations which are therapeutically unacceptable (Fig. 8.1). The persistence of *Pseudomonas* infections in patients with compromised antibacterial defences has encouraged the development of aminoglycosides with greater activity against this species. Tobramycin is more active against many

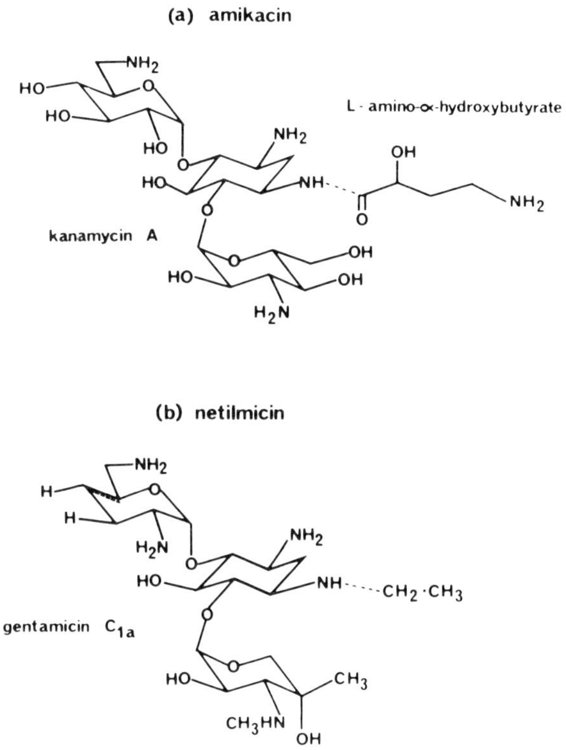

(a) amikacin

L - amino-α-hydroxybutyrate

kanamycin A

(b) netilmicin

gentamicin C$_{1a}$

Fig. 8.2
(a) Structure of amikacin, a semi-synthetic derivative of kanamycin A.
(b) Structure of netilmicin, a semi-synthetic derivative of gentamicin C$_{1a}$.

Pseudomonas strains including some which are gentamicin-resistant but against most other Gram-negative bacteria tobramycin is equivalent to gentamicin (Neu, 1976b). Amikacin also is active against some gentamicin-resistant pseudomonas strains.

Carbenicillin and the aminoglycosides have synergistic anti-pseudomonal activity in vitro (Riff and Jackson, 1972) and accordingly they are often used together in therapy. The concurrent use of carbenicillin has however been shown to reduce the serum concentrations of gentamicin measured by microbiological assay (Hull and Sarubbi, 1976) and there is some uncertainty about the value of the synergism in vivo (Smith, 1971).

Low therapeutic index

With the introduction of each new aminoglycoside the hope for diminished toxicity is renewed. There appears however to be a roughly parallel relationship between antibacterial potency and toxicity. Gentamicin and tobramycin are more potent in terms of inhibitory concentrations than streptomycin, kanamycin or amikacin; they are accordingly prescribed at one-third or one-quarter of the dose. Nevertheless ototoxicity is still observed in patients predisposed by impairment of kidney function demonstrating that the margin of safety remains very narrow. The preliminary data on netilmicin suggests that this may offer a greater margin of safety (Rahal et al, 1976) but it is necessary to await the results of prospective, comparative clinical studies.

Although differing in antibacterial and toxic potency the various aminoglycosides are very similar in the way they are handled in the body.

PHARMACOKINETICS

The small handling differences between the aminoglycosides become insignificant when the large differences between patients are considered. The same drugs are given to neonates weighing a few kg and to full grown adults, to the elderly and to patients with gross renal impairment. The between-patient differences in drug elimination rate produce almost a hundred-fold variation in daily dosage requirements.

Absorption from the site of injection appears to be complete as would be expected from the high water solubility of the aminoglycosides (Fig. 8.2), although the rate of absorption may be slowed by accidental subcutaneous injection or repeated use of the same injection site (Winters, Litwack and Hewitt, 1971). Variation in the proportion of a prescribed dose which is actually absorbed is probably caused primarily by variability in injection technique and by difficulties in the calculation or measurement of injection volumes corresponding with awkward doses.

When absorption is very rapid as after intravenous injection, the apparent initial volume of distribution is only a little larger than the vascular compartment and it is necessary to postulate a two compartment open system to explain the double exponential decay of serum aminoglycoside concentration (Dobbs and Mawer, 1976). In other circumstances (intramuscular injection or slow intravenous infusion) however a single compartment open system is an adequate model. Most authors have assumed this and have expressed volumes of distributions as litres per kg of body weight (Table 8.1, a). The impressive feature of this data is its relative lack of variation; differences between aminoglycosides appear to be less than differences between laboratories. The aminoglycoside distribution volume in the adult is usually about one quarter of the body weight (0.25 l/kg). Orme and Cutler (1969) working with kanamycin and Gyselynck, Forrey and Cutler (1971) working with gentamicin found no significant difference between the aminoglycoside distribution volume and the inulin space. Relatively large distribution volumes were found in the elderly by Lumholtz et al (1974), in the newborn (Milner et al, 1972) and in patients with severe renal failure (Gyselynck et al, 1971).

Table 8.1 Pharmacokinetic characteristics of aminoglycoside antibiotics

Aminoglycoside	a Distribution volume (l/kg)	b Clearance ratio*	c Half-time $T_{1/2}$ (h)	Comment	Reference
Kanamycin	0.19	0.60	2.1	Mean $T_{1/2}$ when $CL_{cr} > 60$ ml/min best fit values	Orme & Cutler, 1969
	0.25	0.65			Mawer et al, 1972
	0.16		2.1	<70 years, serum creatinine <133 μmol/l	Lumholtz et al, 1974
Amikacin	0.26	0.47	3.3	Mean $T_{1/2}$ when $CL_{cr} > 60$ ml/min	Pijck et al, 1976
	0.21	0.71	1.4	$CL_{cr} > 80$ ml/min per 1.73 m^2	Plantier et al, 1976
Gentamicin	0.24	0.85	2.0	Mean $T_{1/2}$ when GFR > 60 ml/min	Gyselynck et al, 1971
	0.16		1.8	<70 years, serum creatinine <133 μmol/l	Lumholtz et al, 1974
	0.28			Best fit values	Mawer et al, 1974
	0.23	0.75	2.5	$T_{1/2}$ for slow decay phase	Dobbs & Mawer, 1976
Tobramycin	0.22		1.8	Normal male volunteers	Geddes et al, 1974
	0.24		2.4	$T_{1/2}$ for slow decay phase	Dobbs & Mawer, 1976
		0.47	1.3	$CL_{cr} > 80$ ml/min per 1.73 m^2	Péchère & Dougal, 1976

*Renal aminoglycoside clearance as proportion of creatinine clearance

This is probably due to the greater proportion of the body weight represented by extracellular water in these patient subgroups.

The recent application of very sensitive assay methods has revealed evidence of deep distribution compartments (Shentag and Jusko, 1977). A proportion of the cumulative dose of aminoglycoside persists in such compartments causing a very slow excretion phase after the bulk of the dose has been eliminated.

Except in patients with gross impairment of kidney function elimination of the aminoglycosides is almost entirely dependent on kidney function. Renal amino-glycoside clearance estimates parallel the clearance of creatinine (Table 8.1, b; Fig. 8.3) and inulin (Orme and Cutler, 1969; Gyselynck et al, 1971) but tend to

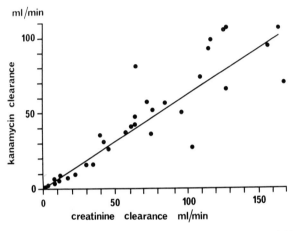

Fig. 8.3   Relationship between renal clearance of kanamycin and creatinine within a population of patients representing a wide range of kidney function. The best fitting line shown has a slope of 0.6 (Orme and Cutler, 1969).

be a little smaller due to association with plasma proteins (20–30 per cent bound). The relationship between aminoglycoside clearance and creatinine clearance is of practical value since the latter can readily be estimated from the serum creatinine concentration in an individual patient and used to predict his dosage requirements (Lumholtz et al, 1974).

The volume of distribution and the clearance together determine the serum concentration half time: published values for the different aminoglycosides do vary (Table 8.1, c) but this variation is probably due mainly to sampling from different patient populations. The half time of gentamicin for example is about 2 h in the older child and young adult (Fig. 8.4). During early life however substantially longer half times are encountered (Milner et al, 1972) particularly in babies with serum creatinine concentrations above the range appropriate to the very young. Similarly the half time is increased in the elderly as would be predicted from the decline in creatinine clearance with age (Lumholtz et al, 1974) but the longest half times which can exceed two days are encountered in patients with severe renal insufficiency (Gyselynck et al, 1971). The persistence of the aminoglycosides in these circumstances necessitates dosage redution to avoid accumulation and toxicity.

Dosage requirements

When the regularly repeated dose is scaled down appropriately to match diminished kidney function it becomes necessary to give a larger loading dose at the start of treatment; otherwise there is a substantial delay extending over three or more half times before the serum concentrations attain the full steady state levels which may be necessary for a therapeutic response. The main factor determining the size of the loading dose is the volume of distribution. This is proportional to body weight or lean body mass (Hull and Sarubbi, 1976) but

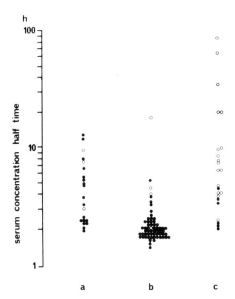

Fig. 8.4 Gentamicin serum concentration half times in patients studied by the author and his colleagues. Children younger than three months (a) showed a wide range, whereas older children (b) commonly had values close to 2 h. The adult population studied (c) was heavily biased towards renal insufficiency. Patients with high serum creatinine concentrations (greater than 80 μmol/1, indicated by open circles) in any age group tended to have longer half times.

also changes in response to salt and water overload or deprivation. Appropriate scaling down of the maintenance dosage rate (mg/day) without prolongation of the dosage interval reduces the difference between peak and trough serum antibiotic concentrations but does not alter the mean concentration ($\overline{C}pss$ mg/l) in the steady state. This is determined only by the repeating dose (Q mg), the interval between doses (I days) and the total clearance of drug from the plasma (CL_d l/day). In the steady state by definition the rate of drug input is equal to the rate of drug output and if complete absorption is assumed:—

$$Q/I = CL_d \times \overline{C}pss \qquad (1)$$

or by rearrangement:—

$$(Q/I)/\overline{C}pss = CL_d \qquad (2)$$

Thus the daily dosage rate for unit mean concentration is equal to the total drug clearance (2). Since the renal clearance of the aminoglycoside is proportional to the creatinine clearance (CL_{cr}) it is to be expected that the daily dosage requirement for a desired mean concentration (x mg/l) will be a linear function of the creatinine clearance.

$$x\,CL_d = a + b\,CL_{cr} \qquad (3)$$

This involves the additional and probably valid assumptions of first order elimination kinetics and a constant or very small non-renal clearance.

In two series of adult patients representing a wide range of kidney function studied by the author and his colleagues (Mawer et al, 1972; Mawer, 1975) the daily dosage requirements for kanamycin and gentamicin correlated more strongly with individual creatinine clearance rate than with other variables such as age or body weight.

The importance of creatinine clearance as a guide to the drug dosage requirements of individual adult patients has been repeatedly emphasised by Dettli (Dettli, Spring and Ryter, 1971) when considering drugs like the aminoglycosides which are eliminated mainly by the kidney. It is probably an equally valid guide in the child.

The individual gentamicin dosage requirements of 100 children (Ashurst et al, 1977) correlated strongly with the ratio of body weight to serum creatinine concentration. Since the rate of urinary creatinine excretion is proportional to the body weight (Counahan et al, 1976) this ratio is an index of creatinine clearance. When the small proportion of children with kidney impairment (serum creatinine concentration greater than 80 μmol/l) had been excluded however, the dosage requirement correlated better with body weight alone.

Thus individual creatinine clearance probably provides the best guide to aminoglycoside maintenance dosage amongst patients with impaired kidney function whereas body weight provides a simpler yet adequate guide for other patients. Kanamycin for example was routinely prescribed at a dose of about 7.5 mg/kg (or 500 mg in a 70 kg patient) every 12 hours. This commonly gave serum concentrations between 15 and 25 mg/l one hour after a dose and allowed virtually complete excretion of the previous dose before the next was given. The same dosage schedule is probably appropriate for amikacin in adults with creatinine clearance values above 60 ml/min (Pijck et al, 1976). Despite its similar handling characteristics a different practice developed with gentamicin; relatively smaller doses (0.8–1.6 mg/kg) were given at shorter (eight hour) intervals. This resulted in serum concentrations one hour after dosage below the minimum (5 mg/l) generally considered desirable (Noone et al, 1974); awareness of underdosage has grown and it is now widely appreciated that doses of 2–3 mg/kg are commonly required for the attainment of adequate concentrations particularly in children. Current dosage recommendations for tobramycin are almost as cautious as they were initially for gentamicin and there is a danger that the underdosage error will be repeated.

Computer models and nomograms

The relative simplicity of aminoglycoside pharmacokinetics has encouraged the development of computer simulations. These have been tested by their ability to predict serum antibiotic concentrations in treated patients and have been used to calculate appropriate dosage schedules for new patients. Jelliffe (1971) in Los Angeles and Mawer et al (1972, 1974), in Manchester were able to predict serum concentrations of kanamycin and gentamicin to a significant extent. Similar results were obtained by Hull and Sarubbi (1976) and by Michelson et al (1976), working with gentamicin but Barza et al (1975), considered that the handling of this drug was not predictable.

Several of these and other investigators who have studied aminoglycoside kinetics in renal failure have produced nomograms as guides to prescribing (Mawer, 1975). At least five such guides have been published for gentamicin alone. They all have similar theoretical foundations and make dosage predictions on the basis of body weight and estimated or measured creatinine clearance. Nevertheless dosage recommendations differ and there is a risk of confusion from the multiplication of nomograms.

Sceptics argue that a large part of individual variation in aminoglycoside handling is not accounted for by differences in body weight and kidney function. Such residual variation may however be less relevant to clinical response than individual differences in the sensitivity of pathogen and host to antibiotic concentration.

CLINICAL RESPONSE

Patients differ not only in their drug handling characteristics but also in their responses to the serum drug concentrations which result. As shown earlier, the various Gram-negative bacteria differ in their sensitivity to aminoglycoside concentration and certain sites of infection, notably the CSF (Newman and Holt, 1971) and the sputum (Morrice et al, 1976), have restricted access which reduces the concentrations to which the bacteria are actually exposed. Cellular and humoral mechanisms of host resistance also influence the outcome.

Tissue penetration and duration of exposure influence host cell toxicity which may also be modified by other drugs; the ototoxicity of the aminoglycosides is potentiated by potent diuretics (Weinstein, 1975) and the nephrotoxicity by certain cephalosporins (Noone et al, 1974).

Effective therapeutic concentration
The previous discussion about aminoglycoside pharmacokinetics has considered the selection of a dosage schedule for an individual patient to give a *desired* mean serum antibiotic concentration. The question of what constitutes a desirable concentration has been deliberately postponed. Each nomogram designer has assumed an answer with the exception of Jelliffe who has left the question open by making the user stipulate his own desired peak concentration. Even Jelliffe however has assumed that it is the *peak* serum concentration which is critical rather than the trough or the mean. Few clinical investigators have designed experiments to answer these questions.

Noone et al (1974) reported that it was necessary to attain 1 h serum gentamicin concentrations of at least 5 mg/l within 72 h of the start of treatment for Gram-negative septicaemia. Four patients with lower concentrations died whereas 10 out of 11 patients in whom this concentration was attained survived. The critical 1 h concentration appeared to be higher (8 mg/l) in patients with Gram-negative pneumonia. Above this level 16 out of 18 patients recovered but below it 3 out of 7 patients did not.

All children studied by Ashurst et al (1977) had steady state peak (1 h) serum gentamicin concentrations of 3 mg/l or more. The duration of fever was longer in children with septicaemia, chest infection, abscess formation and infection by highly resistant organisms; surgical drainage of pus predictably shortened its duration but after each of these clinical factors had been allowed for there was no significant relationship between therapeutic response and peak, trough or mean serum gentamicin concentration. One possible explanation is that the antibiotic concentration must exceed a threshold level for a minimum time and that above this the concentration is irrelevant to the therapeutic response.

Gentamicin dosage schedules consistent with their nomogram (Mawer et al, 1974) gave serum concentrations 2 h after dosage within a range of 3–10 mg/l. Other schedules gave a wider range of concentrations which extended down to 1 mg/l. This prompted a clinical trial of nomogram doses against acute febrile episodes in patients with leukaemia, lymphoma or aplastic anaemia (Wilkinson et al, 1977). Patients were allocated randomly to gentamicin at a fixed dose of 80 mg every 8 h or to the dosage schedule generated by the nomogram; clindamycin was given concurrently to both patient groups to combat anaerobic infections. A successful response to treatment was defined as disappearance of fever which was sustained for not less than seven days. The response rate amongst patients with proven bacterial sepsis was significantly better with nomogram based dosage (9/12 episodes) than with fixed dosage (5/16 episodes).

The experience of Anderton, Hanson and Raeburn (1976) with the nomogram of Chan, Benner and Hoeprich (1972) was similar. Patients with impaired kidney function and serious Gram-negative sepsis were treated with a fixed dose of 80 mg gentamicin at extended intervals or with more finely adjusted doses based on the nomogram. Infection was eradicated more frequently (17/20 episodes) in the nomogram treated group than in the fixed dose group (20/35 episodes).

McAllister and Tait (1976) determined the minimum inhibitory concentration (MIC) of tobramycin in serum against the causal organisms of infective episodes in 11 patients with urological conditions. The peak serum concentration (45 min after im and 20 min after iv injection) during treatment was compared with the MIC and the clinical response. The organism was eradicated in 10 patients who experienced peak concentrations between 2.5 and 12 mg/l and in whom the peak always exceeded the MIC. Infection persisted in one patient despite a peak of 4.8 mg/l when the MIC was substantially greater (16 mg/l). The urinary tobramycin concentrations were greater by more than ten-fold but it has been shown for gentamicin in the dog that the concentration in the renal lymph resembles plasma rather than urine (Gingell et al, 1969). Thus urinary concentrations are probably irrelevant when infection involves the renal parenchyma.

Serum concentrations for a therapeutic response to tobramycin are probably the same as for gentamicin. Making this assumption Tobias et al (1977) have shown that a nomogram for gentamicin dosage (Mawer et al, 1974) is equally applicable to tobramycin and the manufacturers have produced a 'Tobragram' which generates the same doses.

A peak (0.5–1 h) serum kanamycin concentration between 10 and 30 mg/l was considered to be therapeutic by Cutler and Orme (1969). Jelliffe provided concentrations up to 30 mg/l on his nomogram and indicated that 20 mg/l was generally suitable. Other authors have accepted these early assumptions without independent verification (Lumholtz et al, 1974; Mawer et al, 1972) but it is difficult to trace the original sources. Cutler and Orme for example do not quote a reference. Probably the desired range was based on the concentrations produced by conventional doses of streptomycin.

The available evidence suggests that therapeutic serum concentrations of amikacin are in the same range. A randomised prospective clinical trial of amikacin (with carbenicillin) against gentamicin (with carbenicillin) has been performed in leukopenic patients with fever and suspected Gram-negative infection (Lau et al, 1977). Individual dosage rates of amikacin were adjusted to give peak serum concentrations of 20–35 mg/l and trough concentrations below 10 mg/l. The corresponding gentamicin concentrations were 4–10 mg/l and 2 mg/l. In each treatment group the standard dosage interval was 8 h. The two treatment regimes proved to be approximately equitherapeutic both in the total patient group and in the sub-group with proven bacterial sepsis. The overall frequency of successful treatment in the latter group was 77 per cent.

There is justified anxiety about acquired resistance to the newer systemic aminoglycosides. Nevertheless more than 80 per cent of strains of *Esch. coli*, *Klebsiella pneumoniae* and *Proteus species* are currently sensitive to kanamycin or amikacin (MIC < 30 mg/l) and to gentamicin or tobramycin (MIC < 8 mg/l) (Moellering et al, 1977). These authors also observed a falling incidence of resistance to streptomycin and kanamycin coinciding with their replacement by the newer amingolycosides in the treatment of severe Gram-negative sepsis. Thus in many such cases it is likely that equitherapeutic effects could be produced by kanamycin or amikacin at peak serum concentrations of 10–30 mg/l and by gentamicin or tobramycin at peak serum concentrations of about one third of these levels.

Safe, non-toxic concentration

Changes in the cochleagram have been observed (Wilson and Ramsden, 1977) within an hour of the intravenous injection of tobramycin but it is not known what relationship if any these changes bear to hair cell damage and permanent deafness. So far as toxicity is concerned recent work has tended to show a correlation with trough serum concentration rather than peak.

Line, Poole and Waterworth (1970) reported that ototoxicity in patients with tuberculosis receiving daily streptomycin injections was associated with a 24 h concentration above 3 mg/l. Similarly Mawer et al (1974) detected ataxia or high frequency hearing loss in 4 out of 5 patients with renal disease who experienced trough gentamicin concentrations greater than 4 mg/l for more than 10 days. Lerner, Seligsohn and Matz (1977) observed raised mean trough concentrations in four patients with ototoxicity due to gentamicin or amikacin whilst the mean *peak* levels were lower than in the 49 patients who showed no evidence of toxicity.

The factors which predispose to aminoglycoside ototoxicity are well established. The likelihood of toxicity is increased by each of the following:— A large total cumulative dose of drug, previous exposure to aminoglycoside antibiotics, a treatment course lasting more than 10 days, concurrent administration of other ototoxic drugs, impairment of kidney function and old age. Several of these associations have been observed repeatedly with the earlier aminoglycosides (Weinstein, 1975) and with tobramycin (Neu and Bendush, 1976) and amikacin (Lane, Wright asd Blair, 1977).

The significance of diminished kidney function whether due to age, kidney disease or extrarenal factors is probably that it results in persistence of the amino-glycosides and higher serum trough concentrations despite dosage adjustment to avoid excessive peaks. It is not difficult in turn to explain the importance for toxicity of raised trough concentrations for the rate of aminoglycoside entry into the inner ear is very slow (Federspil, Schätzle and Tiesler, 1976). In the guinea-pig there is a delay of 4–6 h after a dose before equilibration between perilymph and

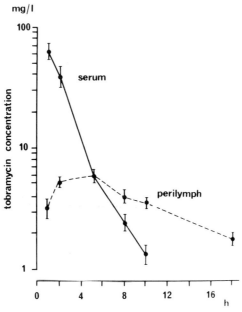

Fig. 8.5 Concentrations of tobramycin in guinea-pig serum and inner ear fluid (perilymph) at intervals after subcutaneous injection of 50 mg/kg. The perilymph concentration rose slowly to equal that in serum 4–6 h after injection. The concentration then decayed more slowly in the perilymph than in the serum (Federspil, Schätzle and Tiesler, 1976).

serum is attained (Fig. 8.5). Thereafter the concentration in the perilymph decays very slowly with a half time of 10–12 h and remains substantially higher than that in the serum. Thus the maximum concentration to which the vulnerable hair cells are exposed is normally limited by the rapid decay of serum aminoglycoside concentration, but when renal elimination is delayed, there is sufficient time for the perilymph concentration to attain relatively high levels. In brief the inner ear fluids exhibit the kinetic properties of a deep compartment.

Nephrotoxicity is difficult to assess since many conditions treated with aminglycosides already carry an increased risk of renal impairment. Similarly drug excretion rate decreases as kidney function deteriorates. Nevertheless it is likely that raised trough concentrations increase the risk of nephrotoxicity (Dahlgren, Anderson and Hewitt, 1975).

CONCLUSIONS

New semi-synthetic aminoglycosides are effective against many Gram-negative bacteria with acquired or natural resistance to the parent aminoglycosides. The biochemical versatility of bacteria has no limits however and it will be prudent to avoid over-exposure of these agents. Reduced host toxicity may ultimately be achieved but in the meantime the margin between toxic dose and effective dose remains narrow.

Aminoglycoside pharmacokinetics is not complex because the drugs show a strong resemblance to each other and to inulin. Distribution is within the extracellular water and elimination is mainly by glomerular filtration. When kidney function is appropriate to body size the serum concentration half time is short, toxic accumulation is not a problem and body weight provides a satisfactory guide for dosage. When kidney function is impaired however the daily maintenance dose must be scaled down; the renal clearance of creatinine provides a practical guide and a loading dose may be needed. Several prescribing aids are available.

Many factors influence the clinical response to treatment in Gram-negative sepsis and no graded concentration/response relationship has been recognised. It is probably necessary however for the *peak* serum antibiotic concentration to exceed a minimum threshold of about 5 mg/l for gentamicin/tobramycin (or 3–4 times this for kanamycin/amikacin). The threshold is also modified by the MIC of the pathogen and the accessibility of the infection site. Toxicity on the other hand appears to relate more to *trough* concentration and it is becoming customary to consider 2 mg/l a safe upper limit for gentamicin/tobramycin (or 3–4 times this for kanamycin/amikacin). The duration of treatment and the use of other drugs are also relevant. In the presence of particularly inaccessible or relatively resistant infection the clinician may give priority to the therapeutic effect and deliberately accept potentially toxic trough concentrations.

REFERENCES

Anderton, J. L., Hanson, E. & Raeburn, J. A. (1976) The use of gentamicin in patients with impaired kidney function. *Chemotherapy* Vol. 4, pp. 121–125. eds. Williams, J. D. & Geddes, A. M. Plenum: London.

Ashurst, A., Houston, I. B., Mawer, G. E. & Sambo-Donga, L. (1977) Factors influencing the therapeutic response to gentamicin treatment in children. *British Journal of Clinical Pharmacology*, **4**, 394P–395P.

Barza, M., Brown, R. B., Shen, D., Gibaldi, M. & Weinstein, L. (1975) Predictability of blood levels of gentamicin in Man. *Journal of Infectious Diseases*, **132**, 165–174.

Chan, R. A., Benner, E. J. & Hoeprich, P. D. (1972) Gentamicin therapy in renal failure: a nomogram for dosage. *Annals of Internal Medicine*, **76**, 773–778.

Counahan, R., Chantler, C., Ghazali, S., Kirkwood, B., Rose, F. & Barratt, T. M. (1976) Estimation of glomerular filtration rate from plasma creatinine concentration in children. *Archives of Diseases of Childhood*, **51**, 875–878.

Cutler, R. E. & Orme, B. M. (1969) Correlation of serum creatinine concentration and kanamycin half life. *Journal of the American Medical Association*, **209**, 539–542.

Dahlgren, J. G., Anderson, E. T. & Hewitt, W. L. (1975) Gentamicin blood levels: a guide to nephrotoxicity. *Antimicrobial Agents and Chemotherapy*, **8**, 58–62.

Davies, J. & Courvalin, P. (1977) Mechanisms of resistance to aminoglycosides. *American Journal of Medicine*, **62**, 868–872.

Dettli, L., Spring, P. & Ryter, S. (1971) Multiple dose kinetics and drug dosage in patients with kidney disease. *Acta Pharmacologica et Toxicologica*, **29**, (Suppl. 3): 211–224.

Dobbs, S. M. & Mawer, G. E. (1976) Intravenous injection of gentamicin and tobramycin without impairment of hearing. *Journal of Infectious Diseases*, **124**, S114–S117.

Editorial (1977) Amikacin. *Lancet*, **2**, 891.

Federspil, P., Schätzle, W. & Tiesler, E. (1976) Pharmacokinetics and ototoxicity of gentamicin, tobramycin and amikacin. *Journal of Infectious Diseases*, **134**, S200–S205.

Geddes, A. M., Goodall, J. A. D., Spiers, C. F., Gillett, A. P., Andrews, J. & Williams, J. D. (1974) Clinical and laboratory studies with tobramycin. *Chemotherapy*, **20**, 245–256.

Gingell, J. C., Chisholm, G. D., Calnan, J. S. & Waterworth, P. M. (1969) The dose, distribution and excretion of gentamicin with special reference to renal failure. *Journal of Infectious Diseases*, **119**, 396–401.

Guerrant, R. L., Strausbaugh, L. J., Wenzel, R. P., Hamory, B. H. & Sande, M. A. (1977) Nosocomial bloodstream infectious caused by gentamicin-resistant Gram-negative bacilli. *American Journal of Medicine*, **62**, 894–901.

Gyselynck, A., Forrey, A. & Cutler, R. (1971) Pharmacokinetics of gentamicin: distribution and plasma and renal clearance. *Journal of Infectious Diseases*, **124**, S70–S76.

Hull, J. H. & Sarubbi, F. A. (1976) Gentamicin serum concentrations: pharmacokinetic predictions. *Annals of Internal Medicine*, **85**, 183–189.

Jelliffe, R. W. (1971) Nomograms for kanamycin and gentamicin therapy. Abstracts 11th Interscience Conference on Antimicrobial Agents and Chemotherapy, p. 63. Atlantic City, N.J.

Klein, J. O., Eickhoff, T. C. & Finland, M. (1964) Gentamicin: activity in vitro and observations in 26 patients. *American Journal of Medical Sciences*, **248**, 528–543.

Lane, A. Z., Wright, G. E. & Blair, D. C. (1977) Ototoxicity and nephrotoxicity of amikacin. *American Journal of Medicine*, **62**, 911–918.

Lau, W. K., Young, L. S., Black, R. E., Winston, D. J., Linné, S. R., Weinstein, R. J. & Hewitt, W. L. (1977) Comparative efficacy and toxicity of amikacin/carbenicillin versus gentamicin/carbenicillin in leukopenic patients. *American Journal of Medicine*, **62**, 959–966.

Lerner, S. A., Seligsohn, R. & Matz, G. J. (1977) Comparative clinical studies of ototoxicity and nephrotoxicity of amikacin and gentamicin. *American Journal of Medicine*, **62**, 919–923.

Line, D. H., Poole, G. W. & Waterworth, P. M. (1970) Serum streptomycin levels and dizziness. *Tubercle, London*, **51**, 76–81.

Lumholtz, B., Kampmann, J., Siersbaek-Nielsen, K. & Mølholm Hanson, J. (1974) Dose regimen of kanamycin and gentamicin. *Acta Medica Scandinavica*, **196**, 521–524.

McAllister, T. A. & Tait, S. (1976) Laboratory findings on tobramycin and their relation to clinical response. *Journal of Infectious Diseases*, **134**, S20–S27.

Mawer, G. E., Knowles, B. R., Lucas, S. B., Stirland, R. M. & Tooth, J. A. (1972) Computer-assisted prescribing of kanamycin for patients with renal insufficiency. *Lancet*, **1**, 12–15.

Mawer, G. E., Ahmad, R., Dobbs, S. M., McGough, J. G., Lucas, S. B. & Tooth, J. A. (1974) Prescribing aids for gentamicin. *British Journal of Clinical Pharmacology*, **1**, 45–50.

Mawer, G. E. (1975) Dosage schedules for aminoglycoside antibiotics. In *Advanced Medicine, Topics in Therapeutics*, ed. Turner, P., Vol. 2, pp. 36–50. Bath: Pitman.

Michelson, P. A., Miller, W. A., Warner, J. F., Ayers, L. W. & Boxenbaum, H. G. (1976) Multiple dose pharmacokinetics of gentamicin in man: evaluation of the Jelliffe nomogram and adjustment of dosage in patients with renal impairment. In *The effect of disease states on drug pharmacokinetics*, ed. Benet, L. Z. pp. 207–245. Washington, D.C.: American Pharmaceutical Association.

Milner, R. D. G., Ross, J., Froud, D. J. R. & Davis, J. A. (1972) Clinical pharmacology of gentamicin in the newborn infant. *Archives of Diseases of Childhood*, **47**, 927–932.

Moellering, R. C., Wennersten, C., Kunz, L. J. & Poitras, J. W. (1977) Resistance to gentamicin, tobramycin, and amikacin among clinical isolates of bacteria. *American Journal of Medicine*, **62**, 873–881.

Morrice McCrae, W., Raeburn, J. A. & Hanson, E. J. (1976) Tobramycin therapy of infections due to *Pseudomonas aeruginosa* in patients with cystic fibrosis; effect of dosage and concentration of antibiotic in sputum. *Journal of Infectious Diseases*, **134**, S191–S193.

Neu, H. C. (1976a) Aminoglycosides: do we need new agents? *Drugs*, **12**, 161–165.

Neu, H. C. (1976b) Tobramycin: an overview. *Journal of Infectious Diseases*, **134**, S3–S19.

Neu, H. C. & Bendush, C. L. (1976) Ototoxicity of tobramycin: a clinical overview. *Journal of Infectious Diseases*, **134**, S206–S217.

Newman, R. L. & Holt, R. J. (1971) Gentamicin in infections of the central nervous system. *Journal of Infectious Diseases*, **119**, 471–475.

Noone, P., Parsons, T. M. C., Pattison, J. R., Slack, R. C. B., Garfield-Davies, D. & Hughes, K.

(1974) Experience in monitoring gentamicin therapy during treatment of serious Gram-negative sepsis. *British Medical Journal*, **1,** 477–481.

Orme, B. M. & Cutler, R. E. (1969) The relationship between kanamycin pharmacokinetics: distribution and renal function. *Clinical Pharmacology and Therapeutics*, **10,** 543–550.

Péchère, J.-C. & Dugal, R. (1976) Pharmacokinetics of intravenously administered tobramycin in normal volunteers and in renal-impaired and haemodialysed patients. *Journal of Infectious Diseases*, **134,** S118–S124.

Pijck, J., Hallynck, T., Soep, H., Baert, L., Daneels, R. & Boelaert, J. (1976) Pharmacokinetics of amikacin in patients with renal insufficiency: relation of half-life and creatinine clearance. *Journal of Infectious Diseases*, **134,** S331–S341.

Plantier, J., Forrey, A. W., O'Neill, M. A., Blair, A. D., Christopher, T. G. & Cutler, R. E. (1976) Pharmacokinetics of amikacin in patients with normal or impaired renal function: radioenzymatic acetylation assay. *Journal of Infectious Diseases*, **134,** S323–S330.

Rahal, J. J., Simberkoff, M. S., Kagan, K. & Moldover, N. H. (1976) Bactericidal efficacy of Sch 20569 and amikacin against gentamicin-sensitive and -resistant organisms. *Antimicrobial Agents and Chemotherapy*, **9,** 595–599.

Riff, L. J. & Jackson, G. G. (1972) Laboratory and clinical conditions for gentamicin inactivation by carbenicillin. *Archives of Internal Medicine*, **130,** 887–891.

Schentag, J. J. & Jusko, W. J. (1977) Renal clearance and tissue accumulation of gentamicin. *Clinical Pharmacology and Therapeutics*, **22,** 364–370.

Smith, I. M. (1971) Supplemental antibiotics to enhance the action of gentamicin in *Pseudomonas* and mixed infections. *Journal of Infectious Diseases*, **124,** S198–S201.

Tobias, J. S., Wrigley, P. F. M., Korde, S. & Shaw, E. J. (1977) Nomogram-assisted dosage of tobramycin. *Journal of Antimicrobial Chemotherapy*, **3,** 305–309.

Weinstein, L. (1975) Antimicrobial agents: streptomycin, gentamicin and other aminoglycosides. In *Pharmacological Basis of Therapeutics*, ed. Goodman, L. S. & Gilman, A. 5th edition, pp. 1167–1182. New York: Macmillan.

Wilkinson, P. M., Gorst, D. W., Tooth, J. A. & Delamore, I. W. (1977) The managements of fever in blood dyscrasis: results of a prospective controlled trial of a prescribing aid for gentamicin. *Journal of Antimicrobial Chemotherapy*, **3,** 297–303.

Wilson, P. & Ramsden, R. T. (1977) Immediate effects of tobramycin on human cochlea and correlation with serum tobramycin levels. *British Medical Journal*, **1,** 259–261.

Winters, R. E., Litwack, K. D. & Hewitt, W. L. (1971) Relation between dose and levels of gentamicin in blood. *Journal of Infectious Diseases*, **124,** S90–S95.

9. Automated and rapid methods for the diagnosis of infectious diseases

S. W. B. Newsom

Laboratory methods for the diagnosis of infection (virology excepted) have remained largely unchanged since their introduction in the 1880s. However today's workload continues to rise, boosted by screening programmes like those for rubella, syphilis and hepatitis B antigen, while the budget (up to 80 per cent of which goes on staff) usually fails to keep pace. An obvious solution would be the purchase of machines to handle a part (mechanisation) or all (automation) of a technique. The biochemistry and haematology laboratories are already mechanised and commercial interest is turning to microbiology; indeed Laboratory Equipment Digest (1977) predicts a European market for £24 000 000 worth of automatic sensitivity test machines by 1980.

Traditional specimen handling depends on the technician's hand, eye and brain. Machines might be able to replace any combination of these three while increasing productivity, reducing drudgery and providing accurate and hopefully speedy results. The latter should improve patient care, and some systems are remarkably quick—Throm et al (1977) for example found that radiometry was three times, and impedance ten times, as fast as conventional cultures for detecting bacteraemia. However the time-cycle of the machine is important—all but the most vital results generated at midnight will be ignored till next day.

Several problems are implicit in mechanisation. First is the motivation of technicians and the danger of converting them to electricians. Then there is the economics of purchasing and running a machine. Multi-national trade may be important here, as the high development costs of sophisticated automatic equipment demand a world-wide market and manual test costs vary greatly. Thus a disc sensitivity test in the U.S.A. may cost double that of one in the U.K. which in turn may be dearer than in a country with cheap labour; so that a machine that is competitive in the U.S.A. may be marginal here and uneconomic elsewhere. Finally the capacity of some machines is such that economic use requires a central laboratory with the attendant problems of logistics and diminution of motivation in the periphery.

Notwithstanding these criticisms there is a lot of interest in mechanisation, and the two International Symposia on Rapid Methods and Automation in Microbiology (Hedén and Illeni, 1975; Johnston and Newsom, 1977) presented a somewhat bewildering array of potential techniques. Few were as yet fully automatic, but some are already developed and proving their worth. The topic will be presented under the somewhat arbitrary headings of Detection and identification of microbes, Antibiotics, Serology and Data handling. A system for growth detection may also measure growth inhibition or stimulation and so be used for identification and antibiotic susceptibility tests.

DETECTION OF MICROBES

A microbe may be detected either directly in a specimen, or by the changes caused by growth or metabolism in a suitable medium. Direct techniques include optical methods and detection of specific antigens or metabolites, or of non-specific microbial components (e.g. endotoxin or ATP) in the specimen. Such methods fail to differentiate living and dead cells, and may be invaluable when the causal organism has already been killed by antibiotics—as in pneumococcal pneumonia,

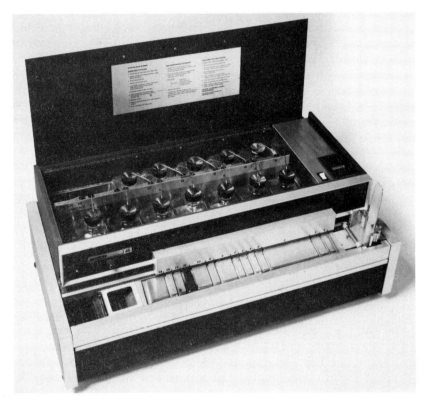

Fig. 9.1   The Ames Haematek adapted for staining acid-fast bacilli (courtesy C. E. D. Taylor)

or cannot be grown in vitro e.g. *Mycobacterium leprae* or hepatitis virus. Microbial growth (or sometimes metabolism) can be signalled by changes in the electrical impedance, radio activity, heat production, chemical composition or optical qualities of the medium. Mechanisation may also be helpful in specimen preparation and culture, particularly for quantitative bacteriology.

Direct demonstration of microbes

Optical methods
Preparation and examination of a gram-stained film is an unlikely candidate for automation in a routine laboratory, although machines like the Haematek (Ames) (Fig. 9.1) might be adapted for staining; Burdash, West and Bannister (1976)

recently evaluated another system—the Microstainer II. Images can be analysed with a flying-spot microdensitometer and image analyser (e.g. the Quantimet). Fluorescence microscopy is easier to automate, because if dark field illumination is used the total light emission should relate to the stained material, and can be measured at reasonable cost with a microfluorometer. Heimer, Joseph and Taylor (1978) have used this as a basis for an automated screen for acid fast bacilli based on the auramine phenol stain.

Particles in suspension will scatter light if the wavelength is similar to their size. The amount of scatter depends on the number of particles, and the proportion scattered at different angles depends on the bacterial shape. Multi-angle light scatter detection forms the basis of two very sophisticated systems. Wyatt (1975) described the Differential III (Science Spectrum) in which the light scatter from a helium-neon laser beam is recorded by a photodetector that traverses around the cuvette and draws a graph so closely related to bacterial shape that two subcultures of the same strain of *Escherichia coli* incubated at different temperatures could be differentiated because one had fimbriae. Wyatt predicted that the machine with its dedicated microcomputer could identify bacteria from a specimen filtrate, and that by re-testing aliquots after perhaps 30 min incubation in different media containing relevant antibiotics—it could produce an antibiogram based on shape changes in sensitive cells. An alternative system currently being developed for cancer research is flow microfluorometry. Microdroplets containing individual cells are stained with a fluorescent dye (e.g. acridine orange for DNA- or FITC-labelled antisera), and then passed through a cell sizing device, followed by an argon-ion laser beam that excites fluorescence. The ratio of cell nucleus to total cell volume can be computed and finally different types of cell can be 'sorted' into separate receivers by being given an electric charge and then being passed through a magnetic field. The Fluorescent Activated Cell Sorter (Bekton Dickenson) (Fig. 9.2) is described in detail by Herzenberg, Sweet and Herzenberg (1976). Cram (1977) reviewed possible microbiological applications which range from detection of PPD-activated lymphocytes and cell fusion due to Newcastle Disease Virus, to use of a multi-angle collector of fluorescent light scatter to differentiate bacteria.

Antigen detection
Microbial antigens can be detected in clinical material. The methods used are all very sensitive and so rely on completely specific antisera devoid of all cross-reactions. The development of antigen-detection was given a major stimulus by the need for an HBag screening programme. Countercurrent immunoelectrophoresis was used initially, because the electric current concentrates the reagents and pushes them together thus providing a quicker and more sensitive result than double diffusion in agar gel. Spencer (1978) has recently reviewed its use to detect pneumococcal, meningococcal and fungal antigens in sputum and cerebrospinal fluid. Reverse passive haemagglutination is a more sensitive method, which uses antibody-coated turkey red cells to detect the antigen The greatest sensitivity (picograms) is provided by radioimmunoassay—which can be fully automated by isolating the immune complexes in drops on a cellulose acetate strip that moves directly into a counter (Bagshawe, 1975); continuous flow methods in tubes are

also under development. The major problems of radio-assays are instability of the reagents and costly apparatus. Engvall and Perlmann (1972) introduced ELISA (enzyme-linked immunosorbent assay) which uses the same principles with stable reagents and cheap apparatus. The reaction between enzyme-linked antibody and antigen is held in solid phase by non-specific adhesion of the reactants to the walls

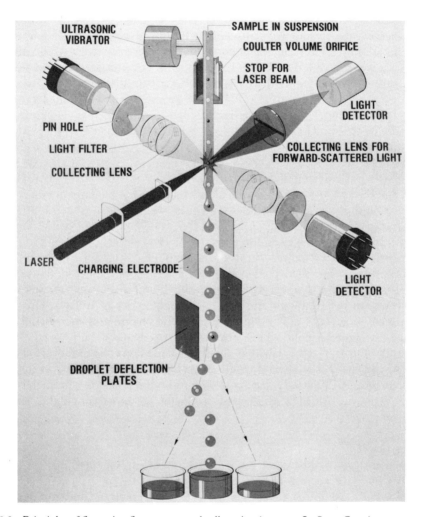

Fig. 9.2   Principles of flow microfluorometry and cell sorting (courtesy L. Scott Cram)

of a microtiter tray. The trays lend themselves to automatic processing and washers, reagent adders and photometers are now available (Dynatech). Organon sell a pre-prepared HBag-detection kit, and ELISA has also been used to detect rotaviruses in faeces.

Finally a new method to detect and measure soluble antigens is the laser nephelometer, a forward light-scatter photometer powered by a helium-neon laser. This detects immune complexes, and as light scatter is proportional to particle numbers, use of standardised antisera (available from the nephelometer makers—Hyland or Boehringer) allows quantitation. To date the nephelometers have only been set up to measure serum proteins, but could doubtless be adapted for soluble microbial antigens.

Detection of microbial materials and metabolites
The presence of bacteria can be inferred from detection of their constituents or metabolites. A simple example is endotoxin which forms a gel with a limulus crab amoebocyte extract. Johnston, Mitchell and Curtis (1976) described an automatic bacteriuria detection system based on measurement of ATP by bioluminescence. Human cellular ATP is liberated with Triton X-100 and destroyed by apyrase— then the bacterial ATP is liberated and causes firefly luciferase to produce a flash that can be measured in a photometer.

Some microbes produce specific metabolites; for example the green pigment of pseudomonas, or the fluorescent red pigment of *Bacteroides melaninogenicus*, which may be detectable in pus. Anaerobes also produce volatile fatty acids, that can be detected by gas/liquid chromatography on pus.

The gas chromatograph may also be used to detect specific bacteria-related gas in the head-space above a culture, for example dimethyl disulphide from *Proteus* spp, and ethanol from *E. coli*, and this has been suggested as a rapid bacteriuria screen (Hayward and Jeavons, 1977).

Impedance
Bacterial growth causes large molecules in the medium to be broken into smaller ones and so lowers the electrical impedance. A sensitive meter can detect changes from an inoculum of 10^5 cells within 2.5 hr (Brown, 1977 personal communication) (Fig. 9.3). The sensing electrodes present a problem, the original ones were gold *and* disposable. Temperature stability to $0.001°C$ is needed, and anaerobic conditions in test cells meant that pseudomonas grew slowly unless the medium contained nitrite. However systems are now being developed with other metal electrodes in tubes of medium to the user's choice. Thirty to 100 or more cultures may be followed using a microcomputer. Such a system would seem ideal for blood cultures and Kagan et al (1977) described its successful use with a lysis-filtration method. Ur (1977) reviewed the prospects and limitations of the process.

Radiometry
Bacterial metabolism releases radioactive carbon dioxide from a radio-labelled source. The Bactec (Johnston laboratories) has been available for blood cultures for some years (Deland and Wagner, 1970). Blood is injected into a sealed ampoule of special medium, which is placed on a machine capable of sampling the head-space gas for radio-activity at hourly intervals. Up to 40 per cent of cultures are positive within the day (by 10 p.m. at least); thereafter cultures are tested daily. Randall (1977) reviewed her experience with the system which detected 98 per cent of positive cultures within 72 hours. Pseudomonas again grows more slowly and recently Strauss, Throm and Friedman (1977) pointed out the need for terminal subcultures as the system did not respond to group *D. streptococci*.

Occasional false positive reactions occur due to metabolism of human cells in the blood.

Microcalorimetry
The minute amounts of heat produced when a culture grows can be detected in a sensitive calorimeter. Microcalorimeters are of two kinds—a static, multichamber instrument in which the thermograms of different strains are measured and stored in a computer, and a flow calorimeter in which the heat already generated by

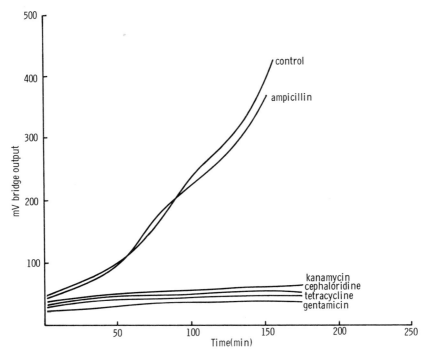

Fig. 9.3   The effect of antibiotics on impedance changes due to growth of *Klebsiella aerogenes* in PPLO broth (courtesy D. F. J. Brown)

a culture is sampled for 3–5 minutes. The graph of heat production has the advantage of being a signature of the strain that produced it, and is readily altered by antibiotics, but it requires a lot of time on an expensive machine. Tests with the flow microcalorimeter (Beezer and Tyrell, 1972) for bacteriuria screening are under way, but so far problems of machine stability and pre-incubation of the urine need to be overcome (Shaw, 1977 personal communication). The subject has been reviewed by Bettelheim and Shaw (1978).

Optical growth detection
The change of optical density in a medium due to bacterial growth can be detected with a photometer. Changes have to be compared with a 100 per cent transmission baseline. Forward light scatter can also be used, and a photodetector placed at 35° to the axis picks up maximal light scatter but, as the baseline reading is now

zero, small changes are detectable. Praglin et al (1975) noted that 45 min incubation of an *E. coli* culture produced a 2 per cent increase in optical density but a 170 per cent change in light scatter. Light scatter can also detect microcolonies and is used in the fully automatic urine culture system developed by McDonnell Douglas (The Automicrobic System). Urines are diluted and plated on a set of selective media. The cultures are scanned at intervals and growth patterns are stored in a computer. Five to 13 hours later the bacteria can be identified and the original numbers computed.

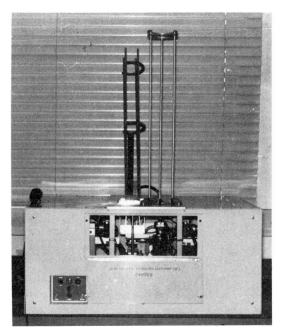

Fig. 9.4   An automatic plate streaking machine

Specimen preparation and handling
Seward laboratories market two small and useful machines: the Stomacher (Sharpe and Jackson, 1972, 1975) and the Droplette (Sharpe and Jackson, 1975). The Stomacher is an efficient blender that works by squeezing a plastic bag containing the sample and diluent. It works well for sputum, and produces much less of an aerosol than conventional blenders (Newsom, 1977), although the safe removal of the sample from the bag presents a problem. The Droplette is a simple and economic means of counting bacteria in drops of agar in a petri dish, which Kelly (1977) adapted for use with anaerobes. Malike (1977) described a somewhat similar 'minidisc' counting method. Plating out can also be automated. Trotman (1972) described a prototype machine, with an electrically-heated wire loop and a turntable, to streak out material from the centre of a plate. The fully developed machine is seen in Figure 9.4 in my laboratory, and includes a system of plate transport and lid removal/replacement powered by compressed air. In addition to saving time the streaks are standardised so the growth pattern relates to the original

inoculum, and the machine has a good technician acceptance value. Campbell (1977) used a similar machine for quantitative food microbiology.

IDENTIFICATION OF MICROBES

Bacterial speciation traditionally requires a mixture of biochemical tests like fermentations and indole production. An Adansonian taxonomy requires the results of as many tests as possible, while the routine laboratory needs a few selected reliable tests. The main advance has been the use of computers to generate taxonomic matrices and define useful tests. The supply of standardised identification kits, backed in some cases (e.g. API) by a substantial worldwide data bank, is invaluable for one-off tests, and allows valid biotypes of common microbes like *E. coli* and *Klebsiella pneumoniae*. However when many strains need testing the cost is excessive and replica plating in plates or trays with automatic inoculators such as those sold by Denley or Dynatech is required.

A 9 cm petri dish contains around 24 ml of agar—this could form a 1 cm ribbon the same depth 75 cm long. The ribbon is much better adapted to automatic handling and Prof. Hedén and his colleagues used this as the basis of their 'Autoline' system (Hedén, 1975). The ribbon is inoculated with a ceramic roller, and chemicals can be applied at defined points. The resulting growth (or inhibition) patterns can be charted by passing the ribbon through a light-scatter system. Kuhn and Hedén (1977) have used the Autoline for 'metabolic fingerprinting' to obtain biotypes of bacteria such as *E. coli*.

The standard identification tests may take several days to complete, although the computer can process the results in picoseconds! Bascomb and Grantham (1975) described a 1.2 hr identification system based on the release of ammonia from various substrates, thus providing a bacterial enzyme profile. This system which uses continuous-flow (Technicon) apparatus is still under active development. Enzyme inhibition profiles may be even more specific.

An alternative technique is analysis of bacterial components. Pyrolysis releases a host of chemicals that can be analysed by mass spectrometry or gas chromatography. Both systems generate a complex chart of peaks that requires computer analysis. Quinn (1977) and Meuzelaar et al (1977) reviewed current progress. The latter use a low voltage four-channel mass spectrometer which can handle the products of Curie point pyrolysis of 20 bacterial colonies per hour. The gas chromatograph can only deal with two specimens per hour and has a lower resolving power. Feltham and Sneath (1977) used electrophoretic trace analysis of bacterial proteins. Finally hybridisation studies with nucleic acids provide useful taxonomic data, but are impractical for routine use.

ANTIBIOTICS

Antibiotic technology is more defined than that needed for isolation and identification of microbes, and so more amenable to mechanisation.

Antibiotic assays
Assays may be needed for three reasons: by drug firms to establish the pharmacokinetics of a new agent, or to quality control a product; and by the users to

monitor patient therapy. The drug firm may warrant an automatic plating machine (Sykes and Evans, 1975) and an automatic plate reader capable of image analysis of zones, and computer comparison of the results with pre-programmed regression lines; or at least a pair of electronic calipers able to turn a zone size into a computer input or digital reading. The user on the other hand does relatively few tests, sometimes at great intervals and so may not warrant automation except on grounds of accuracy; radioimmunossays can be used if an antiserum is available, and presumptively ELISA too.

Susceptibility tests

Two approaches to susceptibility tests are currently being explored: the multi-well tray (with replicator) and the fully automatic machine. A simple approach with multi-well trays or agar plates containing antibiotic dilutions allows the screening of many strains with ease and economy (Fung and Hartman, 1975, Newsom, 1975). Inoculum reproducibility is an important property of multi-point inoculators, and can be tested by measuring the carry-over of methylene blue—either as drops onto blotting paper, or in a colorimeter set at 535 nm. I found that the eyes of No. 11 Needles in a home made inoculator transferred 0.001 ml ± 21 per cent SD, which seemed acceptable. Tilton et al (1973) tested a commercial model which had an SD of ± 320 per cent, which was clearly unsatisfactory and caused variable MIC results.

Two commercial micro-tray options are now available: ready made trays primed with dried antibiotic (Seward laboratories) or user-filled trays from a special dispenser teamed up with an inoculator and a reading unit—as in the MIC 2000 (Dynatech) or the Autotiter IV (Canalco). Pre-prepared trays are cheap and standard; machines are expensive and rely on the user's ability to make accurate dilutions, but allow flexibility in the choice of agents tested, and the addition of identification tests if required. Antibiotic deterioration may occur in either system, and the medium used and inoculum size make a considerable difference to the results. Micro-trays are economic in terms of technician time, medium and incubator space (1500 tests need 150 ml and occupy $20 \times 13 \times 8$ cm); furthermore they allow subsequent measurement of bactericidal levels; a parameter currently of increasing interest.

Automation of susceptibility testing might mean quick, reproducible results with minimal effort. Although impedance, microcalorimetry and radiometry might be developed—particularly for slow-growers like *Mycobacterium tuberculosis*, optical sensors are already in use. Praglin et al (1975) described the Autobac (Pfizer)—a semi-automatic system based on forward light-scatter. The test strain is inoculated into a tube of special medium, standardised in a photometer, and added to a tube of Eugon broth used to feed the 13 chambers of a multi-well cuvette. Twelve chambers are loaded with antibiotic discs, and the last is a control. The cuvette is placed in a shaking incubator which holds 30 tests, and when the user notes adequate growth (a minimum of three generation times) he returns it to the photometer. The time required is usually three hours—but *Pseudomonas* spp. take up to five. The logarithm of the light scatter produced by the control culture is compared with that of the initial inoculum, and if adequate the machine measures a 'light scatter index' relating the growth in the antibiotic containing wells with that of the control; and then computes sensitivity to pre-determined break points.

The Abbot/Akromedic MS—2 kinetic analysis system (Spencer et al, 1977) (Fig. 9.5) is fully automatic, but still undergoing proving tests. A multi-well cuvette loaded with antibiotic discs is used, and the inoculum reservoir is separated from the wells by a membrane. After inoculation the cuvette is put on a shaking incubator/analyser module and from then on the process is automatic. Each module holds eight cuvettes and is fitted with light emitting diodes with matched, sensitive, photodetectors. Each diode lights every 5 minutes, and the optical density readings are fed into a Motorola microcomputer capable of monitoring seven modules, i.e. 56 cultures, at a time. The readings are sorted and used to generate individual growth curves which can be printed out or stored on magnetic tape.

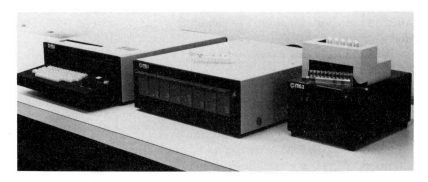

Fig. 9.5   The Abbot/Akromedic MS 2. The computer is on the left, analyser/incubator in the centre, and antibiotic disc dispenser on the right (courtesy of H. J. Spencer)

Once the inoculum goes into log-phase growth, suction is applied and the culture is distributed into ten antibiotic-containing wells plus a control. The microcomputer compares the different growth rates with the control, and when the latter is adequate for differentiation—sensitivity test results are computed in relation to pre-programmed 'break points'.

Mitchell, Curtis and Johnston (1977) also used an optical density detector in their continuous-flow system for testing rapid-growing clinical isolates. They used an automatic sampler linked to a peristaltic pump that fed samples through an incubated 155 min delay coil to a colorimeter set to detect optical density at 425 nm.

The Autobac is the only system to date in worldwide use after thorough trials (Thornsberry et al, 1975) in comparison with disc tests. A seven-centre study gave reproducible results with a 90 per cent agreement with disc tests using 13 agents; only nitrofurantoin gave the low correlation of 77 per cent. The system has been adapted for anaerobes, using a larger inoculum, and for haemophilus with the aid of small carbon dioxide generators.

Most Autobac tests are finished within three hours, although pseudomonas requires up to five. The main discrepancy in the tests was an Autobac-sensitive result, with disc-resistant. This raises some general points relevant to *all* rapid sensitivity tests—namely which gives the correct answer—a reading at 5–8 hrs or an overnight one? Some resistant strains grow more slowly in the presence of the relevant antibiotic—possibly because the resistance is due to inducible enzymes. Such resistance will be missed by a reading at three hours although the control is fully grown, but may be picked up at say five hours. Misleading optical patterns have also been found with the Autobac—although presumptively applicable to all machines based on optical measurements. False sensitivity may be the result of bacterial cells clumping and leaving a clear supernatant (e.g. enterobacter in the presence of ampicillin). False resistance and variable results with ampicillin were noted by Waterworth (1976) to be due to swelling of ampicillin-damaged cells prior to lysis—later readings gave a correct answer.

SEROLOGY

Serology is easily automated as it encompasses large numbers of defined tests. Microtiter trays (Cooke) and the associated dispenser/diluters (Dynatech, Flow) make for simplified handling and economic use of reagents. Other accessories include the Microcompupet (Warner) based on a finely adjustable eight-channel peristaltic pump that can suck or blow; and manually operated multi-tip micro-pipettes. The Autotiter IV (Canalco) and the Bioreacteur (Engelbrecht, 1975) are alternatives for mechanisation of tube tests and Kwantes (1977) reviewed the whole topic.

The Blood Transfusion Service probably has the country's heaviest serological workload, and uses 1 out of a 15-channel continuous flow (Technicon) system for the Carbon VDRL, in which the result appears as drops on an absorbent paper tape. A moving tape also forms the basis of the 'Autotape' machine (Gower, 1977) developed by the Central Veterinary Laboratories, Weybridge in conjunction with Vickers Ltd. The Autotape does 1200 brucella agglutinations per hour. The test, which takes two minutes, is done in a droplet that is carried on the tape through a humidified incubator, past a reading device into a bowl of glutaraldehyde. Such a machine can only be justified in a large central laboratory, but its use alleviated boredom and fatigue in technicians and produced more standardised results.

Enzyme-linked immunosorbent assay (ELISA) is a simple and highly sensitive antibody-detection technique, particularly valuable for use with difficult antigens like helminths or protozoa. Voller described several tests, e.g. Voller and Bidwell (1975) and Denmark and Chessum (1978) detail practical aspects of a reference toxoplasma antibody service. Now that suitable enzyme-linked anti-human globulin is available the test may be put to a wider use, but more data is needed on how antigens adhere to microtiter trays; and just how consistent the adhesion is.

DATA HANDLING

Computers for microbiology have had a slow start. The original grand plans for a computerised hospital record system with direct laboratory input have not materialised and the main value to date has been for classification and identification schemes such as that developed by the National Collection of Type Cultures at Colindale. However the cost of computers has decreased to an incredible degree.

A machine costing $20 million in 1962 can now almost be equalled by one costing $1000, and by 1985 possibly by a $100 unit (Holton, 1977). Thus the laboratory possibilities are vastly increased. Machines already exist with integral micro-computers (e.g. the MS-2) and more may be expected. Goodwin (1976) described the problems and successful introduction of electronic data handling in Northwick Park; Gaya and Thirlwall (1977) described a self-assembly system for under £20,000.

However owning the equipment is one thing—using it is quite another. Pro-grammes are needed, and the right data must be collected and entered. This may create problems, especially if as is usual request forms are badly completed.

CONCLUSION

Mechanical microbiology is an expanding field. I have only been able to outline the possibilities and give some key references. A fuller bibliography was drawn up by Palmer and Le Quesne (1976), and individual chapters will be found in the 'Methods in Microbiology' series (Ed. Norris and Ribbons) and in the 'Technical Reports' of the Society for Applied Bacteriology—all published by Academic Press.

What will actually happen in the routine diagnostic laboratory? The traditions of wire loop and Petri dish will die hard; even so I predict an increasing use of micro trays both for identification/sensitivity testing and for serology—particularly ELISA, and I think that bacteraemia detection by impedance looks very promising —time will tell!

REFERENCES

Bagshawe, K. D. (1975) Computer controlled automated radioimmunoassay. *Laboratory Practice*, **24**, 573–575.

Bascomb, S. & Grantham, C. A. (1975) Automated identification of bacteria. In *Some Methods for Microbiological Assay*, ed. Board, R. G., Lovelock, D. W., pp. 30–55. London: Academic Press.

Beezer, A. E. & Tyrell, H. J. V. (1972) Microcalorimetry. *Science Tools*, **19**, 13–16.

Bettelheim, K. A. & Shaw, E. J. (1978) Microcalorimetry in diagnostic medical microbiology. In *Biological Uses of Microcalorimetry*, ed. Beezer, A. S. London: Academic Press.

Burdash, N. M., West, M. E. & Bannister, E. R. (1976) Automatic gram-staining with the Microstainer 11. *Health Laboratory Sciences*, **13**, 1.

Campbell, J. E. (1977) Estimation of microbial density through pattern recognition. In *Rapid Methods and Automation in Microbiology*, ed. Johnston, H. H. & Newsom, S. W. B., p. 87. Oxford: Learned Information.

Cram, L. S. (1977) Rapid cell analysis and automation of disease diagnosis using flow microfluorometry. In *Rapid Methods and Automation in Microbiology*, ed. Johnston, H. H. & Newsom, S. W. B., pp. 215–221. Oxford: Learned Information.

Deland, F. H. & Wagner, H. N. (1970) Automated radiometric detection of bacterial growth in blood culture. *Journal of Laboratory and Clinical Medicine*, **75**, 529–534.

Denmark, J. R. & Chessum, B. S. (1978) Standardization of enzyme-linked immunosorbent assay (ELISA) and the detection of toxoplasma antibody. *Medical Laboratory Sciences*, **35**, 227–232.

Engelbrecht, E. (1975) The Bioreacteur—a robot technician in *Automation in Microbiology and Immunology*, ed. Hedén, C.-G. & Illeni, T., pp. 411–429. New York: Wiley.

Engvall, E. & Perlmann, P. (1972) Enzyme-linked immunosorbent assay, ELISA. *Journal of Immunology*, **109**, 129–135.

Feltham, R. K. A. & Sneath, P. H. A. (1977) Electrophoretic trace analysis. In *Rapid Methods and Automation in Microbiology*, ed. Johnston, H. H. & Newsom, S. W. B., p. 53. Oxford: Learned Information.

Fung, D. & Hartmann, P. A. (1975) Miniaturized microbiological techniques for rapid characterisation of bacteria. In *New Approaches to the Identification of Microorganisms*, ed. Hedén, C.-G. & Illeni, T., pp. 349–370. New York: Wiley.

Gaya, H. & Thirlwall, J. (1977) Data handling in clinical microbiology in rapid methods and automation in microbiology, eds. Johnston, H. H. & Newsom, S. W. B., pp. 301–306. Oxford: Learned Information.

Goodwin, C. S. & Smith, C. (1976) Computer printing and filing of microbiology reports. *Journal of Clinical Pathology*, **29**, 543–560.

Gower, S. G. M. (1977) Automated serum testing. In *Rapid Methods and Automation in Microbiology*, eds. Johnston, H. H. & Newsom, S. W. B., p. 251. Oxford: Learned Information.

Hayward, N. H. & Jeavons, T. H. (1977) Assessment of a technique for rapid detection of *E. coli* and *proteus* in urine by head-space gas-liquid chromatography. *Journal of Clinical Microbiology*, **6**, 202–206.

Hedén, C.-G. (1975) The modular approach to automation of microbiological routines. In *New Approaches to the Identification of Microorganisms*, ed. Hedén, C.-G. & Illeni, T., pp. 13–39. New York: Wiley.

Hedén, C.-G. & Illeni, T. (1975) *Automation in Microbiology and Immunology*. New York: Wiley.

Heimer, G. V., Joseph, N. & Taylor, C. E. D. (1978) Staining clinical specimens for acid-fast bacilli by means of a mechanical conveyor system. *Journal of Clinical Pathology* (at press).

Herzenberg, L. A., Sweet, R. G. & Gerzenberg, A. (1976) Fluorescence-activated cell sorting. *Scientific American*, **234**, 108–116.

Holton, W. C. (1977) The large scale integration of microelectronic circuits. Ibid, **237**, 82–90.

Johnston, H. H., Mitchell, C. J. & Curtis, G. D. W. (1976) Automated test for the determination of significant bacteriuria. *Lancet*, **ii**, 400–402.

Johnston, H. H. & Newsom, S. W. B. (1977) *Rapid Methods and Automation in Microbiology*. Oxford: Learned Information.

Kagan, R. L., Schuette, W. H., Zierot, C. H. & Maclowry, J. D. (1977) Rapid automated diagnosis of bacteraemia by impedance detection. *Journal of Clinical Microbiology*, **5**, 51–57.

Kelly, M. J. (1977) Aerobic and anaerobic mixture of human pathogens, a rapid 4-plate counting technique. *British Journal of Experimental Pathology*, **58**, 478–483.

Kuhn, I. & Hedén, C.-G. (1977) From biotyping to metabolic fingerprinting. In *Rapid Methods and Automation in Microbiology*, eds. Johnston, H. H. & Newsom, S. W. B., pp. 173–177. Oxford: Learned Information.

Kwantes, W. (1977) Automation in serology. Ibid pp. 197–202.

Laboratory Equipment Digest (1977) Editorial, **15**, 1.

Malik, K. M. (1977) Rapid surface colony counts with three new minituarised techniques. *Zentrall Blatt fur Bakteriologie—Reihe A*, **237**, 415–423.

Meuzellar, H. L. C., Kistemaker, P. G., Eshuis, W. & Engel, H. W. B. (1977) Progress in automated computerised characterisation of microorganisms by pyrolysis mass spectrometry. In *Rapid Methods and Automation in Microbiology*, eds. Johnston, H. H. & Newsom, S. W. B., pp. 225–230. Oxford: Learned Information.

Mitchell, C. J., Johnston, H. H. & Curtis, G. D. W. (1977) Antimicrobial sensitivity testing by a continuous-flow method. Ibid, p. 77.

Newsom, S. W. B. (1975) Easy economic typing of enterobacteria. In *New Approaches to the Identification of Microorganisms*, eds. Heden, C.-G. & Illeni, T., pp. 435–444. New York: Wiley.

Newsom, S. W. B. (1977) In *Laboratory Infections*, pp. 254–256. MD Thesis, Cambridge University.

Palmer, W. J. & Lequesne, S. (1976) *Rapid Methods and Automation in Microbiology and Immunology*. A Bibliography. London: Information Retrieval.

Praglin, J., Curtis, A. C., Longhenry, D. K. & McKie, J. C. (1975) Autobac—A 3-hour automated antimicrobial susceptibility system. In *Automation in Microbiology and Immunology*, eds. Hedén, C.-G. & Illeni, T., pp. 197–209. New York: Wiley.

Quinn, P. (1977) Identification of organisms by pyrolysis. In *Rapid Methods and Automation in Microbiology*, eds. Johnston, H. H. & Newsom, S. W. B., pp. 178–187. Oxford: Learned Information.

Randall, E. (1977) Radiometric detection of microorganisms in blood. Ibid, pp. 144–147.

Sykes, D. A. & Evans, C. J. (1975) An automatic plating-cut machine for microbiological assays. In *Some Methods for Microbiological Assay*, eds. Board, R. D. & Lovelock, D. W., pp. 57–62. London: Academic Press.

Sharpe, A. N. & Jackson, A. K. (1972) Stomaching—a new concept in bacteriological sample preparation. *Applied Microbiology*, **24**, 175.

Sharpe, A. N. & Jackson, A. K. (1975) Two inexpensive instruments for speeding microbiological analysis. In *Automation in Microbiology and Immunology*, eds. Hedén, C.-G. & Illeni, T., pp. 125–138. New York: Wiley.

Spencer, H. J., Stockert, P., Welaj, R., Wilburn, R. & Price, P. (1977). In *Rapid Methods and Automation in Microbiology*, eds. Johnston, H. H. & Newsom, S. W. B., pp. 262–263. Oxford: Learned Information.

Spencer, R. C. (1978) Application of gel diffusion techniques in bacteriology. In *Modern Topics in Infection*, ed. Williams, J. D. London: Heinemann.

Strauss, R. R., Throm, R. & Friedman, H. (1977) Radiometric detection of bacteraemia. Requirement for terminal subcultures. *Journal of Clinical Microbiology*, **5**, 145–148.

Thornsberry, C., Gavan, T. L., Sherris, J. C., Balows, A., Matsen, J. M., Sabath, L. B., Schoernknecht, F., Thrupp, L. D. & Washington, J. A. (1975) Laboratory evaluation of a rapid automated susceptibility testing system—report of a collaborative study. *Antimicrobial Agents and Chemotherapy*, **7**, 466–472.

Throm, R., Strauss, S., Specter, S. & Friedman, H. (1977) Automated blood culture testing using radioisotope and electrical impedance monitoring equipment. In *Rapid Methods and Automation in Microbiology*, eds. Johnston, H. H. & Newsom, S. W. B., pp. 21–23. Oxford: Learned Information.

Tilton, R. C., Lieberman, L. & Gerlach, E. H. (1973) Microdilution antibiotic susceptibility tests—examination of certain variables. *Applied Microbiology*, **26**, 658–665.

Trotman, R. E. (1972) Automatic methods in diagnostic bacteriology. In *Automation, Mechanization and Data Handling in Microbiology*, eds. Baillie A. & Gilbert, R. J., pp. 211–221. London: Academic Press.

Ur, A. (1977) Prospects and limitations of the impedance technique. In *Rapid Methods and Automation in Microbiology*, eds. Johnston, H. H. & Newsom, S. W. B., pp. 245–247. Oxford: Learned Information.

Voller, A. & Bidwell, D. E. (1975) A simple method for detecting antibodies to rubella. *British Journal of Experimental Pathology*, **56**, 338–339.

Waterworth, P. (1976) Automated sensitivity tests. *Journal of Antimicrobial Chemotherapy*, **2**, 104.

Wyatt, P. J. (1975) Automation of differential light scattering for antibiotic susceptibility testing. In *Automation in Microbiology and Immunology*, eds. Hedén, C.-G. & Illeni, T., pp. 267–291. New York: Wiley.

ACKNOWLEDGEMENTS

I am grateful to C. E. D. Taylor for Fig. 9.1, Dr L. Scott Cram for Fig. 9.2, D. F. J. Brown for Fig. 9.3 and Dr H. J. Spencer for Fig. 9.5.

10. Antibiotic policies

Ian Phillips

An antibiotic policy is a set of rules that determines the circumstances under which antibacterial chemotherapeutic agents may—and may not—be prescribed in a given community. It assumes rational chemotherapy for the individual patient: that the antibiotic chosen is likely to cure or prevent his infection; that the pathogen is sensitive to it in vitro; that the risk of side effects is minimised; and that pharmacological and pharmaceutical properties are appropriate. It then superimposes on the definition of rational treatment several other considerations that

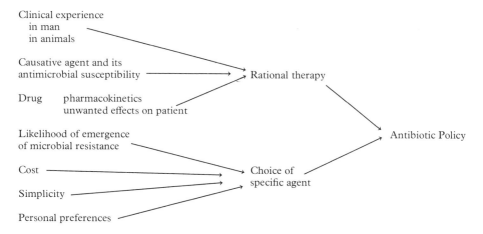

Fig. 10.1   Factors to be assessed in the formulation of an Antibiotic Policy

lead to a suggestion as to which agent, among the several that are rational, should actually be used: the need to prevent the emergence of antibiotic resistance; the need to simplify treatment and its laboratory control; and the need to minimize costs (Fig. 10.1). Because decisions on what is rational depend upon local circumstances and the choice of an individual drug depends upon the personal preferences of the small group of enthusiasts who drew it up, a policy usually has local validity only. Even so, its application by the doctor in charge of the patient is essentially voluntary, and it may be rejected if, in his opinion, circumstances demand it.

The first policies came into being with the emergence of the multiply-resistant 'hospital' staphylococcus. For example, at St Thomas' Hospital in 1959 the new 'Sepsis Committee' set up 'to review hospital infection and to suggest methods for its prevention' soon turned its attention to antibiotics, and following the recommendations of Mary Barber (Barber et al, 1960; Barber, 1963) suggested 'that erythromycin should not be used alone, but always in combination . . . (to) delay the emergence of antibiotic resistance'. Very soon the use of erythromycin, even in combination, was restricted, as was that of methicillin when it became available. Such policies became commonplace for the treatment of all staphylococcal infections.

The problem did not confine itself to staphylococci. With increasing use of antibiotics and changes in medical practice the Gram-negative bacilli became more prevalent and in their turn acquired resistance (Finland, Jones and Barnes, 1959; Barber, 1963; Finland, 1970). This led to the introduction of yet more antibiotics and created confusion as to which agent, among many similar to each other, was best—the second major determinant of the need for a policy for antibiotic use.

The original concept of an antibiotic policy has now been stretched to include not only problems of resistance and problems of choice among appropriate agents, both in and out of hospitals, but also the fundamental problems of rational therapy.

Individual policies have varied in their approach: some have advocated *restriction*, even to the point of total abstinence, while others have suggested *diversification* almost to the point of random use. Other approaches include use of two or three agents in *rotation*, or the use of certain agents only in *combination* (Williams et al, 1960).

Are guides to the use of antibiotics needed? Most microbiologists would say that they are, though some clinicians deny it. Only a few years after the introduction of antibiotics Garrod (1955) drew attention to their indiscriminate use, a theme to be later echoed by many others. Facts on abuse have been slow to emerge, but the subject has recently received renewed attention, especially in the United States. Scheckler and Bennett (1970), Roberts and Visconti (1972), and Kunin, Tupasi and Craig (1973) working in a variety of hospitals, all tell a similar story of clear overuse and abuse of antibiotics. Simmons and Stolley (1974) suggest that 'hundreds of thousands of patients may be unnecessarily exposed to the hazards of antibiotics because of their inappropriate use . . .', and recently Castle et al (1977) at Duke University Medical Center found that one third of all their patients received antibiotics; in 64 per cent of cases they were either not indicated or inappropriately administered. Hospital Accreditation in the U.S.A. now requires a regular review of antimicrobial usage in hospitalised patients (Counts, 1977). There have been few U.K. studies along these lines—perhaps we are less confident than out American colleagues about labelling someone else's treatment inappropriate—but a recent study from Glasgow (Lawson and MacDonald, 1977) suggests that we too may have similar problems.

THE DESIGN OF AN ANTIBIOTIC POLICY

Rational chemotherapy

It is not the purpose of this account to discuss in detail the factors that lead to decisions on rational chemotherapy. There are many guides, including textbooks such as those of Garrod, Lambert and O'Grady (1973) and Smith (1977) as well as shorter accounts such as the Therapeutic Guide (1972) in *Drugs* and those recently published by Bint and Reeves (1978), Geddes (1978) and Wise (1977). Another approach is the series of 'Audits of Antimicrobial Usage' produced for the U.S. Veterans' Administration by Kunin (1977b). However, a brief account of some of the problems in defining rational chemotherapy is appropriate, as this is, at least, the essential foundation of an antibiotic policy, if not a component of it.

The cure and prevention of infection
The fundamental requirement to cure or prevent infection is, except with a few diseases, the most difficult to assess. Most infectious diseases run a variable course and very careful assessment is needed to arrive at the conclusion that a patient has been cured by chemotherapy. The second problem is that in some clinical situations that might give the answer most readily, ethical constraints make clinical trials almost impossible.

Despite these problems there is information on the efficacy of antibiotics in many conditions, ranging from that obtained in formal clinical trials to that from personal experience. Gonorrhoea is often cited as the one disease in which the choice of drug can be shown in comparative clinical trials to determine success or failure. It is thus possible to determine not only which antibiotics cure the patients, but to distinguish between the success rates of closely similar dosage regimens. At the other extreme, in infections for which results in man are not available or difficult to assess, the wise clinician will take note of the results of animal experiments and will follow the difficult path of giving them neither too little nor too much attention (O'Grady, 1976).

As both kinds of clinical information, from therapeutic trials and personal experience, and the results of animal experiments are considered in the discussion as to what constitutes rational therapy, the 'style' of an individual or circumstances in an institution are often dominant, making antibiotic policies overall more suitable for local rather than universal use.

The causative organism
The first important need is the demonstration of what organisms are associated with particular diseases (McGowan and Finland, 1974a). Next is the determination of their in vitro antibiotic susceptibility. The standard parameters are the minimum inhibitory concentration (MIC) and, in certain cases, minimum bactericidal concentration (MBC) of the antibiotic in liquid or solid medium for a reasonable inoculum of the organism. The method of testing affects the results considerably and technical problems must be taken into account in any assessment of the value of the investigation.

The case for the clinical relevance of high-level resistance seems relatively clear, although local concentration of antibiotic, as in the bile or in the urine, may result in seeming anomalies. The importance of low-level in vitro resistance is much more difficult to assess.

Another problem arises with the assessment of agents that are destroyed or inactivated by bacterial enzymes. It seems reasonable to choose agents in any particular class that are resistant to them but the argument continues as to whether a minor degree of inactivation has any clinical relevance. Greater susceptibility such as that of benzylpenicillin to gonococcal β-lactamase clearly does matter because treatment of gonorrhoea caused by such an organism is unsuccessful with penicillin.

It has been suggested that the use of MICs and MBCs is naïve and that they have little to do with infection in patients. Several workers have used in vitro models that allow a more dynamic approach to the problem. It seems possible that continuous observations on the behaviour of cultures might tell us more about the dynamics of infection, but whether it is a better guide to the choice of an antibiotic is still debatable.

The information gleaned from in vitro determinations of antibiotic sensitivity is used in two ways. The first is in the drawing up of tables of resistance that determine rational therapy in general: if 80 per cent of isolates of *Staph. aureus* are penicillin resistant it is probably irrational to use benzylpenicillin for the treatment of patients with severe staphylococcal infections of undetermined sensitivity. The second use is in the management of an individual patient's infection: if his staphylococcus has been shown to be one of the few penicillin-sensitive strains, it is now rational to use benzylpenicillin.

Pharmacokinetics

It is reasonable to suggest that a policy for treatment should indicate the use of an agent that reaches the site of infection in adequate concentrations. The antibiotic must clearly be absorbed from its site of administration and must then be carried in the blood, where its concentration can be measured, to the site of infection. The clinical relevance of binding to plasma proteins remains another matter for debate.

If the infection is in the bile, urine, eye, or meninges, or results in the accumulation of an exudate as in the pleural or peritoneal cavities or joints, or even if there is an accumulation of pus in the tissues, it is relatively easy to find out whether the antibiotic is present in sufficient concentration. But it is usually impossible to determine the antibiotic concentration at the actual site of infection in the tissues. Thus another of the foundation stones of rational chemotherapy requires very careful assessment and judgement.

Unwanted effects on patients

Unwanted effects of antibiotics, which are said to occur in about 5 per cent of hospitalised patients who receive them (Simmons and Stolley, 1974), include toxicity, hypersensitivity, and superinfection as well as difficulties in administration arising from irritant effects on tissues. Such unwanted effects of antibiotics are a major determinant of their clinical use. Major limitation of use is usual where severe toxicity is predictable even though rare. Thus in the U.K., chloramphenicol is largely reserved for the treatment of enteric fever and meningitis, and possibly infections due to organisms resistant to other agents in vitro. If toxicity is dose related, usually declaring itself most readily in patients with excretory failure, any antibiotic policy that suggests the use of a particular toxic agent must give guidance on its prevention, as for example with aminoglycosides. Finally, rational therapy must include an assessment of the importance of hypersensitivity to given antibiotics, both in terms of their general incidence, and of the management of the individual known to be hypersensitive to a given drug.

Choice of antibiotic

Having made the difficult decisions on what constitutes rational chemotherapy for specific types of infection and for particular infected patients, the clinician now turns to the other aspect of antibiotic policy that will guide him to a specific choice. As has already been stated, this is largely based on four factors, which will now be considered in more detail.

Emergence of resistance

It has already been suggested that the emergence of multiple antibiotic resistance in *Staphylococcus aureus* was the first stimulus to the drawing up of antibiotic policies. Did these policies actually prevent resistance? Mary Barber and her colleagues at the Postgraduate Medical School (Barber et al, 1960) clearly felt that by restricting the use of all antibiotics to patients in whom there was a prospect of benefit, the total withdrawal of penicillin, and the use of antibiotics in combination (along with measures to control cross infection) they reversed resistance trends in *Staphylococcus aureus*. Ridley and his colleagues at St Thomas' Hospital (Ridley et al, 1970) came to similar conclusions. The St Thomas' results which are now available up to 1977 are worth examination in detail (Table 10.1). In 1958, with no concerted policy in operation, but with measures to limit cross-infection, 80 per cent of *Staph. aureus* isolates were resistant to penicillin and 20 per cent resistant also to streptomycin, tetracycline and usually erythromycin. The first policy was one of restriction: erythromycin was largely withdrawn (only a tenth as much was used in 1959 as in 1958) and erythromycin resistance fell to under 5 per cent. On the introduction of methicillin this too was restricted and at the same time the combined use of erythromycin and novobiocin was recommended. About 5 kg of novobiocin were used in the hospital in 1961. By 1962 about 20 per cent of staphylococci were again erythromycin resistant: the policy of use of combinations may have delayed, but did not seem to prevent this. By the end of 1965 it had become clear that the predicted increase in methicillin resistance had not occurred and erythromycin, novobiocin and the newly available sodium fusidate were restricted to patients hypersensitive to penicillins or infected with methicillin-resistant staphylococci, and infections were treated either with penicillin or methicillin or cloxacillin. The consumption of erythromycin was only about 0.5 kg per year between 1966 and 1968 and that of novobiocin declined to 50 mg in 1968: like McGowan and Finland (1974b) we have demonstrated that a policy of restriction actually results in a decline in the use of an antibiotic. After 1969, erythromycin resistance remained at low levels, and at the same time combined resistance to streptomycin and tetracycline declined markedly. It is of interest that during this period chloramphenicol resistance in staphylococci occurred mainly in a ward in which a senior surgeon used the antibiotic extensively, and it disappeared when he retired. Methicillin resistance became gradually more prevalent until 1968–69 after which it hovered between 1 and 2 per cent among all isolates and then it too declined, so that in 1977 there was only one isolate. After 1970, clindamycin and fusidic acid were used more often, and re-

Table 10.1 St Thomas' Hospital policy and resistance of *Staphylococcus aureus*

% isolates resistant to	1958	1959	1960	1961	1962	1963	1964	1965	1966	1967	1968	1969	1970	1971	1972	1973	1974	1975	1976	1977
Year																				
P	80	62	75	63	72	63	72	75	62	73	75	72	78	74	79	82	81	79	85	83
PST	20	32	35	25	31	32	18	24	14	9	5	7	7	8	5	4	3	0.4	Not tested	
M	Not tested							0.1	0.2	0.5	1	2	1	1	1	2	1	0.4	0.4	<.05
E	18	4	4	2	20	24	15	17	4	3	4	9	3	3	2.5	5	4.5	5	6	7
L	Not tested													0	0.3	0.3	1	0.5	0.4	0.5
F	Not tested												0	2	2.5	2	2	2.6	3.4	4
Total number of isolates	202	771	629	762	1089	1133	1240	1397	957	973	935	1109	1128	1414	1759	1476	1441	1348	1748	2305
Antibiotic policy	None	erythromycin restricted	i. penicillin; ii. erythromycin plus novobiocin; iii. methicillin or cloxacillin						i. penicillin; ii. methicillin or cloxacillin; ENvF restricted					gradual relaxation of policy: increased use of clindamycin and fusidic acid			decreasing use of clindamycin		

*P penicillin, S streptomycin, T tetracycline, M methicillin, E erythromycin, L lincomycin/clindamycin, F fusidic acid, Nv novobiocin sistance to them climbed to about 1–2 per cent in 1974: clindamycin resistance then declined somewhat associated with a dramatic decrease in the use of the drug, while the incidence of resistance to erythromycin and fusidic acid continued to increase gradually, associated with their more widespread use.

Can we therefore conclude that our antibiotic policies, which have involved restriction, combined use and rotation, have actually worked in terms of preventing the emergence of resistance? The evidence is fairly convincing that this was so for erythromycin and chloramphenicol, and others (Kirby and Ahern, 1953; Lepper et al, 1954; Lowbury, 1955; Shooter, 1957; Hinton and Orr, 1957; Barber et al, 1958; Goodier and Parry, 1959; Wallmark and Finland, 1961) noted similar results for these drugs. The rise, albeit slight, in the incidence of resistance to methicillin, clindamycin and fusidic acid might also have been a direct result of our policies. But what are we to make of the subsequent decline of methicillin resistance in the face of ever-increasing use of penicillins, and the continuing decline since 1963 of multiple resistance to such an extent that the 'hospital staphylococcus' has largely disappeared even from the hospital that contributed significantly to its invention? The latter might be due to a more conservative use of streptomycin and tetracycline, as was offered as an explanation of similar findings in the U.S.A. (Bulger and Sherris, 1968) and in Denmark (Rosendal et al, 1977). Others have suggested that it is the staphylococcus that has quite spontaneously declined (Parker, 1971), though it is worthy of note that the phenomenon is not universal: Ayliffe et al (1977) have reported convincing multiple-resistance problems in dermatology and burns units.

Policies for the treatment of infections due to other organisms, particularly Gram-negative bacilli, emerged when they started to increase in prevalence and in antibiotic resistance in the 1960s. Finland, Jones and Barnes (1959) and later Finland (1970) have given detailed accounts of this increase and blamed it on the use of antibiotics, among other factors. Mouton and his colleagues (Mouton, Glerum and Van Loenen, 1976) have recently followed the emergence of resistance of Staph. aureus, Klebsiella spp., Esch. coli and Proteus spp., and have found more complex relationships with the usage of various antibiotics, some direct but some paradoxical. Their paper includes a useful summary of the work of the others on the subject.

There are few parallels of the detailed work on staphylococci to assess the effects of antibiotic policies on the control of resistance in Gram-negative organisms. Price and Sleigh (1970) imposed total restriction of antibiotic use to eradicate Klebsiella aerogenes and Lowbury, Babb and Roe (1972) restricted carbenicillin totally, and to a lesser extent ampicillin, cephaloridine, tetracycline and kanamycin, and eradicated carbenicillin-resistant Ps. aeruginosa. It is as yet too early to know whether policies restricting the use of the new cephalosporins and aminoglycosides will preserve their usefulness.

Cost
The first requirement is that therapy should be needed: unnecessary treatment is unnecessarily expensive (Kunin, Tupasi and Craig, 1973). When the need for treatment has been established, and despite statements that cost should not be a limiting factor in prescribing, it has always been reasonable to ask clinicians to use

the cheapest among a group of equally effective agents. But cost consciousness should not be carried to extremes: unless a product actually contains the stated amount of the drug, unchanged and unadulterated, there is no true benefit.

The real problem, however, lies in the requirement for equal efficacy, and even this is not absolute. It may be reasonable to use a drug less likely to be effective if the patient is not severely ill and such a trial is without significant risk. A sulphonamide is often suggested for the treatment of cystitis in a domiciliary context although the more expensive co-trimoxazole, with a broader spectrum, might be preferable if a favourable response is more important, as for example if the patient has pyelonephritis. If the patient has septicaemia, it might be reasonable to substitute gentamicin, at considerable cost.

Simplicity

Over 20 years ago Garrod (1955), regretting that so many antibiotics had been discovered, suggested that 'the choice is now so wide, and the indications are so complex, that few clinicians can keep fully abreast of knowledge about them'. Multiplicity of antibiotics is now vastly more confusing, particularly in the context of β-lactam antibiotics and aminoglycosides. How is the average clinician, having decided to use a cephalosporin, to decide between cephaloridine, cephalothin, cephalexin, cephradine, cefamandole, cefuroxime and cefoxitin, assuming that a given organism is sensitive to all? Even when the various routes of administration have been sorted out, a wide choice remains. Either by a process of reasoning, taking into account all the factors involved in rational chemotherapy, or by tossing a coin (does it matter which?) a decision can be made to use, say, one parenteral and one oral preparation.

There is another consideration however, that will often over-ride this, and that is the need for simplicity in the laboratory. Few clinical microbiologists will be anxious to include in their basic sensitivity testing scheme more than one or two similar agents. Furthermore, they will also be disinclined to establish assay systems for all the members of a given drug family. For many years we have discouraged the use of kanamycin and encouraged the use of gentamicin for this reason.

Finally, the pharmacist requires simplicity. It is unreasonable to expect him to stock large numbers of infrequently-used antibiotics with very similar properties.

Personal preferences

It would be reassuring if we could state that personal preferences are firmly based on factors relevant only to the treatment of the patient. However, they are also influenced by the persuasive powers of others, perhaps especially those of the pharmaceutical firms, whose activities vary from the direct to the highly subtle depending on circumstances. It is not my intention to denigrate the pharmaceutical industry, but merely to underline their need to sell a product and their legitimate use of all the skills of advertising to do so. We require equal skill to assess what they tell us and it is particularly regrettable that decisions based on their information are often left in the hands of doctors not competent to assess it.

Examples of antibiotic policies

The basic principles of restriction, rotation, diversification and use in combination have resulted in a bewildering array of suggestions on which particular antibiotics should be used in given circumstances. Detailed discussion of each of them would be fruitless but the conclusions reached by one group (Lowbury et al, 1975) will serve as an example of a well-balanced policy. They advocate basing antibiotic policies on locally-determined patterns of resistance, and give examples of different policies for different hospitals in one city. They suggested that antibiotics should be placed in three categories: the first consists of antibiotics for unrestricted prescription for sensitive organisms—for one hospital, penicillin, sulphonamides, nitrofurantoin and tetracycline; the second has antibiotics that should be prescribed with restraint (because of resistance or toxicity)—ampicillin, streptomycin, kanamycin, cloxacillin, novobiocin, cephalosporins, nalidixic acid, colistin and chloramphenicol; the third has antibiotics to be used only on a consultant's recommendation, for severe infection, for organisms resistant to other agents, and for blind therapy of severe infection—gentamicin, carbenicillin, fucidin, rifamycins, vancomycin, lincomycin and co-trimoxazole. Following the same principles a second hospital in the same group emerged with rather different lists, and furthermore these had almost completely changed in 1974.

MANAGEMENT OF ANTIBIOTIC POLICIES

The antibiotic committee

An account of the setting up of a sepsis committee in 1959 in St Thomas' has already been given. In 1960, after less than two years, it suggested the creation of a second committee to 'consider, continually review, recommend and give information on antibiotic policy in the hospital'. Thus the St Thomas' Antibiotic Committee came into existence. Its first document recommended the formulation of a general policy of uniform use of antibiotics to which infecting organisms were susceptible, an avoidance of topical therapy, and the reservation of newly-introduced antibiotics.

In the U.S.A. Kunin (1977a) suggests that the guidelines on antimicrobial usage drawn up by the Veterans' Administration (Kunin, 1977b) should be used in arriving at a policy for individual hospitals after the guidelines have been thoroughly reviewed and debated by staff. Whatever the basis, discussion is essential.

An Antibiotic Committee, which may be a sub-committee of a Pharmacy or Therapeutics Committee, is useful in initiating such discussions. It should have among its members a microbiologist, a physician, a surgeon and a pharmacist, and, if they are available, an infectious diseases specialist and a clinical pharmacologist. When the time seems ripe, a general practitioner might be added—we have just taken this step, necessary in our view when the extent of antibiotic prescribing in general practice is realised (Skegg, Doll and Perry, 1977). The members of the committee should be senior and respected, and thus more likely to be able to persuade errant clinical colleagues to comply. It should be properly constituted within the committee framework of a Health District, and should meet about twice a year unless circumstances dictate more frequent meetings.

Enforcement of policy
Having decided on an antibiotic policy on the results of an assessment of the factors discussed above, the Committee is faced with the task of dissemination of information and the enforcement of the policy.

Dissemination of the information has received considerable attention. Our own initial efforts consisted of two cyclostyled sheets submitted first to the whole Medical Committee and then widely distributed in the hospital. It contained the current policy for treating staphylococcal infections and notes on recommended available penicillins, colomycin and fucidin. By 1963 it contained recommendations on the avoidance of topical therapy and the treatment of urgent, bacteriologically undiagnosed cases, recommending the combined use of cloxacillin and ampicillin, as well as antistaphylococcal treatment and notes on ampicillin. From these simple beginnings there evolved in gradual stages the first privately-printed booklet for internal use in St Thomas' Hospital in 1966. Many others have produced similar guides for limited local use. There have also been publications designed for more general use such as *A Pocket Guide to Antimicrobial Chemotherapy* (Ridley, 1971) and *Clinicians Guide to Antibiotic Therapy* (Noone, 1977). *A Guide to the Use of Antimicrobial Drugs* (South East Thames Regional Health Authority, 1977) produced by a Region's microbiologists is a new type of collaboration. However, as already suggested, the more generalised a publication becomes the less useful, in certain ways, it becomes. It cannot, for example, take full account of differences between institutions. As Lowbury et al (1975) pointed out 'in Dudley Road (Birmingham) in 1971 a severe wound infection with a *Klebsiella* could be treated with kanamycin: in the Burns Unit of Birmingham Accident Hospital, kanamycin would be an incorrect choice . . .' But, perhaps most important, it cannot rely on the personal authority of the authors among their own colleagues. There would seem then still to be a case for local publications instead of or as a supplement to general publications.

Enforcement of antibiotic policies and assessments of clinicians' compliance have been given less attention than dissemination of information. Education of the prescriber is an important prerequisite (Counts, 1977). Neu and Howrey (1975) have described self-assessment and learning techniques, and Kunin (1977a, b) has set out the U.S. Veterans' Administration's programme of audits on antimicrobial therapy, which educate the prescriber and then test standards of prescribing in some detail. Lockwood (1974) has suggested the setting up of 'Antibiotics Anonymous' groups to control the syndrome of Compulsive Antibiotic Prescribing (CAP).

The very first St Thomas' policy charged the microbiologist with recommending which antibiotic was most suitable—a most important innovation in the context of policy enforcement, which has evolved into our present system of selective reporting of antibiotic sensitivities coupled with, or sometimes replaced by, a direct recommendation. For example, only three antibiotics, penicillin, flucloxacillin and erythromycin, out of the eight routinely tested, are reported to the clinician in the case of *Staph. aureus*, and for *Strep. pyogenes* we merely print 'penicillin recommended' unless the organism is resistant to tetracycline, in which case this fact is reported along with the recommendation.

The work of McGowan and Finland (1974b, 1976) in Boston has demonstrated that requiring justification before antibiotic treatment starts can have a profound effect on prescribing. Kunin et al (1973) in the U.S.A. and more recently Perry and Guyatt (1977) in Canada have also advocated discussions of this kind, demonstrating the importance in their context of the involvement of infectious diseases consultants and the provision of a good laboratory service. The two functions are often combined in this context in Britain and the *Lancet* (1974) has suggested that the prerequisite for any successful antibiotic and infection control policy is an active, clinically orientated medical microbiology department. Extensive 'peer review' of antibiotic prescribing is unfortunately not yet possible in most hospitals in Britain. Our approach to the problem at St Thomas' Hospital may be of interest. We confine ourselves to restricted antibiotics: if one of these is prescribed we are informed by the pharmacy, and a microbiologist then discusses the prescription with the clinician.

Other possible approaches to control are the omission of drugs from formularies, a requirement for written justification, the use of automatic limitations of duration of treatment, and a requirement for bacteriological confirmation of infection (Counts, 1977).

Consultation, between clinicians and microbiologists, involving the assessment and updating of all the factors that lead to sound antibiotic prescribing, is essential. If antibiotic policies ensure that these discussions take place, we have a good case for continuing them.

REFERENCES

Ayliffe, G. A. J., Green, W., Livingston, R. & Lowbury, E. J. L. (1977) Antibiotic-resistant *Staphylococcus aureus* in dermatology and burns wards. *Journal of Clinical Pathology*, **30**, 40.

Barber, M. (1963) Antibiotics and hospital infection in *Infection in Hospitals*, eds. Williams, R. E. O. & Shooter, R. A., p. 289. Oxford: Blackwell.

Barber, M., Csillag, A. & Medway, A. J. (1958) Staphylococcal infection resistant to chloramphenicol, erythromycin and novobiocin. *British Medical Journal*, **ii**, 1377.

Barber, M., Dutton, A. A. C., Beard, M. A., Elmes, P. C. & Williams, R. (1960) Reversal of antibiotic resistance in hospital staphylococcal infections. *British Medical Journal*, **i**, 11.

Bint, A. J. & Reeves, D. S. (1978) A guide to new antibiotics. *British Journal of Hospital Medicine*, **19**, 335.

Bulger, R. J. & Sherris, J. C. (1968) Decreased incidence of antibiotic resistance among *Staphylococcus aureus*. *Annals of Internal Medicine*, Vol. 69, 6.

Castle, M., Wilfert, C. M., Cate, T. R. & Osterhout, S. (1977) Antibiotic use at Duke University Medical Center. *Journal of American Medical Association*, **237**, 2819.

Counts, G. W. (1977) Review and control of antimicrobial usage in hospitalized patients. *Journal of American Medical Association*, **238**, 2170.

Finland, M. (1970) Changing ecology of bacterial infections as related to antibacterial chemotherapy. *Journal of Infectious Diseases*, **122**, 419.

Finland, M., Jones, W. K. & Barnes, M. W. (1959) Occurrence of serious bacterial infections since the introduction of antibacterial agents. *Journal of American Medical Association*, **170**, 2188.

Garrod, L. P. (1955) Present position of the chemotherapy of bacterial infections. *British Medical Journal*, **ii**, 756.

Garrod, L. P., Lambert, H. P. & O'Grady, F. (1973) *Antibiotics and Chemotherapy*. Edinburgh: Churchill Livingstone.

Geddes, A. M. (1978) Antibacterial chemotherapy. *Medicine* (3rd series), **3**, 155.

Goodier, T. W. & Parry, W. R. (1959) Sensitivity of clinically important bacteria to six common antibacterial substances. *Lancet*, **i**, 356.

Hinton, N. A. & Orr, J. H. (1957) Studies on the incidence and distribution of antibiotic-resistant staphylococci. *Journal of Laboratory and Clinical Medicine*, **49**, 566.

Kirby, W. M. M. & Ahern, J. J. (1953) Changing patterns of resistance of staphylococci to antibiotics. *Antibiotics and Chemotherapy*, **3**, 831.

Kunin, C. M. (1977a) Guidelines and audits for use of antimicrobial agents in hospitals. *Journal of Infectious Diseases*, **135**, 335.

Kunin, C. M. (1977b) Audits of Antimocrobial Usage. *Journal of American Medical Association*, **237**, 1001, 1134, 1241, 1366, 1481, 1605, 1723, 1859, 1967.

Kunin, C. M., Tupasi, T. & Craig, W. A. (1973) Use of antibiotics. A brief exposition of the problem and some tentative solutions. *Annals of Internal Medicine*, **79**, 555.

Lancet (1974) Antibiotics for disease (Leader) *Lancet*, **ii**, 1054.

Lawson, D. H. & MacDonald, S. (1977) Antibacterial therapy in general wards. *Postgraduate Medical Journal*, **53**, 306.

Lepper, M. H., Moulton, B., Dowling, H. F., Jackson, G. G. & Kofman, S. (1954) Epidemiology of erythromycin-resistant staphylococci in a hospital population. *Antibiotic Annual, 1953–54*, p. 308.

Lockwood, W. R. (1974) Antibiotics anonymous. *New England Journal of Medicine*, **290**, 465.

Lowbury, E. J. L. (1955) Cross-infection of wounds with antibiotic resistant organisms. *Lancet*, **i**, 985.

Lowbury, E. J. L., Babb, J. R. & Roe, E. (1972) Clearance from a hospital of Gram-negative bacilli that transfer carbenicillin resistance to *Pseudomonas aeruginosa*. *Lancet*, **ii**, 941.

Lowbury, E. J. L., Ayliffe, G. A. J., Geddes, A. M. & Williams, J. D. (1975) *Control of Hospital Infection*. London: Chapman and Hall.

McGowan, J. E. & Finland, M. (1974a) Infection and antibiotic usage at Boston City Hospital: changes in prevalence during the decade 1964–73. *Journal of Infectious Diseases*, **129**, 421.

McGowan, J. E. & Finland, M. (1974b) Use of antibiotics in a general hospital: effects of requiring justification. *Journal of Infectious Diseases*, **130**, 165.

McGowan, J. E. & Finland, M. (1976) Effects of monitoring the usage of antibiotics: an inter-hospital comparison. *Southern Medical Journal*, **69**, 193.

Mouton, R. P., Glerum, J. H. & Van Loenen, A. C. (1976) Relationship between antibiotic consumption and frequency of antibiotic resistance of four pathogens—a seven-year study. *Journal of Antimicrobial Chemotherapy*, **2**, 9.

Neu, H. C. & Howrey, S. P. (1975) Testing the physician's knowledge of antibiotic use: self-assessment and learning via videotape. *New England Medical Journal*, **293**, 1291.

Noone, P. (1977) *A clinician's guide to Antibiotic Therapy*. Oxford: Blackwell.

O'Grady, F. (1976) Animal models in the assessment of antimicrobial agents. *Journal of Antimicrobial Chemotherapy*, **2**, 1.

Parker, M. T. (1971) Current national patterns: Great Britain. In *Nosocomial Infections*, eds. Brachman, P. S. & Eickhoff, T. C. Chicago: American Hospitals Association.

Perry, T. L. & Guyatt, G. H. (1977) Antimicrobial drug use in three Canadian general hospitals. *Canadian Medical Association Journal*, **116**, 253.

Price, D. J. E. & Sleigh, J. D. (1970) Control of infection due to *Klebsiella aerogenes* in a neurosurgical unit by withdrawal of all antibiotics. *Lancet*, **ii**, 1213.

Ridley, M. (1971) *A pocket guide to antimicrobial chemotherapy*. London: Medical Illustrations and Publications.

Ridley, M., Barrie, D., Lynn, R. & Stead, K. (1970) Antibiotic-resistant *Staphylococcus aureus* and hospital antibiotic policies. *Lancet*, **i**, 230.

Roberts, A. W. & Visconti, J. A. (1972) The rational and irrational use of systemic antimicrobial drugs. *American Journal of Hospital Pharmacy*, **29**, 828.

Rosendal, K., Jessen, O., Betzon, M. W. & Bülow, P. (1977) Antibiotic policy and spread of *Staphylococcus aureus* strains in Danish hospitals, 1969–1974. *Acta pathologica et microbiologica Scandinavica*, Section B, **85**, 143.

Scheckler, W. E. & Bennett, J. V. (1970) Antibiotic usage in seven community hospitals. *Journal of American Medical Association*, **213**, 264.

Shooter, R. A. (1957) The problem of resistant organisms and chemotherapeutic sensitivity in surgery. *Proceedings of Royal Society of Medicine*, **50**, 158.

Simmons, H. E. & Stolley, P. D. (1974) This is medical progress? Trends and consequences of antibiotic use in the United States. *Journal of American Medical Association*, **227**, 1023.

Skegg, D. C. G., Doll, R. & Perry, J. (1977) Use of medicines in general practice. *British Medical Journal*, **i**, 1561.

Smith, H. (1977) *Antibiotics in clinical practice*. Tunbridge Wells: Pitman Medical.

South-East Thames Regional Health Authority (1977) *A guide to the use of antimicrobial drugs.*

Therapeutic Guide (1972) A guide to the selection of a systemic antibacterial agent. *Drugs*, **4,** 132.

Wallmark, G. & Finland, M. (1961) Phage types and antibiotic susceptibility of pathogenic staphylococci. Results at Boston City Hospital 1949–1960 and comparison with previous years. *Journal of American Medical Association*, **175,** 886.

Williams, R. E. O., Blowers, R., Garrod, L. P. & Shooter, R. A. (1960) In *Hospital Infection, Causes and Prevention*, p. 213. London: Lloyd-Luke.

Wise, R. (1977) Rational choice of antibiotics. *Practitioner*, **219,** 449.

11. Enzymes which modify aminoglycoside antibiotics

A. V. Reynolds and J. T. Smith

Aminoglycoside antibiotics are widely used in the treatment of bacterial infections. However, as their use has increased, so too has bacterial resistance. This problem is exacerbated by two factors. First, transmissible drug resistance plasmids are usually responsible for the insensitivity of clinical bacteria to these drugs. Second, the resistance conferred by plasmids is complex in that, depending on the plasmid concerned, a bewildering variety of cross-resistance patterns occur.

Before 1965 it was believed that plasmid-mediated resistance to aminoglycoside antibiotics resulted from impermeability which prevented the drugs from reaching their target site. This hypothesis was based on two observations; firstly, cell-free protein synthesis systems derived from resistant bacteria were still sensitive to the drug and secondly, when resistant cells were incubated with the drug, inactivation did not seem to occur. However, Okamoto and Suzuki (1965) were able to show that cell-free extracts of amioglycoside resistant organisms *did* inactivate the antibiotics provided that appropriate co-factors were added. The cell-free extracts were shown to contain enzymes responsible for the inactivation. Since then the enzymic mechanisms of aminoglycoside-resistance have been extensively elucidated, in particular by groups of workers led by H. Umezawa, J. Davies, S. Mitsuhashi and F. Le Goffic. They have shown that there are three basic ways in which resistant organisms modify these antibiotics; O-phosphorylation and O-adenylylation, where the co-factor is ATP, and N-acetylation, where the co-factor is acetyl coA. Several reviews have been written on this subject (for example, Benveniste and Davies, 1973a; Umezawa, 1974, 1975; Haas and Dowding, 1975) and a rational system of nomenclature has also been proposed (Mitsuhashi, 1975). However, several new enzymes have been discovered since then. This review attempts to describe enzymes responsible for aminoglycoside resistance, clarify their nomenclature and discuss clinical implications. The nomenclature proposed by Mitsuhashi (1975) is based on resistance phenotypes. However, as described below, resistance can be dependant on the strain producing the enzyme, and therefore the nomenclature used here is based on the properties of the enzymes themselves. Table 11.1 lists the enzymes described to date, and where appropriate, the corresponding trivial name. Table 11.2 shows the substrate profiles of these enzymes with some other relevant properties.

Aminoglycoside antibiotics can be divided into two main groups, those based on L-glucose (such as streptomycin) and those based on D-glucose (such as kanamycin). Enzymes that modify antibiotics containing L-glucose do not attack those containing D-glucose and vice versa; therefore this review has been divided on these lines.

Table 11.1   Enzymes which modify aminoglycoside antibiotics

Rational name		Trivial name
Aminoglycoside 6'-N-acetyltransferase-I	(AAC (6')-I)	Kanamycin acetyltransferase
Aminoglycoside 6'-N-acetyltransferase-II, -III, -IV	(AAC (6')-II, -III, -IV)	—
Aminoglycoside 2'-N-acetyltransferase	(AAC (2'))	Gentamicin acetyltransferase II
Aminoglycoside 3-N-acetyltransferase-I	(AAC (3)-I)	Gentamicin acetyltransferase I
Aminoglycoside 3-N-acetyltransferase-II	(AAC (3)-II)	—
Aminoglycoside 3-N-acetyltransferase-III	(AAC (3)-III)	Gentamicin acetyltransferase III
Aminoglycoside 2"-O-nucleotidyltransferase	(ANT (2"))	Gentamicin adenylyl synthetase
Aminoglycoside 4'-O-nucleotidyltransferase	(ANT (4'))	Tobramycin adenylyl transferase
Aminoglycoside 3'-O-phosphotransferase-Ia	(APH (3')-Ia)	Neomycin-Kanamycin phosphotransferase I
Aminoglycoside 3'-O-phosphotransferase-Ib	(APH (3')-Ib)	—
Aminoglycoside 3'-O-phosphotransferase-II	(APH (3')-II)	Neomycin-Kanamycin phosphotransferase II
Aminoglycoside 3'-O-phosphotransferase-III, -IV	(APH (3')III, -IV)	—
Aminoglycoside 2"-O-phosphotransferase	(APH (2"))	—
Aminoglycoside 5"-O-phosphotransferase	(APH (5"))	—
Aminoglycoside 3"-O-adenylyltransferase	(AAD (3"))	Streptomycin-spectinomycin adenylyltransferase
Aminoglycoside 6-O-adenylyltransferase	(AAD (6))	—
Aminoglycoside 3"-O-phosphotransferase	(APH (3"))	Streptomycin phosphotransferase
Aminoglycoside 6-O-phosphotransferase	(APH (6))	—

Table 11.2   Substrate specificity profiles of enzymes modifying D-aminoglycoside antibiotics

Antibiotic	AAC 6' I	AAC 6' II	AAC 6' III	AAC 6' IV	AAC 2' (†)	AAC 3 I (†)	AAC 3 II (†)	AAC 3 III (†)	ANT 2"	ANT 4'	APH 3' Ia	APH 3' Ib	APH 3' II	APH 3' III	APH 3' IV	APH 2"	APH 5"
Kanamycin A	+	+	+	+	–	–	(+)	+	+	+	+	+	+	+	+	+	O
Kanamycin B	+	O	+	+	(+)	(+)	+	+	+	+	+	+	+	+	+	+	O
Kanamycin C	O	⊕	O	O	+	–	+	ND	+	⊕	+	+	+	(+)	+	⊕	O
Dideoxy Kanamycin B	+	+	+	⊕	+	–	+	ND	+	O	O	O	O	O	O	⊕	O
Tobramycin	+	+	+	+	+	(+)	+	+	+	+	O	O	O	O	O	+	O
Amikacin	+	+	–	+	–	–	–	–	–	+	–	–	–	–	–	+	O
Gentamicin C₁	–	⊖	–	–	+	+	+	+	+	O	O	O	O	O	O	+	O
Gentamicin C₁A	+	+	+	+	+	+	+	⊕	+	O	O	O	O	O	O	+	O
Gentamicin C₂	+	ND	ND	–	+	+	+	⊕	+	O	O	O	O	O	O	+	O
Gentamicin A	O	O	O	O	–	–	+	ND	+	O	(+)	(+)	+	ND	+	+	O
Gentamicin B	+	⊕	⊕	+	+	–	+	⊕	+	O	+	+	+	⊕	+	+	O
Sisomicin	+	⊕	+	+	+	+	+	+	+	O	O	O	O	O	O	+	O
Netilmicin	+	+	+	⊕	–	–	+	ND	+	O	O	O	O	O	O	+	O
Neomycin B or C	O	O	O	O	+	–	ND	+	O	+	+	+	+	+	+	O	⊕
Paromomycin	O	O	O	O	+	–	–	ND	O	+	+	+	+	+	+	O	⊕
Lividomycin A	O	O	O	O	+	–	+	+	O	+	+	+	–	+	+	O	⊕
Butirosin A or B	+	ND	–	+	–	–	–	–	O	+	–	–	+	+	+	O	ND
Ribostamycin	+	⊕	⊕	(+)	(+)	–	+	ND	O	+	+	+	+	+	+	O	+
Iso-electric point	5.1	7.5	–	5.7	–	7.4	6.4	–	5.1	5.1	6.4	6.7	4.7	–	4.9	5.8	–

Key

+ = Rate is >21% of the rate obtained with kanamycin A

(+) = Rate is 11–20% of the rate obtained with kanamycin A

– = Rate is <10% of the rate obtained with kanamycin A

(†) = As above but taking rate with gentamicin C1 as 100%

⊕ and ⊖ = inspired guesses

O = The substrate lacks the substituent necessary for that modification

ND = Not done

ENZYMES THAT MODIFY D-AMINOGLYCOSIDE ANTIBIOTICS

Acetyl transferases

Aminoglycoside 6'-N-acetyltransferase (AAC (6'))
The aminoglycoside modifying enzyme specified by the R-factor R5 was first described by Okamoto and Suzuki (1965). Umezawa and co-workers further studied this enzyme and showed that kanamycin A (but not kanamycin C, neo-mycin or paromomycin) was inactivated by a cell-free extract in the presence of acetyl CoA (Okanishi et al, 1967). The site of modification was shown to be the 6'-amino group of the D-glucosamine ring, see Fig. 11.1a (Umezawa et al, 1967a).

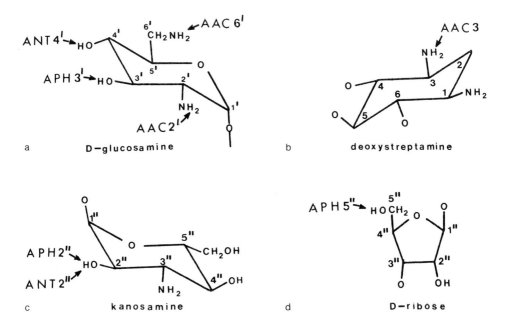

Fig. 11.1   Representative structures to illustrate the sites of modification of D-aminoglycoside antibiotics.

Benveniste and Davies (1971a) studied enzymes from strains of *Escherichia coli* harbouring R5 or NR 79, using the now classical phosphocellulose paper binding assay, with radioactive co-factors. These workers found that kanamycins A and B, neomycin, tobramycin and gentamicin C_{1a} and C_2 were acetylated. Paromomycin, which has a hydroxyl group at C6', and gentamicin C_1 which has a secondary amino group at this position lack the specific site for attack by this enzyme and therefore are not substrates for it. With the exception of kanamycin A and ribostamycin it would seem that all the other antibiotics when acetylated at the 6' amino group still retain significant antibiotic activity (Benveniste and Davies, 1973b). Thus when dealing with these enzymes care must be taken to distinguish between modification and inactivation. Indeed the title of this review was deliberately chosen to encompass aminoglycosidic modifications by bacterial enzymes that do not result in antibiotic inactivation as well as those that do cause loss of antibiotic potency.

Another enzyme which acetylates the 6' amino group of aminoglycoside antibiotics has been found by Kawabe, Naito and Mitsuhashi (1975) and Yagisawa et al (1975) in *Pseudomonas aeruginosa*. However, unlike strains of *E. coli* producing this type of enzyme, the *Ps. aeruginosa* was, in addition to being kanamycin-resistant, also resistant to amikacin, kanamycin B, tobramycin, dideoxykanamycin B, butirosin and gentamicin C_{1a}. This would correspond to the AAC (6')-IV phenotype of Mitsuhashi (1975), whereas *E. coli* harbouring R5 or NR 79 would be of type AAC (6')-I, despite the enzymes produced by these strains being of similar substrate profile. Haas et al (1976) has termed this enzyme type as AAC (6')-I, and their nomenclature is adopted here. These results, and those of others (Davies, 1975; Jacoby, 1975) show that the resistance determined by a particular plasmid can be influenced by the host bacterium. This may be related to differences in the permeability of the strains to the antibiotics, as has been demonstrated for strains of *Ps. aeruginosa* by Bryan, van den Elzen and Shahrabadi (1975) and Mills and Holloway (1976). R-factor mediated enzymes with substrate profiles similar to AAC (6')-I have also been detected in *Klebsiella pneumoniae* and *Enterobacter cloacae* (Minshew et al, 1974).

Kanamycin-tobramycin-amikacin resistant strains of *Moraxella* species also produce an enzyme that acetylates the 6-amino group of certain aminoglycosides, but which was claimed to differ from AAC (6')-I in a number of parameters, and, despite a substrate profile similar to AAC (6')-I, was therefore termed AAC (6')-II (Le Goffic and Martel, 1974). The enzyme from *Moraxella* sp. acetylated gentamicin C_{1a} and tobramycin more rapidly at pH 5.3 than 6.5, whereas the type I enzyme acetylated gentamicin C_{1a} more efficiently at pH 7.6 than 5.3, while tobramycin was an equally good substrate at both pH values. The K_m values for tobramycin, kanamycin and amikacin for the two enzymes were reported to be different, as were the iso-electric points (pH 5.4 for the type I from *E. coli* harbouring R5 and pH 7.6 for the enzyme from *Moraxella* sp.).

Davies (1975) and Kawabe et al (1975) described an enzyme from strains of *Ps. aeruginosa* that differs from the type I and II enzymes in that it did not acetylate butirosin or amikacin, both of which have the 1-amino moiety substituted with a 4-amino-2-hydroxy butyryl group. This enzyme has been tentatively termed AAC (6')-III by Haas et al (1976).

Recently Le Goffic et al (1977a) and Dowding (1977) have described strains of *Staphylococcus aureus* resistant to 4,6-glycosidically linked 2-deoxystreptamine containing D-aminoglycosides, but sensitive to those D-aminoglycosides that are substituted at 4,5-positions of 2 deoxystreptamine. These strains synthesised APH (2″) (see below) and another variant of AAC (6'). Unlike other AAC (6') enzymes described above, neomycin and ribostamycin are poor substrates for this enzyme, which has an iso-electric point of pH 5.7 and a molecular weight of 28 000 (Le Goffic et al, 1977a). Logically this enzyme should be ACC (6')-IV.

At present it is difficult to be dogmatic as to whether these four types of AAC (6') are indeed different, as no direct comparison of them has been undertaken in the same laboratory at the same time. However, Haas et al (1976) compared the type I enzyme produced by *E. coli* R5/W677 and *Ps. aeruginosa* GN 315 with the type III from *Ps. aeruginosa* 3796 and showed these were different with respect to substrate profiles. As mentioned above, Le Goffic and Martel (1974) compared the type I and type II enzymes and found these were different by a number of parameters.

Aminoglycoside 2′-N-acetyltransferase (AAC (2′))

Strains of *Providencia stuartii* are often resistant to gentamicin but sensitive to kanamycin (Reynolds, Hamilton-Miller and Brumfitt, 1974). Such strains produce enzymes that acetylate a wide range of aminoglycosides but not amikacin or kanamycin A (Chevereau et al, 1974; Yamaguchi and Mitsuhashi, 1974); the site of acetylation being the 2′-amino group of the D-glucosamine ring, see Fig. 11.1a. In the case of gentamicins the glucosamine ring is usually called the purpurosamine ring. This enzyme may also be present in strains of *Proteus* that show the same resistance pattern (Chevereau et al, 1974; Price, Godfrey and Kawaguchi, 1974). Mitsuhashi (1975) listed two phenotypes of this enzyme, the type I being gentamicin-resistant only. However, the type I enzyme was ascribed to a preliminary observation by Le Goffic and Davies quoted by Benveniste and Davies (1973a). In a later paper (Chevereau et al, 1974) this phenotype was omitted and now it has also been deleted from the rational nomenclature proposals (Kawabe, personal communication, 1977).

Aminoglycoside 3-N-acetyletransferase (AAC (3))

Three enzymes have been described which acetylate the 3-amino group of the deoxystreptamine ring (see Fig. 11.1b) of D-aminoglycosides, but which differ in their substrate specificities. AAC (3)-I acetylates C-type gentamicins and sisomicin while kanamycin B and tobramycin are relatively poor substrates (Brzezinska et al, 1972). This enzyme is the first aminoglycoside modifying enzyme to be purified to homogeneity, and has been found to be a tetrameric protein of molecular weight 63 000 (Williams and Northrop, 1976). Strains which produce this enzyme are phenotypically gentamicin-resistant but tobramycin and kanamycin-sensitive. This enzyme has been detected in *Ps. aeruginosa* (Brzezinska et al, 1972; Holmes et al, 1974) *E. coli, Klebsiella* sp, *Enterobacter* sp and *Serratia* sp (Witchitz, 1972).

Le Goffic, Martel and Witchitz (1974) described a strain of *E. coli* which had received an R-factor from a gentamicin-tobramycin-kanamycin resistant strain of *Klebsiella*. The enzyme produced by this strain acetylated C-type gentamicins, sisomicin, gentamicin B, tobramycin and kanamycin B; kanamycin A was a relatively poor substrate. Amikacin, neomycin and paromomycin were not acetylated. The iso-electric point for this enzyme, termed AAC (3)-II, was 6.4 compared to pH 7.4 for AAC (3)-I.

A third enzyme of this type produced by *Ps. aeruginosa* modifies a broader substrate range than the other two (Biddlecombe et al, 1976). The gentamicin C group, sisomicin, kanamycins A and B, neomycin, paromomycin and tobramycin are all good substrates for the enzyme, whereas amikacin and butirosin are not attacked. Although neomycin is an excellent substrate, possession of this enzyme does not lead to significant resistance to this antibiotic. It may be that 3-N-acetyl neomycin retains some antibiotic activity as shown for 6′-N-acetyl neomycin (see above).

Nucleotidyltransferases

Aminoglycoside 2″-0 nucleotidyltransferase (ANT) 2″))

Benveniste and Davies (1971b) described the transfer of an R-factor from a gentamicin-resistant strain of *Klebsiella pneumoniae* to *E. coli*. This R-factor specified an enzyme that utilised ATP as co-factor and inactivated by adenylylation the gentamicin group of antibiotics. Kanamycin A but not neomycin was modified. Naganawa et al (1971) showed that the 2″-hydroxy group of the kanosamine ring (see Fig. 11.1c) was the site of attack by this enzymic type. By analogy it would seem that the garosamine ring would be the site of attack in gentamicins. This enzyme has also been found in gentamicin-resistant strains of *Ps. aeruginosa* (Kobayashi et al, 1971; Kabins, Nathan and Cohen, 1974) and *Enterobacter aerogenes* (Witchitz and Chabbert, 1971).

Aminoglycoside 4′-0-nucleotidyltransferase (ANT (4′))

This enzyme, so far found only in strains of *S. aureus* and *S. epidermidis*, inactivates by adenylylation a wide range of D-aminoglycosides, but none of the gentamicin C complex (Le Goffic et al, 1976a, b; Kayser, Santanam and Biber, 1976). The site of attack is the 4′-hydroxyl group of the D-glucosamine ring (see Fig. 11.1a), ATP being the co-factor. Although amikacin and lividomycin are also substrates for the enzyme, only moderate resistance to these antibiotics is conferred on bacteria that produce it (Le Goffic et al, 1976b).

Phosphotransferases

Aminoglycoside 3′-0-phosphotransferase (APH (3′))

Umezawa et al (1967b) were the first to describe an enzyme that phosphorylated kanamycin, using ATP as a co-factor. The site of attack is the 3′-hydroxyl group of the D-glucosamine ring, see Fig. 11.1a (Kondo et al, 1968). This enzyme, later termed APH (3′)-Ia (Le Goffic et al, 1977b), also modifies and gives resistance to neomycin, ribostamycin and lividomycin, but not butirosin. Lividomycin, which lacks a 3′-hydroxyl substituent, is phosphorylated at the 5″ position of the ribose ring. Molecular models have shown that the 3′ and 5″ hydroxyl groups in ribostamycin, which structurally is similar to lividomycin, lie very close to one another and it may be possible for the enzyme to phosphorylate either substituent (Umezawa et al, 1973). Matsuhashi et al (1975) studied three type Ia enzymes from *E. coli* and *Ps. aeruginosa* and showed that they had different molecular weights (54 000, 62 000 and 27 000), pH optima and K_1 values for 3′, 4′-dideoxykanamycin B. From the work of Kobayashi et al (1973) and Davies (1975) it is apparent that this enzyme can also be found in staphylococci.

Recently Le Goffic et al (1977b) described a variant of the type I enzyme, which they termed type Ib, from *Haemophilus parainfluenzae*. Kanamycin A and gentamicin A were poorer substrates for this enzyme than type Ia. In addition, tobramycin inhibits the phosphorylation of all substrates of the type Ia enzyme, but does not inhibit the modification of kanamycin A and gentamicin A by the type Ib enzyme. The molecular weight of the type Ia enzyme specified by R112 was 17 000, compared with the value of 54 000 reported by Matsuhashi et al (1975) for the same enzyme. These values can only be reconciled by proposing the enzyme to be composed of sub-units. The molecular weight of the type Ib enzyme was 27 000. The iso-electric point of the type Ia and Ib enzymes were similar, pH 6.4 and 6.7, respectively.

An enzyme produced by *E. coli* JR66/W677, termed APH (3′)-II could be distinguished from the type I enzymes because it inactivated butirosin but not lividomycin (Yagisawa et al, 1972). Type II ezymes produced by this strain of *E. coli* and *Ps. aeruginosa* H9 appear to be identical on the basis of molecular weight, pH optima, K_m and K_i values (Matsuhashi et al, 1975).

An enzyme produced by a strain of *Ps. aeruginosa* which phosphorylated lividomycin *and* butirosin, but not paromomycin has been termed type III (Umezawa et al, 1975). Kanamycin A and ribostamycin exhibit substrate inhibition at low concentrations whereas butirosin and lividomycin do not. Substrate inhibition has been observed with kanamycin A, ribostamycin and lividomycin with the type I enzyme (Matsuhashi et al, 1975).

Strains of *S. aureus* and *S. epidermidis* have been described which produce a fourth variant of APH (3′). Unlike the types described above, this enzyme (termed APH (3′)-IV), phosphorylates amikacin, and like the type III enzyme, both lividomycin and butirosin are modified (Kayser, Devaud and Biber, 1976; Courvalin and Davies, 1977). Production of this enzyme, however, does not result in resistance to amikacin, a paradox that can be explained by the much slower rate of amikacin modification compared with that of kanamycin A (Courvalin and Davies, 1977). Previous reports have shown the presence of APH (3′) enzymes in staphylococci which were termed types I and II. However, from the data presented it remains unclear whether this is so or whether, in reality they were of the type IV mentioned above (Davies, 1975).

Aminoglycoside 2″-0-phosphotransferase (APH (2″))

All strains of staphylococci which produce AAC (6′)-IV (see above) studied so far also produce an enzyme which phosphorylates the 2″-hydroxyl group of the kanosamine and garosamine rings (Fig. 11.1c) of 4,6-disubstituted 2-deoxystreptamine-containing aminoglycosides (Dowding, 1977; Le Goffic et al, 1977a). Aminoglycosides that are 4,5-substituted on the deoxystreptamine ring are not modified. All these strains are resistant to kanamycin, tobramycin, gentamicin and sisomicin, and have a higher than normal minimum inhibitory concentration to amikacin, but are sensitive to butirosin, lividomycin, neomycin and paromomycin. The enzyme has a high specificity for the gentamicin group of antibiotics (gentamicin C1, C1a, C2, B and sisomicin) while the kanamycin group (kanamycin A and B, amikacin and tobramycin) were much poorer substrates (Le Goffic et al, 1977a).

Aminoglycoside 5″-0-phosphotransferase (APH (5″))

Kida et al (1974) reported a strain of *Ps. aeruginosa* that produced an enzyme which preferentially phosphorylated the 5″-hydroxyl group of the ribose ring (Fig. 11.1d) of ribostamycin. The 3′-hydroxy group of the glucosamine ring was also phosphorylated, but to a much lesser degree. The activity of this enzyme against other aminoglycosides has not been reported, but it can be postulated that those antibiotics with a 5"- hydroxyl group (neomycin, lividomycin and paromomycin) would also be substrates.

Yamaguchi et al (1972) also reported an enzyme which they claimed inactivated by phosphorylation the 5"-hydroxyl group of lividomycin, paromomycin and neomycin. A crude extract of the strain producing this enzyme less efficiently phosphorylated kanamycins A, B and C, but a partially purified preparation was devoid of this activity. It is probable that overall loss of enzyme during purification gave an apparent loss of activity against kanamycin compared with that against lividomycin, paromomycin and neomycin. However, other work with the same organism has clearly shown it to produce APH (3')-Ia (Umezawa, 1974) and so the status of the claim that this organism produces APH (5") is in doubt.

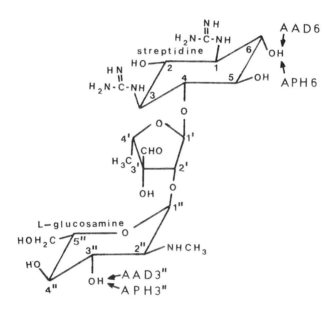

Fig. 11.2   Structure of streptomycin to show the sites of modification.

ENZYMES WHICH MODIFY L-AMINOGLYCOSIDES

Phosphotransferases

Aminoglycoside 3"-0-phosphotransferase (APH (3"))
E. coli harbouring R-factor JR35 produces an enzyme that inactivates streptomycin by phosphorylation. The position of modification is the 3"-hydroxyl group (Fig. 11.2) of the L-glucosamine ring (Ozanne et al, 1969, Kawabe et al, 1971). Spectinomycin, an aminocyclitol, is not a substrate for this enzyme (Benveniste, Yamada and Davies, 1970) although it is attacked by AAD (3") (see below). Bluensomycin and dihydrostreptomycin are inactivated by this enzyme, which has also been found in strains of *Ps. aeruginosa* (Kobayashi et al, 1972).

Aminoglycoside 6″-0-phosphotransferase
The strain of *Ps. aeruginosa* reported to produce APH (5″) (see above), also produces an enzyme that phosphorylates streptomycin and dihydrostreptomycin at the 6-hydroxyl group (Fig. 11.2) of the streptidine ring (Kida et al, 1975). Spectinomycin, which lacks an analogous hydroxy group is not a substrate for this enzyme.

Adenylyltransferases

Aminoglycoside 3″-0-adenylyltransferase (AAD (3″))
Inactivation of streptomycin by adenylylation was first reported by Umezawa et al (1968) by an R-factor carrying strain of *E. coli*. The site of attack is the 3″-hydroxyl group (Fig. 11.2) of the L-glucosamine ring, ATP being the co-factor

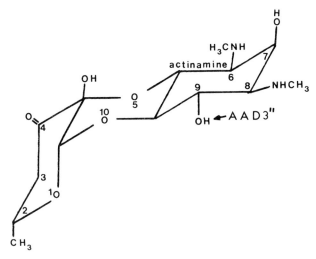

Fig. 11.3   Structure of spectinomycin to show the site of modification.

(Takasawa et al, 1968; Yamada, Tipper and Davies, 1968). Spectinomycin is also modified and inactivated by this enzyme, the C9 hydroxyl group (Fig. 11.3) of the actinamine ring being the site of modification (Benveniste, Yamada and Davies, 1970). This enzyme also confers resistance to dihydrostreptomycin and bluensomycin.

Aminoglycoside 6″-0-adenylyltransferase (AAD (6))
Kawabe and Mitsuhashi (1971) and Kawabe, Inoue and Mitsuhashi (1974) have reported strains of staphylococci that are streptomycin and spectinomycin resistant, streptomycin-resistant and spectinomycin sensitive, or spectinomycin-resistant and streptomycin sensitive. In strains that were resistant to both anti-biotics the resistance could be dissociated by transduction (Kawabe et al, 1974). Streptomycin has been shown to be adenylylated at the 6-hydroxyl group (Fig. 11.2) of the streptidine ring by the enzyme produced by streptomycin-resistant strains; spectinomycin was not a substrate for this enzyme (Suzuki et al, 1975). Spectinomycin-resistant bacteria inativate the drug by adenylylation, but the site

of modification has not yet been determined. Streptomycin is not attacked by the spectinomycin adenylyltransferase. Other workers have also reported similar adenylyltransferase of narrow substrate specificity against either streptomycin or spectinomycin, again from strains of staphylococci (Davies, 1975; Dowding, 1977).

DOES INACTIVATION EXPLAIN RESISTANCE?

One puzzle remains concerning these aminoglycoside-modifying enzymes: where inactivation accompanies modification the rate of loss of antibiotic potency is usually extremely slow (Diedrichsen, Bang and Heding, 1977). Unpublished results of ours show that with R-factor mediated ampicillin or chloramphenicol resistance (*via* β-lactamase and acetylation respectively) MIC values in μg closely approximate the weight of drug in μg destroyed per minute per 10^9 bacteria. However, similar calculations made with bacteria resistant to streptomycin via $3''$ phosphorylation or adenylylation show that the rates of inactivation are derisory, being lower by 3 to 4 orders of magnitude. In addition, we have shown that there is an upper limit in the resistance level that can be obtained by R-factors mediating $3''$ adenylylation of streptomycin, and postulated that this limitation is probably due to ATP utilisation being an energetic constraint (Pinney and Smith, 1974). Another curiosity regarding aminoglycoside inactivating enzymes is that when bacteria that possess them have grown in drug-containing media little or no diminution in the level of drug can be detected. Thus it would seem that the mechanism cannot be ascribed simply to drug inactivation. However, because there is no doubt that drug modification by these enzymes does cause resistance it has been suggested that the inactive drug derivative acts by blocking cellular uptake of unmodified drug (Davies and Benveniste, 1974 and Bryan et al, 1975). This type of resistance mechanism, being a combination of plasmid-mediated drug modification and bacterial impermeability, would by definition be affected by relationships between host bacteria and the plasmid-mediated enzymes they produce. Indeed we have already commented on the differences in resistance pattern seen when the same plasmid is harboured by *E. coli* or by *Pseudomonas* species and it is well known that these two genera exhibit gross differences in their cell wall architecture.

POSSIBLE ORIGINS OF ENZYMES THAT MODIFY
AMINOGLYCOSIDE ANTIBIOTICS

Except in rare instances (Bobrowski et al, 1976) R-factor resistance determinant genes generally have no homology with the chromosomal genes of clinically-isolated drug-resistant bacteria. It has been suggested that the origin of R-factor resistance genes could be in the organisms that produce antibiotics. A number of aminoglycoside-acetylating and phosphorylating enzymes have been detected in such bacteria that have similar (though as yet not identical) substrate specificity profiles to those enzymes found to be mediated by R-factors (for review see Dowding and Davies, 1975). This hypothesis has been strengthened by the demonstration that the gene coding for an aminoglycoside phosphotransferase from a butirosin-producing *Bacillus circulans* can be expressed in *E. coli* which also becomes resistant to a number of aminoglycoside antibiotics (Courvalin, Weisblum and Davies, 1977). In addition to the enzymes detected so far in pathogenic bacteria (see Table 11.2) yet more different enzymes have been detected in the bacteria that produced aminoglycoside antibiotics (Majumdar and Majumdar, 1970 and Kojuma, Inouye and Niida, 1973). If the above hypothesis regarding the origin of aminoglycoside-inactivating enzymes in clinical bacteria is true then the antibiotic-producing organisms are a potential reservoir of genetic information from whence even more aminoglycoside resistance can devolve.

DISTRIBUTION AND FREQUENCY OF AMINOGLYCOSIDE-MODIFYING ENZYMES

Before the widespread use of gentamicin Smith (1969) reported that enzymes that cause 3′ phosphorylation were more common than those that cause 6′ acetylation of D-aminoglycosides. Perhaps it is significant that the former enzymes also conferred a broader spectrum of resistance to aminoglycoside antibiotics in *E. coli*. The 3′-phosphotransferases are still very common and widely distributed (Price et al, 1974). Of the enzymes that confer gentamicin resistance ANT (2″) seemed to occur most frequently, being distributed among many genera (Reynolds et al, 1976). Moreover, they found that it was very common to find bacteria producing not only ANT (2″) but also an APH (3′) enzyme. Such bacteria hence exhibited a very broad range of aminoglycosidic resistance. AAC (2) was found to be restricted to *Proteus* and *Providencia* which again results in a very broad spectrum of resistance (Price et al, 1974). However, they found AAC (6′), which only confers resistance to a restricted range of aminoglycoside antibiotics in *E. coli*, to be extremely rare.

A significant number of clinical isolates mentioned in these two references above have been found to exhibit resistance profiles which could not be ascribed to any enzyme or combination of enzymes described at that time. It is possible that some of these strains may have been resistant to some of the drugs via simple impermeability (i.e. and not due to inactivation) which is a mechanism common in *Pseudomonas* (Bryan, Haraphongse and Van den Elzen, 1976). Indeed there is some indication that this resistance mechanism may even be mediated by R-factors (Maliwan, Grieble and Bird, 1975 and Kono and O'Hara, 1977).

CLINICAL IMPLICATIONS

Table 11.2 shows there are at present as many as 21 different enzymes from pathogenic bacteria, of which 17 modify D-aminoglycoside antibiotics and 4 which modify the streptomycin group. Kanamycin A, which virtually exclusively comprises the commercial product, is a substrate for 14 of these enzymes and this probably accounts for the widespread resistance to this antibiotic so drastically reducing its efficacy as a front line drug. Gentamicin, which is still regarded as a drug of choice for the treatment of serious bacterial infections (Reeves, 1974) is ominously attacked by 10 enzymes, which it should be realised also attack sisomicin. However, the four AAC (6′) acetylating enzymes do not usually confer complete gentamicin resistance because gentamicin C1, which comprises about a third of the commercial drug is not a substrate for them. With the exception of AAC(3)-I, all the other enzymes which attack gentamicins also confer tobramycin-resistance. A tobramycin resistant, gentamicin-sensitive phenotype is seen in staphylococci that produce ANT (4′).

At present information is incomplete regarding resistance to netilmicin (a sisomicin anologue) conferred by these enzymes. It is known that strains producing AAC (2′) or AAC (6′)-I are resistant to this antibiotic (Miller et al, 1976; Phillips et al, 1977). Bacteria that produce an AAC (3) enzyme show variable sensitivity to netilmicin. Although netilmicin is modified by bacteria producing ANT 2″ they remain sensitive to it (Miller et al, 1976) possibly because the adenylylated drug may retain antimicrobial activity (Devaud, Kayser and Huber, 1977).

In contrast to the drugs mentioned above, amikacin is modified by only six enzymes of which three (APH (2″), ANT (4′) and APH (3)-IV) confer but moderate resistance in staphylococci (Le Goffic et al, 1976b, 1977a; Courvalin and Davies, 1977; Kayser et al, 1976). The relative insensitivity of amikacin to enzymic modification is reflected by the low incidence of amikacin-resistant isolates from clinical specimens (for example, Draser et al, 1976; Moellering et al, 1977).

Paradoxically enzymes that modify aminoglycoside antibiotics have also been cleverly exploited to the benefit of man. They have been put to use to estimate aminoglycoside antibiotics in sera not only in order to preclude over-dosage and attendant toxicity but also to ensure adequate serum levels are attained during therapy. This is accomplished by coupling the drug to radioactive co-factors and estimating the amount of drug-bound radioactivity (for examples, Smith, van Otto and Smith, 1972; Broughall and Reeves, 1975; Santanam and Kayser, 1976). Such assays can be completed within an hour.

In conclusion many enzymes have been described which modify aminoglycoside antibiotics. Each antibiotic can be modified by more than one enzyme and each enzyme can modify more than one antibiotic, and hence resistance profiles are complex. However, modification does not always result in resistance, as some modified drugs retain substantial antimicrobial activity and in some other cases the rate of modification seems insufficient to prevent the drug from reaching its target site on the ribosome. In view of the recent demonstration that genes from non-pathogenic aminoglycoside-producing organisms can be expressed in bacteria of clinical importance, it can be postulated that in future new enzymes conferring aminoglycoside resistance should be expected in pathogenic bacteria. Moreover, the fact that the vectors of these drug resistance enzymes are conjugally trans-mitted R-factors in Gram-negative bacteria (and probably in streptococci) and are drug resistance plasmids which are transmitted between staphylococci by transduction, augers an increasing spread of drug resistance in clinical bacteria. Indeed hospitals are reporting increased isolation of gentamicin-resistant organisms among nearly all species of Gram-negative bacteria (Richmond et al, 1975; Draser et al, 1976; Moellering, Wennersten and Kunz, 1976). Outbreaks of gentamicin-resistant staphylococci are also occurring (Soussy et al, 1975; Porterhouse et al, 1976; Speller et al, 1976). To add to our problems it is becoming increasingly common to find clinical isolates harbours not one but several plasmids each conferring different aminoglycoside-modifying enzymes.

Therefore the aminoglycoside antibiotics, which are an important part of the clinician's armoury should be prescribed with circumspection so that by reducing the selective pressures associated with indiscriminant usage their effective life can be prolonged.

REFERENCES

Benveniste, R. & Davies, J. (1971a) Enzymatic acetylation of aminoglycoside antibiotics by *Escherichia coli* carrying an R factor. *Biochemistry*, **10**, 1787–1796.

Benveniste, R. & Davies, J. (1971b) R-factor mediated gentamicin resistance: a new enzyme which modifies aminoglycoside antibiotics. *FEBS letters*, **14**, 293–296.

Benveniste, R. & Davies, J. (1973a) Mechanisms of antibiotic resistance in bacteria. *Annual Reviews of Biochemistry*, **42**, 471–506.

Benveniste, R. & Davies, J. (1973b) Aminoglycoside inactivating enzymes in actinomyctes similar to those present in clinical isolates of antibiotic-resistant bacteria. *Proceedings of the National Academy of Science (U.S.A.)*, **70**, 2276–2280.

Benveniste, R., Yamada, T. & Davies, J. (1970) Enzymatic adenylylation of streptomycin and spectinomycin by R-factor-resistant *Escherichia coli*. *Infection and Immunity*, **1**, 109–119.

Biddlecombe, S., Haas, M., Davies, J., Miller, G. H., Rane, D. F. & Daniels, P. J. L. (1976) Enzymatic modification of aminoglycoside antibiotics: a new 3-N-acetylating enzyme from a *Pseudomonas aeruginosa* isolate. *Antimicrobial Agents and Chemotherapy*, **9**, 951–955.

Bobrowski, M. M., Matthew, M., Barth, P. T., Datta, N., Grinter, N. J., Jacob, A. E., Kontonmichalou, P., Dale, J. W. & Smith, J. T. (1976) Plasmid-determined β-lactamase indistinguishable from the chromosomal β-lactamase of *Escherichia coli*. *Journal of Bacteriology*, **125**, 149–157.

Broughall, J. M. & Reeves, D. S. (1975) The acetyltransferase enzyme method for the assay of serum aminoglycoside concentrations and a comparison with other methods. *Journal of Clinical Pathology*, **28**, 140–145.

Bryan, L. E., Haraphongse, R. & Van den Elzen, H. M. (1976) Gentamicin resistance in clinical-isolates of *Pseudomonas aeruginosa* associated with diminished gentamicin accumulation and no detectable enzymatic modification. *Journal of Antibiotics*, **29**, 743–753.

Bryan, L. E., Van den Elzen, H. M. & Shahrabadi, M. S. (1975) The relationship of aminoglycoside permeability to streptomycin and gentamicin susceptibility of *Pseudomonas aeruginosa*, pp. 475–490. In *Microbial drug resistance*, eds. Mitsuhashi, S., Hashimoto, J. Baltimore: University Park Press.

Brzezinska, M., Benveniste, R., Davies, J., Daniels, P. J. L. & Weinstein, J. (1972) Gentamicin resistance in strains of *Pseudomonas aeruginosa* mediated by enzymatic N-acetylation of the deoxystreptamine moiety. *Biochemistry*, **11**, 761–766.

Chevereau, M., Daniels, P. J. L., Davies, J. & Le Goffic, F. (1974) Aminoglycoside resistance in bacteria mediated by gentamicin acetyl transferase II, an enzyme modifying the 2'-amino group of aminoglycoside antibiotics. *Biochemistry*, **13**, 598–603.

Courvalin, P. & Davies, J. (1977) Plasmid mediated aminoglycoside phosphotransferase of broad substrate range that phosphorylates amikacin. *Antimicrobial Agents and Chemotherapy*, **11**, 619–624.

Courvalin, P., Weisblum, B. & Davies, J. (1977) Aminoglycoside-modifying enzyme of an antibiotic-producing bacterium acts as a determinant of antibiotic resistance in *Escherichia coli*. Proceedings of the National Academy of Sciences (U.S.A.), **74**, 994–1003.

Davies, J. (1975) Some aspects of antibiotic resistance in bacteria, pp. 121–128. In *Drug inactivating enzymes and antibiotic resistance*, eds. Mitsuhashi, S., Rosival, L. & Krcmery, V. Prague: Avicenum.

Davies, J. & Benveniste, R. E. (1974) Enzymes that inactivate antibiotics in transit to their targets. *Annals of the New York Academy of Sciences*, **235**, 130–136.

Devaud, M., Kayser, F. H. & Huber, U. (1977) Resistance of bacteria to the newer aminoglycoside antibiotics: an epidemiological and enzymatic study. *Journal of Antibiotics*, **30**, 655–664.

Diedrichsen, A., Bang, J. & Heding, H. (1977) A new type of inactivation of streptomycin by *E. coli*. *Journal of Antibiotics*, **30**, 83–87.

Dowding, J. E. (1977) Mechanisms of gentamicin resistance in *Staphylococcus aureus*. *Antimicrobial Agents and Chemotherapy*, **11**, 47–50.

Dowding, J. & Davies, J. (1975) Mechanisms and origins of plasmid-determined antibiotic resistance, pp. 179–186. In *Microbiology—1974*, ed. Schlessinger, D. Washington: American Society for Microbiology.

Drasar, F. A., Farrell, W., Maskell, J. & Williams, J. D. (1976) Tobramycin, amikacin, sissomicin, and gentamicin resistant Gram-negative rods. *British Medical Journal*, **2**, 1284–1287.

Haas, M. J. & Dowding, J. E. (1975) Aminoglycoside-modifying enzymes. *Methods in Enzymology*, **43**, 611–628.

Haas, M., Biddlecombe, S., Davies, J., Luce, C. E. & Daniels, P. J. L. (1976) Enzymatic modification of aminoglycoside antibiotics: a new 6'-N-acetylating enzyme from a *Pseudomonas aeruginosa* isolate. *Antimicrobial Agents and Chemotherapy*, **9**, 945–950.

Holmes, R. K., Minshew, B. H., Gould, K. & Sanford, J. P. (1974) Resistance of *Pseudomonas aeruginosa* to gentamicin and related aminoglycoside antibiotics. *Antimicrobial Agents and Chemotherapy*, **6**, 253–262.

Jacoby, G. A. (1975) R plasmids determining gentamicin or tobramycin resistance in *Pseudomonas aeruginosa*, pp. 287–295. In *Drug inactivating enzymes and antibiotic resistance*, eds. Mitsuhashi, S., Rosival, L. & Krcmery, V. Prague: Avivencum.

Kabins, S., Nathan, C. & Cohen, S. (1974) Gentamicin-adenylyltransferase activity as a cause of gentamicin resistance in clinical isolates of *Pseudomonas aeruginosa*. *Antimicrobial Agents and Chemotherapy*, **5**, 565–570.

Kawabe, H. & Mitsuhashi, S. (1971) Inactivation of dihydrostreptomycin by *Staphylococcus aureus*. *Japanese Journal of Microbiology*, **15**, 545–548.

Kawabe, H., Naito, T. & Mitsuhashi, S. (1975) Acetylation of amikacin, a new semisynthetic antibiotic, by *Pseudomonas aeruginosa* carrying an R factor. *Antimicrobial Agents and Chemotherapy*, **7**, 50–54.

Kawabe, H., Kobayashi, F., Yamaguchi, M., Utahara, R. & Mitsuhashi, S. (1971). 3''-phosphoryldihydrostreptomycin produced by the inactivating enzyme of *Pseudomonas aeruginosa*. *Journal of Antibiotics*, **24**, 651–652.

Kawabe, H., Inoue, M. & Mitsuhashi, S. (1974) Inactivation of dihydrostreptomycin and spectinomycin by *Staphylococcus aureus*. *Antimicrobial Agents and Chemotherapy*, **5**, 553–557.

Kawabe, H., Kondo, S., Umezawa, H. & Mitsuhashi, S. (1975) R factor-mediated aminoglycoside antibiotic resistance in *Pseudomonas aeruginosa*: a new aminoglycoside 6'-N-acetyltransferase. *Antimicrobial Agents and Chemotherapy*, **7**, 494–499.

Kayser, F. H., Devaud, M. & Biber, J. (1976) Aminoglycoside 3'-phosphotransferanse IV: a new type of aminoglycoside phosphorylating enzyme found in staphylococci. *Microbios. Letters*, **3**, 63–68.

Kayser, F. H., Santanam, P. & Biber, J. (1976). Genetic basis and mode of resistance to aminoglycosides in *Staphylococcus aureus* and *Staphylococcus epidermidis*. *Zentrablatt fur Bakteriologie, Parasitenkunde, Infektionskranheinten und Hygiene. I. Abt.*, Supplement 5, 275–286.

Kida, M., Igarasi, S., Okutani, T., Asako, T., Hiraga, K. & Mitsuhashi, S. (1974) Selective phosphorylation of the 5''-hydroxy group of ribostamycin by a new enzyme from *Pseudomonas aeruginosa*. *Antimicrobial Agents and Chemotherapy*, **5**, 92–94.

Kida, M., Asako, T., Yoneda, M. & Mitsuhashi, S. (1975) Phosphorylation of dihydrostreptomycin in *Pseudomonas aeruginosa*, pp. 441–448. In *Microbial Drug Resistance*, eds. Mitsuhashi, S. & Hashimoto, H. Baltimore: University Park Press.

Kobayashi, F., Yamaguchi, M., Eda, J., Higashi, F. & Mitsuhashi, S. (1971) Enzymatic inactivation of gentamicin C components by cell-free extract from *Klebsiella pneumoniae*. *Journal of Antibiotics*, **24**, 719–721.

Kobayashi, F., Yamaguchi, M., Sato, J. & Mitsuhashi, S. (1972) Purification and properties of dihydrostreptomycin-phosphorylating enzyme from *Pseudomonas aeruginosa*. *Japanese Journal of Microbiology*, **16**, 15–19.

Kobayashi, F., Koshi, T., Eda, J., Voshimura, Y. & Mitsuhashi, S. (1973) Lividomycin resistance in staphylococci by enzymatic phosphorylation. *Antimicrobial Agents and Chemotherapy*, **4**, 1–5.

Kojuma, M., Inouye, S. & Niida, T. (1973) Biconversion of ribostamycin (SF-733). I. Isolation and structure of 3 (or 1)-N-carboxymethylribostamycin. *Journal of Antibiotics*, **26**, 246–248.

Kondo, S., Okanishi, M., Utamara, R., Maeda, K. & Umezawa, H. (1968) Isolation of kanamycin and paromomine inactivated by *E. coli* carrying R factor. *Journal of Antibiotics*, **21**, 22–29.

Kono, M. & O'Hara, K. (1977) Kanamycin-resistance mechanism of *Pseudomonas aeruginosa* governed by an R-plasmid independantly of inactivating enzymes. *Journal of Antibiotics*, **30**, 688–690.

Le Goffic, F. & Martel, A. (1974) La résistance aux aminosides provoquée par une isoenzyme la kanamycine ácetyltransférase. *Biochimie*, **56**, 893–897.

Le Goffic, F., Martel, A. & Witchitz, J. (1974) 3-N enzymatic acetylation of gentamicin, tobramycin and kanamycin by *Escherichia coli* carrying an R factor. *Animicrobial Agents and Chemotherapy*, **6**, 680–684.

Le Goffic, F., Baca, B., Soussy, C. J., Dublanchet, A. & Duval, J. (1976a) ANT (4′) I: une nouvelle nucléotidyltransférase d'aminoglycosides isolée de *Staphylococcus aureus. Annales de Microbiologie (Institut Pasteur)*, **127A**, 391–399.

Le Goffic, F., Martel, A., Capmau, M. L., Baca, B., Goebel, P., Chardon, H., Soussy, C. J., Duval, J. & Bouanchaud, D. H. (1976b) New plasmid-mediated nucleotidylation of aminoglycoside antibiotics in *Staphylococcus aureus. Antimicrobial Agents of Chemotherapy*, **10**, 258–264.

Le Goffic, F., Marel, A., Moreau, N., Capmau, M. L., Soussy, C. J. & Duval, J. (1977a) 2″-O-phosphorylation of gentamicin components by a *Staphylococcus aureus* strain carrying a plasmid. *Antimicrobial Agents and Chemotherapy*, **12**, 26–30.

Le Goffic, F., Moreau, N., Siegrist, S., Goldstein, F. W. & Acar, J. C. (1977b) La resistance plasmidque de *Haemophilus* sp. aux antibiotiques aminoglycosidque isolement et etude d'une nouvelle phosphotransferase. *Annales de Microbiologie (Institut Pasteur)*, **128A**, 388–391.

Majumdar, M. K. & Majumdar, S. K. (1970) Isolation and characterization of three phosphoamidoneomycins and their conversion into neomycin by *Streptomyces fradiae. Biochemical Journal*, **120**, 271–278.

Maliwan, N., Grieble, H. G. & Bird, T. J. (1975) Hospital *Pseudomonas aeruginosa*: surveillance of resistance to gentamicin and transfer of aminoglycoside R factor. *Antimocrobial Agents and Chemotherapy*, **8**, 415–420.

Matsuhashi, Y., Yagisawa, M., Kondo, S., Takeuchi, T. & Umezawa, H. (1975) Aminoglycoside 3′-phosphotransferases I and II in *Pseudomonas aeruginosa. Journal of Antibiotics*, **28**, 442–447.

Miller, G. H., Arcieri, G., Weinstein, M. J. & Waitz, J. A. (1976) Biological activity of netilmicin, a broad-spectrum, semisynthetic aminoglycoside antibiotic. *Antimicrobial Agents and Chemotherapy*, **10**, 827–836.

Mills, B. J. & Holloway, B. W. (1976) Mutants of *Pseudomonas aeruginosa* that show specific hypersensitivity to aminoglycosides. *Antimicrobial Agents and Chemotherapy*, **10**, 411–416.

Minshew, B. H., Holmes, R. K., Sanford, J. P. & Baxter, C. R. (1974) Transferable resistance to tobramycin in *Klebsiella pneumoniae* and *Enterobacter cloacae* associated with enzymatic acetylation of tobramycin. *Antimicrobial Agents and Chemotherapy*, **6**, 492–497.

Mitshuhashi, S. (1975) Proposal for a rational nomenclature for phenotype, genotype and aminoglycoside-aminocyclitol modifying enzymes, pp. 269–275. In *Drug Action and Resistance in Bacteria*, ed. Mitsuhashi, S. Baltimore: University Park Press.

Moellering, R. C. Jr., Wennersten, C. & Kunz, L. J. (1976) Emergence of gentamicin-resistant bacteria: experience with tobramycin therapy of infections due to gentamicin-resistant organisms. *Journal of Infectious Diseases*, **134**, Suppl. 40–49S.

Moellering, R. C. Jr., Wennersten, C., Kunz, L. J. & Poitras, J. W. (1977) Resistance to gentamicin, tobramycin, and amikacin among clinical isolates of bacteria. *American Journal of Medicine, Amikacin Symposium*, 30–38.

Naganawa, H., Yagisawa, M., Kondo, S., Takeuchi, T. & Umezawa, H. (1971) The structure determination of an enzymatic inactivation product of 3′, 4′ dideoxykanamycin B. *Journal of Antibiotics*, **24**, 913–914.

Okamoto, S. & Suzuki, Y. (1965) Chloramphenicol-, dihydrostreptomycin-, and kanamycin-, inactivating enzymes from multiple drug-resistant *Escherichia coli* carrying episome 'R'. *Nature*, **208**, 1301–1303.

Okanishi, M., Kondo, S., Suzuki, Y., Okamoto, S. & Umezawa, H. (1967) Studies on inactivation of kanamycin and resistances of *E. coli. Journal of Antibiotics*, **20**, 132–135.

Ozanne, B., Benveniste, R., Tipper, D. & Davies, J. (1969) Aminoglycoside antibiotics: inactivation by phosphorylation in *Escherichia coli* carrying R factors. *Journal of Bacteriology*, **100**, 1144–1146.

Phillips, I., Smith, A. & Shannon, K. (1977) Antibacterial activity of netilmicin, a new aminoglycoside antibiotic, compared with that of gentamicin. *Antimicrobial Agents and Chemotherapy*, **11**, 402–406.

Pinney, R. J. & Smith, J. T. (1974) Antibiotic resistance levels of bacteria harbouring more than one R factor. *Chemotherapy*, **20**, 296–302.

Porthouse, A., Brown, D. F., Smith, R. G. & Rogers, T. (1976) Gentamicin resistance in *Staphylococcus aureus. Lancet*, **1**, 20–21.

Price, K. E., Godfrey, J. C. & Kawaguchi, K. (1974) Effect of structural modifications on the biological properties of aminoglycoside antibiotics containing 2-deoxystreptamine. *Advances in Applied Microbiology*, **18**, 191–307.

Price, K. E., Pursiano, T. A., De Furia, M. D. & Wright, G. E. (1974) Activity of BB-K8 (amikacin) against clinical isolates resistant to one or more aminoglycoside antibiotics. *Antimicrobial Agents and Chemotherapy*, **5**, 143–152.

Reeves, D. S. (1974) Gentamicin therapy. *British Journal of Hospital Medicine*, **12**, 837–850.

Reynolds, A. V., Hamilton-Miller, J. M. T. & Brumfitt, W. (1974) Newer aminoglycosides-amikacin and tobramycin: an in vitro comparison with kanamycin and gentamicin. *British Medical Journal*, **3**, 778–780.

Reynolds, A. V., Hamilton-Miller, J. M. T. & Brumfitt, W. (1976) In vitro activity of amikacin and ten other aminoglycoside antibiotics against gentamicin-resistant bacterial strains. *Journal of Infectious Diseases*, **134**, Supplement S291–S296.

Richmond, A. S., Simberkoff, M. S., Rahal, J. J. Jr. & Schaefler, S. (1975) R factors in gentamicin-resistant organisms causing hospital infections. *Lancet*, **2**, 1176–1178.

Santanam, P. & Kayser, F. H. (1976) Enzymatic adenylylation by aminoglycoside 4′-adenylyltransferase and 2″-adenylyltransferase as a means of determining concentrations of aminoglycoside antibiotics in serum. *Antimicrobial Agents and Chemotherapy*, **10**, 664–667.

Smith, D. H. (1969) R factors for aminoglycoside antibiotics. *Journal of Infectious Diseases*, **119**, 378–380.

Smith, D. H., Van Otto, B. & Smith, A. L. (1972) A rapid chemical assay for gentamicin. *New England Journal of Medicine*, **286**, 583–586.

Soussy, C. J., Bouanchaud, D. H., Fouace, J., Dublanchet, A. & Duval, J. (1975). A gentamycin resistance plasmid in *Staphylococcus aureus*. *Annales de Microbiologie (Institut Pasteur)*, **126B**, 91–94.

Speller, D. C., Raghunath, D., Stephens, M., Viant, A. C., Reeves, D. S., Wilkinson, P. J., Broughall, J. M. & Holt, H. A. (1976) Epidemic infection by a gentamicin-resistant *Staphylococcus aureus* in three hospitals. *Lancet*, **1**, 464–466.

Suzuki, I., Takahashi, N., Shirato, S., Kawabe, H. & Mitsuhashi, S. (1975) Adenylylation of streptomycin by *Staphylococcus aureus*: a new streptomycin adenylyltransferase, pp. 463–473. In *Microbial Drug Resistance*, eds. Mitsuhashi, S. & Hashimoto, M. Baltimore: University Park Press.

Takasawa, S., Utahara, R., Okanishi, M., Maeda, K. & Umezawa, H. (1968) Studies on adenylylstreptomycin, a product of streptomycin inactivated by *E. coli* carrying the R factor. *Journal of Antibiotics*, **21**, 477–484.

Umezawa, H. (1974) Biochemical mechanism of resistance to aminoglycosidic antibiotics. *Advances in Carbohydrate Chemistry and Biochemistry*, **30**, 183–225.

Umezawa, H. (1975) Biochemical mechanism of resistance to aminoglycoside antibiotics, pp. 221–248. In *Drug Action and Resistance in Bacteria*, Vol. 2. ed. Mitsuhashi, S. Baltimore: University Park Press.

Umezawa, H., Okanishi, M., Utamari, R., Maeda, K. & Kondo, S. (1967a). Isolation and structure of kanamycin inactivated by a cell free system of kanamycin-resistant *E. coli*. *Journal of Antibiotics*, Series A, **20**, 136–141.

Umezawa, H., Okanishi, M., Kondo, S., Hamana, K., Utahara, R., Maeda, K. & Mitshuhashi, S. (1967b) Phosphorylative inactivation of aminoglycoside antibiotics by *Escherichia coli* carrying R factor. *Science*, **157**, 1559–1561.

Umezawa, H., Takasawa, S., Okanishi, M. & Utahara, R. (1968) Adenylylstreptomycin, a product of streptomycin inactivated by *E. coli* carrying R factor. *Journal of Antibiotics*, **21**, 81–82.

Umezawa, H., Yamamoto, H., Yagisawa, M., Kondo, S., Takeuchi, T. & Chabbert, Y. A. (1973) Kanamycin phosphotransferase I: mechanism of cross resistance between kanamycin and lividomycin. *Journal of Antibiotics*, **26**, 407–411.

Umezawa, Y., Yagisawa, M., Sawa, T., Takeuchi, T., Umezawa, H., Matsumoto, H. & Tazaki, T. (1975) Aminoglycoside 3′-phosphotransferase III, a new phosphotransferase resistance mechanism. *Journal of Antibiotics*, **28**, 845–853.

Williams, J. W. & Northrop, D. B. (1976) Purification and properties of gentamicin acetyltransferase I. *Biochemistry*, **15**, 125–131.

Witchitz, J. L. (1972) Plasmid-mediated gentamicin resistance not associated with kanamycin resistance in Enterobacteriaceae. *Journal of Antibiotics*, **25**, 622–624.

Witchitz, J. L. & Chabbert, Y. A. (1971) High level transferable resistance to gentamicin. *Journal of Antibiotics*, **24**, 137–139.

Yagisawa, M., Yamamoto, H., Naganawa, H., Kondo, S., Takeuchi, T. & Umezawa, H. (1972) A new enzyme in *Escherichia coli* carrying R-factor phosphorylating 3′-hydroxyl of butirosin A, kanamycin, neamine and ribostamycin. *Journal of Antibiotics*, **25**, 748–750.

Yagisawa, M., Kondo, S., Takeuchi, T. & Umezawa, H. (1975) Aminoglycoside 6′-N-acetyltransferase of *Pseudomonas aeruginosa*: structural requirements of substrate. *Journal of Antibiotics*, **28**, 486–489.

Yamada, T., Tipper, D. & Davies, J. (1968) Enzymatic inactivation of streptomycin by R factor-resistant *Escherichia coli*. *Nature*, **219**, 288–291.

Yamaguchi, M., Koshi, T., Kobayashi, F. & Mitsuhashi, S. (1972) Phosphorylation of lividomycin by *Escherichia coli* carrying an R factor. *Antimicrobial Agents and Chemotherapy*, **2**, 142–146.

Yamaguchi, M., Mitsuhashi, S., Kobayashi, F. & Zenda, H. (1974) A 2′-N-acetylating enzyme of aminoglycosides. *Journal of Antibiotics*, **27**, 507–515.

12. Recent advances in non-gonococcal urethritis

G. L. Ridgway

Non-gonococcal urethritis (NGU) is now the commonest sexually transmitted disease in men. Upwards of 70 000 each year are notified in England, whilst in the United States, where reporting is not undertaken, estimates of over 2 000 000 cases annually are made. The degree of symptoms varies considerably, from a purulent urethritis clinically indistinguishable from gonococcal urethritis, to minimal or absent symptoms. On examination of the urethra, the meatus may appear hyperaemic. Examination of the discharge by Gram's stain demonstrates the absence of gonococci, though this finding should be confirmed by failure to isolate this organism on suitable media. The polymorphonuclear leucocyte count (PNL) in the stained smear should exceed an average of 10 cells per high power field ($\times 100$ oil objective). A first catch specimen of urine will show the presence of threads, which if examined microscopically will be seen to consist of PNL. Patients with minimal symptoms should be examined for the presence of significant numbers of PNL in an early morning smear, and a first catch urine held in the bladder overnight should also be inspected. Post gonococcal urethritis (PGU) appears to be due to an associated NGU revealed after specific therapy for *Neisseria gonorrhoeae*. The previous use of the term non-specific urethritis to describe NGU is no longer tenable, as a cause has now been established for over 50 per cent of the cases. Reiters' disease, epididymitis, prostatitis and urethral stricture may all be associated with NGU, but space does not allow the consideration of these conditions.

It is apparent that NGU is multifactorial in aetiology. Many organisms have been implicated, but few have survived rigorous investigation. King (1964) discussed the evidence for and against *Trichomonas vaginalis*, quoting isolation figures of from 5.5 per cent to an improbable 68 per cent. Jeansson and Molin (1971) reported the isolation of *Herpesvirus hominis* from five men with NGU, without other manifestations of herpes infection. However, Holmes et al (1975) in a classic study were unable to implicate *T. vaginalis*, *H. hominis*, *Mycoplasma hominis*, or cytomegalovirus (CMV) as aetiological agents in NGU. It is probable that a few cases may be associated with bacterial infections of the bladder or kidney, or secondary to urethral stricture. These, and cases associated with *H. hominis*, *T. vaginalis*, *M. hominis*, or CMV may account for at most 10 per cent of NGU (King and Nicol, 1975). Holmes et al (1975) were also unable to demonstrate an aetiological role for the ureaplasmas, but this is the subject of some controversy. Only one organism has been conclusively demonstrated to be a cause of NGU, namely *Chlamydia trachomatis*.

THE ROLE OF *C. TRACHOMATIS* IN NGU

Isolation and epidemiological studies

Early isolation techniques involved the inoculation of the yolk sac of embryonated hen's eggs. These methods are cumbersome, and of lower sensitivity than the more recent cell culture techniques. There have been a number of advances in the cell culture technique, based largely on chemical treatment of cell monolayers, in contrast to the earlier methods of irradiation. The following agents have been used, cytochalasin B (Sompolinsky and Richmond, 1974), 5-iodo-2-deoxyuridine (Wentworth and Alexander, 1974; Reeve, Owen and Oriel, 1975), and cycloheximide (Tribby, Friis and Moulder, 1973). Hobson et al (1974) have described a method using non-treated cells, which seems to rely on a reduced density of host cells, compared with other cell culture techniques. The principle of the cell culture techniques involves two important procedures. Firstly, the competition between host cell and *Chlamydia* for nutrients in the media must be weighted in favour of the parasite, either by rendering the host cells into a stationary phase (using irradiation or chemical treatment), or by reduction in the numbers of host cells present, as in the technique of Hobson et al. Secondly, centrifugation of the inoculum onto the cell monolayer is necessary. The particular cell line used, be it McCoy, Hela 229, or BHK does not seem to be of major importance.

The development of simple cell culture techniques resulted in facilities for the isolation of *C. trachomatis* becoming available in a number of centres involved in clinical studies on NGU. In 1972, reports were published from Bristol (Richmond, Hilton and Clarke, 1972), and London (Oriel et al, 1972). The Bristol study concerned the prevalance of chlamydiae in men with NGU or gonorrhoea, and a control group without urethritis. Specimens were collected from the endo-urethra using cotton-wool tipped swabs, which were found to be more convenient than a curette. Chlamydiae were isolated from 39 per cent of the men with NGU, 32 per cent with gonorrhoea, and 5 per cent of control patients. Patients with a urethral discharge of more than seven days duration yielded a significantly higher number of chlamydial isolates. In the gonorrhoea group, 31 per cent developed PGU after treatment with penicillin, a significant number of these being initially *Chlamydia* positive. In the discussion of the results, the question of latency was mentioned. Latency is known to occur in infections of birds and mammals, including man, with *C. psittaci*, and Hanna et al (1968) demonstrated inclusion bodies of *C. trachomatis* in the eyes of patients not exhibiting clinical conjunctivitis. Richmond et al commented that latent infection might not be revealed by cell culture if the chlamydiae persisted in the non-infectious intracellular form. They argued that if *C. trachomatis* is a primary urethral pathogen, the recovery rate from men with NGU should be higher than in men with gonorrhoea. Since in their study, the isolation rates in the two groups were similar, they suggested that *C. trachomatis* is seldom the primary pathogen, but generally a sexually aquired commensal in the genital tract. In other words, it was suggested that the gonococcus, or an unknown agent activates latent chlamydial infection to give respectively PGU or NGU.

Oriel et al (1972) isolated *Chlamydia* from 38 per cent of men with NGU, and from none of a control group. It is of particular note that early morning urethral smears were examined to exclude minimal urethritis in the controls. These workers concluded that *Chlamydia* was *not* a commensal in the male urethra. An attempt was made to identify the primary contacts of the *Chlamydia*-positive patients, and chlamydiae were isolated from seven out of eight women in this category. Oriel et al (1974) reported the isolation of chlamydiae from the cervix of 33 per cent of the female contacts of NGU, and from 32 per cent of women with gonorrhoea. A control group of women with no history of contact with NGU, and no clinical or microbiological evidence of gonorrhoea, yielded an isolation rate for *Chlamydia* of 2 per cent. Simultaneously, Hilton et al (1974) also reported on the prevalence of *Chlamydia* in the female cervix. Contacts of men with NGU yielded positive isolates in 34 per cent, whilst patients with gonorrhoea yielded 62 per cent. It was concluded that the high isolation rate of *C. trachomatis* in the presence of gonorrhoea was due to reactivation of latent chlamydial infection by the gonococcus, as previously postulated in the male (Richmond et al, 1972). The interaction of *Chlamydia* with other organisms is well known, particularly in ocular disease. Darougar et al (1977) using a cat model found that the ocular infection was far more severe in the presence of *Chlamydia* and a *Streptococcus* species, than with either infective agent alone.

An epidemiological study of over 1600 patients by Schacter et al (1975) demonstrated *C. trachomatis* in over 57 per cent of men with NGU with frank discharge, and from 11 per cent with concurrent gonorrhoea. Asymptomatic men did not yield chlamydial isolates from the urethra.

Application of serological techniques

Until 1971, serological investigations had depended largely on the lympho-granuloma venereum complement fixation test. This test is insensitive, and lacks specificity. The development of a micro-immunofluorescence (MIF) technique has allowed the classification of *C. trachomatis* into 15 serotypes, as well as the monitoring of antibody production in infections (Wang and Grayston, 1971). Reeve et al (1974) used both MIF and a radio-immunoprecipitation (RIP) test to investigate patients with NGU, finding the MIF test more specific than RIP. Over 80 per cent of the men yielding *C. trachomatis* isolates had antibodies demonstrable in the MIF-IgG test. An extension of the MIF test by Wang and Grayston (1974) demonstrated a type-specific response in 79 per cent of patients with NGU. They were able to demonstrate that the initial antibody produced was of the IgM class, being replaced subsequently by IgG. Studies in monkeys suggested that on reinfection with a different serotype, the IgG to the *previous* serotype is first recalled, followed by IgM, and subsequently IgG of the new serotype. They therefore stressed that in patients with a history of multiple chlamydial infections, with differing serotypes, a serological response to a single type specific antigen might not be obtained. The full MIF test is technically difficult to perform, and too complicated for use in routine screening. Others have attempted to simplify the technique, using either pooled antigens (Treharne, Darougar and Jones, 1977), or a single cross reacting antigen (Richmond and Caul, 1975; Thomas, Reeve and Oriel, 1976). These workers have been unable to confirm the highly specific responses found by Wang et al, but would seem to be in overall agreement as to the demonstration of an antibody response in the presence of positive chlamydial cultures. The significance of raised antibody levels in *Chlamydia* culture-negative urethritis is uncertain.

Definitive evidence for the role of *C. trachomatis* **in NGU**
The study by Holmes et al (1975) involved three groups of men. Those with NGU, those with gonorrhoea, and a group with no urethritis. The groups were matched for demographic details, and sexual activity. *C. trachomatis* was isolated from 42 per cent of the NGU group, 19 per cent of the gonorrhoea group, and 7 per cent of the controls. All of the *Chlamydia*-positive controls could have represented asymptomatic urethritis on the criteria used. Where symptoms of urethritis were present for more than one week, the isolation rate of *C. trachomatis* rose to 56 per cent. This finding was confirmed by Oriel et al (1976a) with an isolation rate of 59 per cent in prolonged symptomatic NGU, compared with an overall isolation rate of 49 per cent for their NGU group. Holmes et al also carried out MIF serological studies. In general, the pattern of immunotype specificity of the serum antibody reflected the pattern of immunotype isolated from these patients. In the gonorrhoea group, 100 per cent of the patients with concurrent *C. trachomatis* infections developed PGU after specific anti-gonococcal therapy with a penicillin, cephalosporin or spectinomycin, all of which have little antichlamydial activity (Ridgway, Owen and Oriel, 1978). This finding is consistent with the work of Oriel et al (1975), Oriel et al (1976b) and Oriel et al (1977), who demonstrated the development of *Chlamydia*-positive PGU in patients whose gonorrhoea was treated with gentamicin, ampicillin or spectinomycin respectively. During the discussion of their results, Holmes et al drew attention to the reservoir of chlamydial infection in the female cervix, and recommended that the treatment of NGU contacts should become standard practice.

In a review of chlamydial infection, Grayston and Wang (1975) noted that a rise in antibody titre was uncommon in *Chlamydia*-negative NGU, suggesting that current methods of isolation reflect the true incidence of *Chlamydia* as a cause of NGU. They conclude that the weight of evidence suggest that *C. trachomatis* infection of the genital tract may be asymptomatic, but produces disease.

The inoculation of the urethra of volunteers has not yet been reported, although the successful infection of the baboon urethra has been described by Digiacomo et al (1975). Since latency is known to occur in chlamydial diseases, more knowledge of the pathogenesis of these diseases will be required before volunteer inoculation can be ethically justified.

THE ROLE OF UREAPLASMAS IN NGU

The role of ureaplasmas in the aetiology of NGU has been the subject of considerable controversy, space does not allow the detailing of the innumerable clinical studies involving this agent, and it is doubtful whether such a review would be of any benefit since the results are contradictory. One problem in the evaluation of the results with ureaplasmas has been the use of inappropriate control groups. An extensive review by McCormack et al (1973) after highlighting the contradictory evidence of comparable studies, concludes by noting the lack of a regularly demonstrable serological response to ureaplasmas in NGU, and suggests that direct challenge of volunteers may prove of value, although natural challenge with these organisms is probably common. They note that prepubertal boys are usually free of genital mycoplasma, whereas an increasing number of adult men become colonised, apparently related to sexual activity. In a carefully controlled study from the same workers (Lee et al, 1976) no difference could be detected between ureaplasmas colonisation of controls, or men with NGU. However, Shepard (1974) had indicated that quantitative studies with ureaplasma might demonstrate a role for this agent. Bowie et al (1977) investigating the role of *C. trachomatis* and ureaplasmas in NGU found that in *Chlamydia*-negative NGU, not only were ureaplasmas more commonly isolated than in *Chlamydia*-positive NGU, but the concentration (colour changing units) of ureaplasmas was significantly higher than in the *Chlamydia*-positive group. Serological studies were performed for complement-fixing, and complement independent ureaplasma antibodies, but with inconclusive results. They noted that previous studies had shown both tetracyclines and erythromycin to be effective in the therapy of NGU, both agents being active against ureaplasmas and *C. trachomatis*. They implied that the use of selectively active antimicrobials could aid the elucidation of the role of ureaplasmas and *C. trachomatis* in NGU. Bowie et al (1976) compared the effect of therapy with sulphisoxazole (predominantly anti-chlamydial activity), with spectinomycin or streptomycin (predominantly anti-ureaplasma activity). They produced evidence that patients with *Chlamydia*-positive NGU responded better to sulphisoxazole, whilst patients with ureaplasma positive, *Chlamydia*-negative NGU responded better to spectinomycin or streptomycin. These findings suggest a role for both agents in NGU.

The intra-urethral inoculation of volunteers was reported by Taylor-Robinson, Csonka and Prentice (1977). Two of the authors inoculated their urethras with cloned strains of ureaplasmas isolated from two cases of *Chlamydia*-negative NGU. They demonstrated multiplication of the organism within the urethra, and a short duration serum metabolism-inhibition antibody was demonstrable. Both men developed urethritis, and one subsequently developed prostatitis. Inoculation of the urethra subsequently with ureaplasma-free growth medium did not produce urethritis.

The position of ureaplasmas remains unclear, but the findings of Bowie and his co-workers, and the experiments of Taylor-Robinson et al would seem to indicate a possible role for this agent in *Chlamydia*-negative NGU. Further, adequately controlled studies with selective therapy and serological investigations are still required.

THERAPY OF NGU

Rational therapy for NGU has been difficult in the past, owing to failure to confirm an aetiological agent for some or all cases. Therapy has been empirical, aided to a considerable extent by spontaneous resolution. Willcox (1972) investigating the effect of a number of antimicrobials for the therapy of NGU, found that 30 per cent of infections responded to a placebo (although duration of follow-up was not stated). It is only now, with a cause for about 50 per cent of cases established, that some rationalisation can be introduced. The advances in cell culture techniques for *C. trachomatis* have allowed the development of in vitro methods for assessing antimicrobial activity (Ridgway, Owen and Oriel, 1976; Treharne et al, 1977). The results of these studies indicate that the empirical experience with tetracyclines has some scientific basis. There have been innumerable studies on the therapy of NGU, demonstrating an apparently beneficial response to tetracyclines (Holmes, Johnson and Floyd, 1967). Previous studies have been conflicting as to duration of therapy and dosage. Comparisons have taken little account of the pharmacokinetics of the tetracyclines. The problems of empirical tetracycline studies were well highlighted by Simopoulos (1977).

The first reported trial of a tetracycline backed by laboratory investigation was by Oriel, Reeve and Nicol (1975). Minocycline was used (100 mg twice daily for 3 weeks). Chlamydial isolations were attempted pre- and post-treatment, and contact tracing and treatment of female partners also carried out. They were unable to detect any difference in response between *Chlamydia*-positive and *Chlamydia*-negative NGU. Prentice, Taylor-Robinson and Csonka (1976) went further with laboratory studies, and looked for ureaplasmas as well as chlamydiae in their patients. This trial also used minocycline therapy, but in addition they were able to use placebo control. A 200 mg loading dose was given, followed by 100 mg twice daily for six days. At seven days, 28.5 per cent of the placebo group were symptom and sign free. The disappearance of symptoms and signs with minocycline correlated well with an initially positive isolation of *C. trachomatis*, but this was not found in the placebo group. Less significance was found between response to antimicrobial therapy and the presence of ureaplasmas.

Handsfield et al (1976) found that recurrence of NGU was higher in *Chlamydia*-negative NGU after one week therapy with oxytetracycline (1G six hourly), than in a similar group with *Chlamydia*-positive NGU. It is not clear from their data whether recurrences are due to relapse or re-infection although this would appear to be important in treatment studies. Further, it has been shown that ureaplasmas have a less predictable in vitro response to tetracyclines than *C. trachomatis* (Spaepen, Kundsin and Horne, 1977), consequently the findings of Handsfield et al could be explained by a differential effect of the treatment on *C. trachomatis* or ureaplasmas, related to the duration of therapy.

Other antibiotics have been tested, largely in empirical studies. In the study of Willcox (1972), the 30 per cent response rate to placebo was similar to that found with ampicillin, nalidixic acid, and novobiocin. Other compounds of questionable value included sulphonamides, penicillin, chloramphenicol, streptomycin, metronidazole and spectinomycin. These findings are reflected in the relative resistance of *C. trachomatis* to these compounds in vitro. Apart from the tetracyclines, rifampicin and erythromycin have high in vitro activity against *C. trachomatis*. Clinical studies of the effect of rifampicin in NGU have not been reported. Erythromycin stearate (500 mg 12 hourly for 14 days) has been shown to be as effective as oxytetracycline (250 mg 6 hourly for 14 days) by Oriel, Ridgway and Tchamouroff (1977), in a laboratory monitored clinical study with *C. trachomatis* isolations.

New antimicrobials are continually being produced, and it is necessary to combine both laboratory and clinical studies to assess their efficiency. The known tendency for latency in chlamydial infections must be borne in mind, particularly as this can be readily demonstrated with antibiotics in vitro (Ridgway et al, 1978). Ideally patients should be subject to prolonged follow-up, although this may prove difficult in view of default or further sexual exposure, before cure is pronounced.

CONCLUSION

Few would now argue that *C. trachomatis* is not a pathogen in some cases of NGU. The evidence for *Ureaplasma urealyticum* is less clear, but the results of volunteer inoculation and quantitative cultures indicate a possible aetiological role. Together, these organisms may be responsible for 60–65 per cent of cases, with a further 10 per cent associated with the other recognised pathogens noted above. This still leaves approximately one quarter of cases to which no pathogen can be ascribed, and for which there would appear to be no likely ascribable pathogen at the present state of our knowledge.

The female sexual partners of men with NGU must also be identified, for a number of reasons. It seems reasonable to identify and treat these contacts in the same manner as gonorrhoea contacts are traced, although there is at present no evidence to support the theory that this would reduce the rate of recurrence. Of greater importance is the development of chlamydial ophthalmia in babies born to mothers with chlamydial colonisation of the cervix. Further, the possible association of chlamydial infection of the cervix with cervicitis and salpingitis must be considered.

REFERENCES

Bowie, W. R., Floyd, J. F., Miller, Y., Alexander, E. R. & Holmes, K. K. (1976) Differential response with sulphasoxizole and spectinomycin. *Lancet*, **ii**, 1276–1278.

Bowie, W. R., Wang, S. P., Alexander, E. R., Floyd, J., Forsyth, P. S., Pollock, H. M., Lin, J-S, L., Buchanan, T. M. & Holmes, K. K. (1977) Etiology of non-gonococcal urethritis. *Journal of Clinical Investigation*, **59**, 735–742.

Darougar, S., Monnickendam, M. A., El-sheikh, H., Treharne, J. D., Woodland, R. M. & Jones, B. R. (1977) Animal models for the study of chlamydial infections of the eye and genital tract. In *Non-gonococcal Urethritis and Related Infections*, eds. Hobson, D. & Holmes, K. K., pp. 186–204. Washington D.C.: American Society for Microbiology.

Digiacomo, R. G., Gale, J. L., Wang, S. P. & Kiviat, M. D. (1975) Chlamydial infection of the male baboon urethra. *British Journal of Venereal Diseases*, **51**, 310–313.

Grayston, J. T. & Wang, S. P. (1975) New knowledge of chlamydiae and the diseases they cause. *Journal of Infectious Diseases*, **132**, No. 1, 87–105.

Handsfield, H. H., Alexander, E. R., Wang, S. P., Pedersen, A. H. & Holmes, K. K. (1976) Differences in therapeutic response of *Chlamydia*-positive and *Chlamydia*-negative forms of NGU. *Journal of the American Venereal Disease Association*, **2**, 5–9.

Hanna, L., Dawson, C. R., Briones, O., Thygeson, P. & Jawetz, E. (1968) Latency in human infections with TRIC agents. *Journal of Immunology*, **101**, 43–50.

Hilton, A. L., Richmond, S. J., Milne, J. D., Hindley, F. & Clarke, S. K. R. (1974) *Chlamydia* A in the female genital tract. *British Journal of Venereal Diseases*, **50**, 1–9.

Hobson, D., Johnson, F., Rees, E. & Tait, I. (1974) Simplified method for diagnosis of genital and ocular infections with *Chlamydia*. *Lancet*, **ii**, 555–556.

Holmes, K. K., Handsfield, H. H., Wang, S. P., Wentworth, B. B., Turck, M., Anderson, J. B. & Alexander, E. R. (1975) Etiology of non-gonococcal urethritis. *New England Journal of Medicine*, **292**, 1199–1205.

Holmes, K. K., Johnson, D. W. & Floyd, T. M. (1967) Double blind comparison of tetracycline hydrochloride and placebo in treatment of NGU. *Journal of American Medical Association*, **202**, 474–476.

Jeansson, S. & Molin, L. (1971) Genital herpes infection and non-specific urethritis. *British Medical Journal*, **2**, 247.

King, A. (1964) In *Recent Advances in Venereology*. Ch. 13, pp. 352–394. London: Churchill Livingstone.

King, A. & Nicol, C. (1975) Non specific genital infection. In *Venereal Diseases*, 3rd edition, p. 256. London: Ballière Tindall.

Lee, Y. H., Tarr, P. I., Schumacher, J. R., Rosner, B., Alpert, S. & McCormack, W. M. (1976) Re-evaluation of the role of T-mycoplasmas in non-gonococcal urethritis. *Journal of the American Venereal Disease Association*, **3**, 25–28.

McCormack, W. M., Braun, P., Lee, Y. H., Klein, J. O. & Kass, E. H. (1973) The genital mycoplasmas. *New England Journal of Medicine*, **288**, 78–89.

Oriel, J. D., Powis, P. A., Reeve, P., Miller, A. & Nicol, C. S. (1974) Chlamydial infections of the cervix. *British Journal of Venereal Diseases*, **50**, 11–16.

Oriel, J. D., Reeve, P., Nicol, C. S. (1975) Minocycline in the treatment of NGU. *Journal of American Venereal Disease Association*, **2**, 17–22.

Oriel, J. D., Reeve, P., Powis, P., Miller, A. & Nicol, C. S. (1972) Isolation of *Chlamydia* from patients with non-specific genital infection. *British Journal of Venereal Diseases*, **48**, 429–436.

Oriel, J. D., Reeve, P., Thomas, J. J. & Nicol, C. S. (1975) Infection with *Chlamydia* group A in men with urethritis due to *N. gonorrhoea*. *Journal of Infectious Diseases*, **131**, 376–382.

Oriel, J. D., Reeve, P., Wright, J. T. & Owen, J. (1976a) Chlamydial infection of the male urethra. *British Journal of Venereal Diseases*, **52**, 568–571.

Oriel, J. D., Ridgway, G. L., Reeve, P., Beckingham, D. C. & Owen, J. (1976b) The effect of ampicillin-probenecid given for genital infections with *N. gonorrhoeae* on associated *C. trachomatis* infections. *Journal of Infectious Diseases*, **133**, 568–571.

Oriel, J. D., Ridgway, G. L. & Tchamouroff, S. (1977) Comparison of erythromycin stearate and oxytetracycline in the treatment of non-gonococcal urethritis. *Scottish Medical Journal*, **22**, 375–379.

Oriel, J. D., Ridgway, G. L., Tchamouroff, S. & Owen, J. (1977) Spectinomycin hydrochloride in the treatment of gonorrhoea: its effect on associated *C. trachomatis* infections. *British Journal of Venereal Diseases*, **53**, 226–229.

Prentice, M. J., Taylor-Robinson, D. & Csonka, G. W. (1976) N.S.U. A placebo controlled trial of minocycline in conjunction with laboratory investigations. *British Journal of Venereal Diseases*, **52**, 269–275.

Reeve, P., Gerloff, R. K., Casper, E., Phillip, R. N., Oriel, J. D. & Powis, P. A. (1974) Serological studies on the role of *Chlamydia* in the aetiology of non-specific urethritis. *British Journal of Venereal Diseases*, **50**, 136–139.

Reeve, P., Owen, J. & Oriel, J. D. (1975) Laboratory procedures for the isolation of *C. trachomatis* from the human genital tract. *Journal of Clinical Pathology*, **28**, 910–914.

Richmond, S. J. & Caul, E. O. (1975) Fluorescent antibody studies in chlamydial infections. *Journal of Clinical Microbiology*, **1**, 345–352.

Richmond, S. J., Hilton, A. L. & Clarke, S. K. (1972) Role of *Chlamydia* sub group A in NGU and PGU. *British Journal of Venereal Diseases*, **48**, 437–444.

Ridgway, G. L., Owen, J. M. & Oriel, J. D. (1976) A method for testing the antibiotic susceptibility of *C. trachomatis* in a cell culture system. *Journal of Antimicrobial Chemotherapy*, **2**, 1, 77–81.

Ridgway, G. L., Owen, J. M. & Oriel, J. D. (1978) The antimicrobial susceptibility of *Chlamydia trachomatis* in cell culture. *British Journal of Venereal Diseases*, **54**, 103–105.

Schachter, J., Hannah, L., Hill, E. C., Massad, S., Sheppard, C. W., Conte, J., Cohen, S. & Meyer, K. F. (1975) Are chlamydial infections the most prevalent venereal disease? *Journal of American Medical Association*, **231**, 1252–1255.

Shepard, M. C. (1974) Quantitative relationship of *Ureaplasma urealyticum* to the clinical course of non-gonococcal urethritis in the human male. *Inserm*, **33**, 375.

Simopoulos, J. C. H. (1977) Tetracycline treatment for non-specific urethritis. *British Journal of Venereal Diseases*, **53**, 230–232.

Sompolinsky, D. & Richmond, S. J. (1974) Growth of *Chlamydia trachomatis* in McCoy cells treated with cytocholosin B. *Applied Microbiology*, **28**, 912–914.

Spaepen, M. S., Kundsin, R. B. & Horne, H. W. (1977) Tetracycline-resistant T-mycoplasmas from patients with a history of reproductive failure. *Antimicrobial Agents and Chemotherapy*, **9**, 1012–1018.

Taylor-Robinson, D., Csonka, G. W. & Prentice, M. J. (1977) Human intra-urethral inoculation of ureaplasmas. *Quarterly Journal of Medicine, New Series*, XLVI, 302–326.

Thomas, B. J., Reeve, P. & Oriel, J. D. (1976) Simplified serological test for antibodies to *C. trachomatis*. *Journal of Clinical Microbiology*, **4**, 6–10.

Treharne, J. D., Darougar, S. & Jones, B. R. (1977) Modification of the MIF test to provide a routine serodiagnostic test for chlamydial infection. *Journal of Clinical Pathology*, **30**, 510–517.

Treharne, J. D., Day, J., Yeo, C. K., Jones, B. R. & Squires, S. (1977) Susceptibility of *Chlamydiae* to chemotherapeutic agents. In *Non-gonococcal Urethritis and Related Infections*, eds. Hobson, D. & Holmes, K. K., pp. 214–222. Washington D.C.: American Society for Microbiology.

Tribby, I., Friis, R. & Moulder, J. (1973) Effect of chloramphenicol, rifampicin and nalidixic acid on *C. psittaci* growing in L cells. *Journal of Infectious Diseases*, **127,** 155–163.

Wang, S. P. & Grayston, J. T. (1971) Classification of TRIC and related strains with microimmunofluorescence. In *Trachoma and Related Disorders caused by Chlamydial Agents*, ed. Nichols, R. L., pp. 305–321. Amsterdam: Excerpta Medica 1971.

Wang, S. P. & Grayston, J. T. (1974) Human serology in *C. trachomatis* infection with microimmunofluorescence. *Journal of Infectious Diseases*, **130,** (4) 388–397.

Wentworth, B. & Alexander, E. R. (1974) The use of IUDR treated cells for the isolation of *C. trachomatis*. *Applied Microbiology*, **27,** 912–916.

Willcox, R. R. (1972) 'Triple Tetracycline' in the treatment of NGU in males. *British Journal of Venereal Diseases*, **48,** 137–140.

13. Quality control in microbiology

E. Joan Stokes

INTRODUCTION

Automation in biochemistry led to a close examination of the reliability of methods because the results from the new machines had to be compared with manual methods and the large number of tests performed made statistical evaluation possible. This revealed important errors in accuracy and precision and demonstrated the need for constant checks. Because of this development biochemistry was the first of the four major pathology disciplines to introduce regular quality control checks; haematology, also highly automated, soon followed.

Antibiotic sensitivity testing was the first procedure in microbiology to be examined for reliability on a large scale in Britain and a high proportion of errors was discovered (A.C.P. Report 1965). It had been suspected for many years that reliability of isolation and identification methods also leave much to be desired and it was known that media prepared in different laboratories, even though materials were obtained from the same manufacturer, could perform very differently (Stokes, 1968). Microbiological methods were therefore also ripe for investigation.

Because biochemistry was first in the field of quality control it was tempting to believe that methods suitable for this discipline could be successfully adapted for the others, and indeed this is true to some extent for haematology. Microbiology is, however, entirely different from these. Instead of monitoring normal values, which change during a disease and return to normal as a result of treatment or recovery, attempts are made to isolate and identify a pathogen often from a site which is laden with commensal microbes, from patients who may, or may not, actually be infected. Or abnormal antibody is sought when nothing less than a four-fold rise or fall in titre is likely to be significant. Having isolated a pathogen it is tested for sensitivity to antimicrobial drugs. Some strains prove to be highly sensitive and some highly resistant. When strains fall between these two extremes it is difficult to predict what the likely outcome of treatment would be. In such a case it is wise, and almost always possible, to use another undoubtedly active drug. The only microbiological investigation which has a biochemical parallel is antibiotic assay which is needed for a small proportion of patients, and even here the degree of precision required is not very great in comparison with biochemical and haematological investigations. What we need to test, therefore, is not great precision and accuracy of measurement but the ability to spread cultures so that single colonies and pure cultures are obtained, the ability to test these cultures appropriately and interpret the results correctly. The judgement as well as the manual skill of the microbiologist is tested repeatedly during these procedures which do not as yet lend themselves to automation.

In microbiology high quality of the media and test reagents is very important and not at all easy to achieve. Fastidious bacteria need media made from biological material which is likely to vary between batches. Moreover, when isolating pathogens from sites with a normal flora selective media must be employed. Some of these media have to be prepared locally and there are numerous sources of error, from the purchase of inferior original ingredients to mishandling in a variety of ways during preparation. For serological tests antigens and immune sera are obtained commercially and vary considerably between manufacturers and from batch to batch from the same manufacturer. There are many different tests of identification and many different methods of performing each of them. Knowledge of the relative merits of these methods is insufficient in most cases for an informed choice to be made. In a particular laboratory the choice is influenced by the training of the director or senior members of the staff, established custom in the laboratory and even the fashion of the moment.

It is clear that the potential for error in microbiology is very great. The fact that there is no stimulus from automation to examine the reliability of methods has not discouraged such tests. Indeed quality control has been practised for some years not only in Britain but also in the United States, in Australasia and in other countries which provide a modern diagnostic bacteriology service. There is some confusion in nomenclature. Quality control is sometimes applied only to testing media and reagents, proficiency testing being the term used for the procedures. In Britain the term quality control is used to include all aspects of the work. It is the quality of the final product, the laboratory report, which needs to be monitored and this is the meaning intended here.

QUALITY CONTROL METHODS

Within-laboratory tests

Routine checks are essential to avoid gross errors. For example, the temperature of incubators and waterbaths must be regularly checked, so must the performance of autoclaves. In-use testing of disinfectants and inoculation cabinets is also important as a safety measure although it is unlikely to affect the quality of the work. In addition the performance of each new batch of medium should be tested in parallel with the previous batch. This is particularly important when preparing selective media. Minor errors in preparation may result in failure to isolate, especially from carriers of intestinal pathogens. It is necessary to test not only for growth of the pathogen but also for inhibition of commensals. Some strains of Salmonella and *Esch. coli* show up deficiencies in media preparation better than others and suitable strains need to be maintained for testing. In short, within-laboratory testing of media is laborious and many laboratories cannot find time to carry it out as they would wish. Reliable commercial suppliers test their products regularly although if they are faced with a choice between failing to supply or sending a below-par batch they probably think the latter is the lesser evil. Since a particular batch may last a hospital laboratory for several months frequent checks should be made and replacement of inferior material demanded. Moreover, unless prepoured plates are purchased, the laboratory needs to check the method of plate preparation. It is possible to ruin good commercial ingredients by mishandling in the laboratory.

When medium is entirely home made tests of efficacy are essential. It is a myth that home made is necessarily best, indeed quality control tests carried out so far indicate that it is often inferior to modern commercially produced media (Table 13.1).

A laboratory check list for daily and weekly tasks is essential in all laboratories but, since pressure of work usually precludes all but the simplest media tests, we are obliged to rely to some extent on commercial quality control.

Table 13.1 Desoxycholate citrate agar. Results of one trial related to source of medium

A Plate to plate variation within batch

Source of medium	Errors	Total tests
Commercial poured locally	9	211
Prepoured commercial	1	45
Home made	6	40
Total laboratories	16	296

B Failure to inhibit *Esch. coli*

Commercial poured locally	17	211
Prepoured commercial	8	45
Home made	11	40
Total laboratories	36	296

National quality control tests

It has been said that to attempt to improve one's performance in laboratory diagnosis by internal quality control only is about as useful as attempting to improve one's game by playing golf against oneself. No diagnostic laboratory can be so self sufficient as to need no outside tests. One reason is that it is impossible for one laboratory to be expert in all aspects of the work. It will perform above average for those microbes in which the director, or another senior member of the staff, takes a particular interest but is liable to do much less well in other areas. Although some specimens may come to a laboratory because of its special reputation most arrive from undiagnosed patients who may be suffering from any infection. It is important for such laboratories to participate in a national scheme not only because, like anyone else, they need to be warned of shortcomings but also because their good performance in their special field will set a standard to which all should aspire.

There are three main purposes of a national quality control service in microbiology.

1. To provide means whereby a laboratory director can assess the performance of his laboratory and the reliability of the reports he sends.
2. To highlight common faults and discover which of the numerous available media and methods are most reliable so that overall performance may improve.
3. To ensure that reports issuing from any laboratory receiving specimens from patients are as reliable as the patient and his doctor have a right to expect.

Organisation of a service

Processing and reporting on simulated specimens is needed to test all aspects of the work. Assessment should include the speed with which a reliable report is achieved. Very meticulous examination taking many days is of little practical use. It is possible to purchase freeze-dried cultures and other material for distribution but quite apart from the cost, which is prohibitive, the material is so unlike specimens usually received that it would not effectively test normal performance. A separate laboratory is needed for the preparation of fresh simulated specimens and such a project is not commercially attractive. It has been necessary therefore to set up a Microbiology Quality Control Laboratory, which is financed by the DHSS and run by the Public Health Laboratory Service, to provide this service. Microbiology is at present the only discipline to have such a laboratory in Britain. The director is advised by a committee composed of practising clinical microbiologists, both within the PHLS and the hospital service, with technical and scientific members representing the various appropriate professional bodies. He is responsible not only for making and distributing most of the specimens but also for assessing and distributing the results. The service is confidential, each laboratory has a number which is known only to the director and the laboratory concerned, not to the committee.

The Quality Control Laboratory began distributions in 1974 when there were about 100 participants. Originally a group of clinical microbiologists interested in establishing a national service were financed by the DHSS to organise preliminary trials (Stokes and Whitby, 1971). At about the same time the PHLS set up its own quality control committee including PHLS members of this group. All those interested ultimately combined and some were original members of the advisory committee. Once the laboratory was established it was possible to invite more participants, a number of whom had been waiting to join. Now there are more than 300 laboratories receiving simulated specimens and any diagnostic laboratory, whether financed by the DHSS or not, can join.

Eighteen distributions were made during 1976. Most of the 59 specimens sent were in Stuart's transport medium containing intestinal pathogens or pyogenic organisms, including anaerobes, but a few were for microscopy and isolation of tubercle bacilli, for examination of water (carried out by public health laboratories only), for virus isolation, fungal isolation, recognition of parasites and antibiotic assay. Experts were called in to prepare these special specimens and to comment on the reports on them. Previously serum was sent for antibody titration but because of the difficulty of supplying sufficient positive human serum this is only rarely possible.

Simulated specimens for culture and identification

Every effort is made to ensure that the bacteria in cultures of these specimens are 'normal'. Commensals are added when appropriate and clinical information is given which is likely to help the participant; some negative specimens are included. Nevertheless it is clear that these are quality control specimens. Inevitably there is a fear that some laboratories will score highly by seeing that these specimens are specially treated instead of going through the normal routine as is intended. Because specimens often contain pathogens of epidemiological importance laboratories must be warned that they are simulated to prevent the institution of control measures. It has been suggested that a clinician should be asked to send the specimens and forward the report to the Quality Control Laboratory. Even if clinicians were prepared to do this it would not solve the problem because, when a dangerous pathogen is suspected, preventive measures are often suggested by the laboratory to save time and, moreover, at a stage when final identification has yet to be confirmed. Extra care with simulated specimens is likely to diminish as quality control becomes more generally accepted but actual performance in microbiology is always likely to be less good than predicted by quality control results because each specimen is individually processed instead of being one of a number in a batch processed in a machine when special treatment is impossible.

The most profitable way of using the quality control service is to process each specimen in duplicate. It should be put through the normal routine and this result should be reported. In addition an experienced member of the staff should also examine it. When he succeeds and the junior fails the error can probably be quickly found and corrected. It is possible that the junior will succeed when the experienced worker fails. It should not then be assumed that this is due to irregular distribution of the pathogen in the specimen. A more likely explanation is that there is batch to batch or even plate to plate variation in the medium, see Table 13.1, and this should be tested forthwith; the senior should also check his own technique critically. When both fail to isolate or identify correctly there is a natural tendency to blame the specimen. Each laboratory discipline embarking on quality control has gone through this stage. Since microbiological specimens are particularly difficult to prepare there are indeed occasional failures and this is discovered when the Quality Control Laboratory re-tests some of the specimens and when all results are returned. It is most unlikely that the specimen is at fault when a poor result is obtained by a small number of laboratories, and every effort should be made to trace the source of error in each laboratory concerned. When identification was at fault tests should be repeated and reagents tested. If the pathogen was not isolated it can be obtained in pure culture from the Quality Control Laboratory and its growth on isolation media checked. Media departments should keep records of dates on which batches of media were used to facilitate subsequent checking. The tendency to blame the specimen disappears when it is realised that, without repeated routine checks, there is no way of knowing how poor performance is, and that in the past most microbiologists have been unduly optimistic about the reliability of methods and what is possible to achieve with them.

Antibiotic sensitivity tests
These are requested on a proportion of pyogenic bacteria sent either in pure or mixed culture in transport medium specimens. At first no guidance was given about the number of tests to be made or which drugs to test. It was left to the microbiologist to do what he would normally do according to the clinical information given. The practice in individual laboratories varied enormously. Moreover it soon became clear, as would be expected, that some drugs, notably the folic acid inhibitors and those sensitive to beta-lactamases, were much more difficult to test than others. If anything is to be discovered about the relative merits of testing

procedures it is necessary to encourage each laboratory to test at least six drugs, even when this might not be clinically necessary, in order to provide sufficient data for analysis. Some laboratories avoid trouble by omitting those drugs which are notoriously difficult to test. Some may do so on the grounds that the tests are unsatisfactory and reliable results are impossible to achieve. They may be right about the methods now popular. If so it is however important to prove this beyond reasonable doubt and to develop better methods, because reliable tests are of clinical value and are likely to become increasingly requested as further bacterial resistance develops. It is therefore necessary to depart from 'normal procedure' to some extent for the evaluation of these methods.

It was also considered that some faults in reporting were particularly dangerous, and that even when the result was correct some reports should be withheld for fear of misuse of the drug. For example, sensitivity to nitrofurantoin or nalidixic acid of *Esch. coli* isolated from blood, or streptomycin sensitivity of *Ps. aeruginosa* when it is also sensitive to gentamicin and carbenicillin which are much more therapeutically active. However, slanting the scoring of results to penalise such errors was not generally agreed. It was however, decided to request laboratories to test six particular drugs on some occasions, and to include in these six some of those most difficult to test. Possibly new simplified methods of estimating minimal inhibitory concentration will prove to be more reliable than disk tests, and need to be introduced for some drugs if performance is to be improved.

Comparison of methods and media
The use of quality control to discover which methods are more successful is of great potential value. Methods employed successfully by workers engaged in research are not necessarily as successful when employed in diagnostic laboratories. This is not because those in hospital laboratories are less able but because they are usually under great pressure, and when a technique requires frequent preparation of reagents, time consuming standardisation of inoculum and other procedures, short cuts are liable to be made. Unlike the research laboratory, where effective controls must be built in if any progress is to be made, the hospital laboratory cannot easily know when short cuts lead to error. Indeed processing known positive quality control specimens is the only way such information can easily be gained. In hospital laboratories the simplest methods are usually the most popular. Often they are reliable, but sometimes a more laborious method is essential to ensure reliability and this can be clearly demonstrated by relating results to the methods employed. Participants are asked to reveal their methods by completing questionnaires.

The reliability of media from different sources can also be investigated. This again demands departure from the normal examination of simulated specimens because possible errors due to technique other than media preparation must be eliminated as far as possible. Pure cultures of a Salmonella and a commensal *Esch. coli* were sent for quantitative assessment of growth on selective and non-selective media prepared for normal use in the laboratories and the results were related to the source of the media and the method of preparation. This trial indicated considerable differences between different brands of desoxycholate citrate agar and methods of preparation (Table 13.1). It is, however, necessary to repeat these tests before firm conclusions about different brands can be drawn because one commercial supplier might have the misfortune to have released a less than average performance batch at the time the test was made and on a subsequent occasion one of his competitors might do so. The results of such tests are useful not only to hospital laboratories but also to the suppliers who have no means of knowing how their product performs in comparison with others in the field.

Results and scoring

Distributors of quality control material do not like to be in the position of saying they are right and anyone obtaining unexpected results is wrong. In practice this is avoided because the majority of laboratories will obtain the expected answer and the distributor has plenty of support. The specimens contain living microbes which may multiply or die during transit but since participants are situated widely over the country, including some abroad, poor performance due to deterioration of the specimen would be easily recognised. There is also the fear that the distribution of microbes within the material distributed might be irregular. Great care is taken by very thorough mixing in a single container before distribution to ensure this does not happen. If it were to happen, for example, in specimens containing tubercle bacilli which are particularly difficult to distribute evenly, statistical analysis of errors would show them to be random and provided a large enough sample of tests were available for analysis the fault would be evident. Indeed random errors, presumably due to occasional faults in specimens or perhaps in typing or entering results, have been noted and these can be distinguished statistically from non-random errors of technique.

One way of convincing laboratories that poor results are not due to faulty specimens has been to send the same strain on more than one occasion for antibiotic sensitivity tests. Results which vary on different occasions can only be due to laboratory error.

Occasionally the majority of laboratories do not obtain the expected result. This happened when the need for modifications of technique for testing staphylococci to methicillin and of interpreting sensitivity tests of *Ps. aeruginosa* to carbenicillin were not widely appreciated. Explanation of the reason for failure and repeated tests was followed by improvement when again the majority obtained the expected result.

There have been objections to the assumption that the majority answer is the right answer, and indeed this would be dangerous if great care were not taken to ensure, as far as possible, that the expected answer is both correct and relevant. Tests of identification are checked when necessary by acknowledged experts in their field, and rapid sensitivity tests employed by most laboratories can be checked by estimation of minimal inhibitory concentration. Clinical relevance is kept in mind by reference to the weekly Communicable Diseases Report when deciding what strains to circulate and by giving clinical details which would be likely to be found on a properly completed request form.

Regional quality control

The great variability in microbiological methods makes national and even supranational distribution desirable because large numbers of results are needed for statistical evaluation. This does not mean, however, that there is no place for effort on a smaller scale. Laboratories making errors are faced with the decision whether to change their method radically or whether greater attention to detail or perhaps purchasing from a different source would be the best course. There is evidence from repeated errors of the same kind that information sent by the Quality Control Laboratory often goes unheeded. Indeed to obtain maximum value from the national scheme time must be given to read and discuss the results in detail and this may not always be possible in individual laboratories. Discussions sponsored in Regions are very valuable and when there is disagreement about the need to change methods small distributions of strains or simulated specimens between local laboratories can settle the question. One such enterprise leading to improved performance was reported from Birmingham (George, 1974).

TECHNICAL INFORMATION FROM QUALITY CONTROL RESULTS

In the absence of regular discussions of quality control results their implication indicating the need for change may go unrecognised. A summary of information gained so far is therefore appropriate.

Antibody tests

Sufficient positive human serum for one national distribution to test the reliability of agglutination tests was obtained. The results revealed fairly wide variation of agglutination titres for antibody to enteric organisms which was not surprising since different antigens and methods were used. The results for Vi antibody tests were, however, disastrous. Five sera were distributed, the expected titres were less than five (two sera), 20, 320, and 1280. Eighty-four laboratories reported and the results ranged from less than five to greater than 5120 for *each* of the five samples. The conclusion must be that this test is not suitable for performance in hospital laboratories, which are seldom requested to do it, and that when necessary sera should be sent to a specialist laboratory familiar with the technique and able to keep the antigen and controls required in a satisfactory condition.

Antibiotic sensitivity tests

It was shown that disk diffusion tests to determine the sensitivity of staphylococci to cephalosporins are unreliable. On two occasions methicillin/cephalosporin-resistant strains of *Staph. aureus* were distributed. The majority of laboratories, knowing that for methicillin-resistant strains of this species cephalosporin resistance can be confidently predicted, did not attempt to test but of those who did half reported sensitive and half resistant on both occasions. The results of the first trial which showed this were published in 1973 (Blowers, Stokes and Abbott), but this did not prevent repetition of the error on the second occasion. This test should no longer be performed.

The inoculum of pyogenic bacteria in simulated pus and urine is aimed at attaining what would be expected in natural specimens. Some laboratories performed primary sensitivity tests from these specimens, as they would normally

Table 13.2   Comparison of all sensitivity tests with primary tests

| | All tests | | Primary tests | |
	Total	Percentage error	Total	Percentage error
All drugs	11,532	5.3	2,423	2.9
Sulphas	367	16.0	60	20.0
Penicillin	175	4.5	72	2.7
Ampicillin	314	13.0	75	5.2
Methicillin	431	13.4	82	12.2

do, to give as quick an answer as possible. When these results were compared with the results of all tests including those with standard inocula there was no evidence that the primary tests were less reliable (Table 13.2), which confirms a report from a single laboratory (Waterworth and del Piano, 1976).

Results from those using controls regularly to help them interpret disk sensitivity tests (which are almost invariably performed by the comparative method or modifications of it in Britain, Broadsheet, 1972) showed, as would be expected, better reliability (Table 13.3).

There is no consensus of opinion as to the optimum disk content of ampicillin for reliable tests. When strains are resistant fewer errors are made with low content disks and when they are sensitive the reverse holds. Comparison of results when ampicillin disks of differing content were employed to test *E. coli* and *Bacteroides fragilis* in simulated specimens other than urine showed that a 10 μg disk gave fewer errors than either a 5 μg disk or a 25 μg disk. The high content disk is suitable for testing urinary pathogens which will be exposed to high levels of the drug but when used for *B. fragilis* false sensitivity was frequently reported. Use of the 5 μg disk led to false reports of resistance of *E. coli* (Blowers et al, 1973).

Table 13.3   Controls for disk diffusion sensitivity tests

| | Methods | | | |
| | A | | B | |
	Errors	Total tested	Errors	Total tested
Methicillin	5 (S)	42	12 (S)	39 *Staph.*
Erythromycin	5 (S)	35	9 (S)	34 *aureus*
Fusidate	0	37	2 (R)	28
Ampicillin	5 (R)	39	3 (R)	36 *Esch.*
Sulphonamide	1 (R)	38	2 (R)	35 *coli*
Total	16	191	28	172

(S) = Sensitivity wrongly reported
(R) = Resistance wrongly reported
Method A Controls cultured daily for comparison with unknown zones
Method B No controls or controls occasionally cultured

Identification tests

Pure cultures of four species of Enterobacteriaceae were distributed in order to test the reliability of identification tests. They were *E. coli, Ent. cloacae, Citrobacter koseri* and *Providencia alcalifaciens*. Many different tests and modifications of them were employed but the results seen in Tables 13.4–6 indicate beyond reasonable doubt that for decarboxylases Moller-like tests were more reliable than Falkow-like tests, that lead acetate papers are unreliable for detecting H_2S production and that indole production testing should be done at 37°C and not at 44°C.

Table 13.4   Tests for decarboxylases

Methods	Arginine		Lysine		Ornithine	
	Errors	Total tested	Errors	Total tested	Errors	Total tested
Moller-like	15	109	11	117	7	108
Falkow-like	39	119	18	130	10	122

For strains tested see text

Table 13.5   Tests for H_2S production

	Errors	Total tests
Lead acetate paper		
expected positive	50	171
expected negative	7	50
TSI		
all strains expected negative	0	63

Table 13.6   Indole production

All tests expected positive		
Incubation temperature	Errors	Total tests
44 C	19	67
37 C	9	393

POOR PERFORMERS

The ultimate aim of all hospital laboratory work and of quality control is to improve the service to patients. It is reasonable to assume that all those engaged in this enterprise have that aim and indeed participation in quality control is evidence that this is so. Statistical analysis of quality control results reveals a small number of laboratories consistently reporting less accurately than others. These are likely to be under-staffed and overworked for a variety of reasons and may not even realise that their performance falls short of what should be possible to achieve; they should therefore be notified. Such notification may help them to overcome whatever difficulty they have, for example, by confirming the need for additional help during prolonged absence of staff. The desired result may then be achieved and the laboratory will emerge from the poor performance category. A very small number of laboratories may fail to improve and may, as a result of notification, cease to participate. In the interest of patients whose doctors use these laboratories something should be done.

Although the Department of Health finances the National Quality Control services it has been agreed that it is entirely the responsibility of the professional bodies concerned to maintain standards of practice, indeed that is one of the main reasons for their existence. Therefore panels have been set up, which are separate from the organisers of the quality control service, whose business it is to satisfy themselves that the evidence for poor performance is valid and to offer help. Each major discipline has its own panel which includes members representing each of the appropriate medical, technical and scientific professional bodies. It is intended that they meet and visit separately but since they have many problems in common they keep in touch with each other. Confidentiality is broken only to make help from the panels possible and the names of the laboratories visited will remain confidential outside the panels.

The organisation for helping poor performers has only recently been set up and no microbiological laboratories have so far been visited. Some participating laboratories are outside the NHS. Nevertheless their staff are part of the professions concerned and help for them, when needed, should not be denied. Moreover, specimens from sick patients arriving in this country from abroad are likely to be processed in them and there is a danger that epidemiologically important pathogens might go unrecognised if their standard too is not maintained.

THE FUTURE OF QUALITY CONTROL

In his report for 1976 Dr Crone, the director of the Microbiology Quality Control Laboratory*, revealed that of results received from more than 300 laboratories, each receiving 59 simulated specimens, the only result correctly achieved by all those reporting was the isolation of a 'coliform' (no detailed identification) from a simulated urine where it alone was present. The material distributed has purposely been straightforward and apart from occasional important pathogens, such as *Corynebacterium diphtheriae* and *Vibrio cholerae*, which laboratories seldom encounter, the specimens have simulated those which laboratories are constantly called upon to deal with. The need for improvement is obvious and it is encouraging that some light has already been thrown on some sources of error. Possibly there has been some improvement but this is unlikely to be noticeable until all laboratories participate. At present any improvement due to quality control education is likely to be diluted by new participants joining who have not had this advantage. Microbiology has almost reached the stage, long passed by biochemistry, when routine examination of quality control specimens is generally regarded as essential to good practice, and undue anxiety about comparative performance

* Address :
Microbiology Quality Control Laboratory, Neasden Hospital, London NW10 8EY.

fades into the background. In the future evidence for or against the reliability of methods will gradually accumulate enabling a logical choice to be made. New methods will be properly evaluated not only in single laboratories but by testing in the field. Because good commercial products will be more easily recognised firms should be stimulated to further effort, and before long we should have evidence of widespread improved performance.

The opinions expressed are those of the author and they may not necessarily be shared by other workers in this field. It is hoped that this account may stimulate further interest and also lead to wider participation in Quality Control.

REFERENCES

Association of Clinical Pathologists, Broadsheet No. 55. Antibiotic sensitivity tests by diffusion methods (revised 1972) by Stokes, E. J. & Waterworth, P.M.

Association of Clinical Pathologists Report (1965) Antibiotic sensitivity test trial organised by the Bacteriology Committee. *Journal of Clinical Pathology*, **18,** 1–5.

Blowers, R., Stokes, E. J. & Abbott, J. D. (1973) Antibiotic sensitivity tests. *British Medical Journal*, **iii,** 46–47.

George, R. H. (1974) Progress towards agreement in reports of antibiotic sensitivity. *Journal of Clinical Pathology*, **27,** 1001–1004.

Stokes, E. J. (1968) Quality control in diagnostic bacteriology. *Proceedings of the Royal Society of Medicine*, **61,** 457–463.

Stokes, E. J. & Whitby, J. L. (1971) Quality control in bacteriology preliminary trials. *Journal of Clinical Pathology*, **24,** 790–797.

Waterworth, P. M. & del Piano, M. (1976) Dependability of sensitivity tests in primary culture. *Journal of Clinical Pathology*, **29,** 179–184.

14. Infections with obligate anaerobes

A. Trevor Willis

Anaerobic bacteria cause a variety of disease processes in man. From the clinical standpoint, anaerobic bacterial diseases exhibit one or another of virtually all the cardinal features of bacterial infection, although they are not communicable from man to man. Botulism stands alone, since it is almost always the result of a pure intoxication that develops in the absence of an infection. At the other extreme are those diseases such as acute ulcerative gingivitis, anaerobic streptococcal myositis and anaerobic necrotizing fasciitis in which bacterial synergism appears to be an essential feature of the infective process.

In the last decade there has been a great resurgence of interest in anaerobic bacteriology among both medical microbiologists and their clinical colleagues. This is due largely to an increasing recognition of the importance of the non-sporing anaerobic bacteria as significant causes of infection in man. In this connection it is pertinent to recall MacLennan's opening remarks in his chapter on infections caused by non-sporing anaerobic bacilli, published in *Recent Advances in Bacteriology* in 1951. 'From a bacteriological point of view this appears to us to be one of the most extraordinary problems in medicine today. Here we have a group of organisms, certainly among the commonest, if not the commonest parasites of man, capable of causing many varied and dangerous infections, and yet so neglected that in standard text-books of the greatest eminence they are for the most part clumped together under the generic name *"Fusiformes"* . . . this must still be regarded as one of the few happy-hunting grounds left for elementary and fundamental studies in bacteriology and infective disease.' And such has proved to be the case.

Clostridial infections of man are essentially wound infections which may develop as a consequence of accidental or surgical trauma because these sporing anaerobes are ubiquitously distributed in nature. The wound infection itself, however, may not be the most prominent feature of the syndrome, for the pathogenic clostridia produce exotoxins which exert their damaging effects systemically. *Clostridium tetani*, for example, produces no tissue-destroying enzymes and is non-invasive, so that lesions infected by it are quite unremarkable, and local symptoms and signs are absent; the soluble tetanospasmin produced by the infecting organisms has a profoundly toxic effect on the central nervous system. In anaerobic myonecrosis there are always overt local pathological changes due to the histotoxic effects of the gas gangrene toxins, but even these are likely to be overshadowed by the accompanying profound systemic toxaemia, a feature of great diagnostic importance.

In contrast to the clostridial diseases, infections due to *Actinomyces israelii*, the anaerobic Gram-negative non-sporing bacilli (incorrectly but conveniently lumped together as the 'bacteroides') and the anaerobic cocci are almost always of endogenous origin, are less acute in their onset and prone to chronicity, and do not commonly produce a severe toxaemia. In general they are lowly pathogens that sometimes produce primary infections, but much more commonly cause disease at sites that have been debilitated or are the seat of some preceding pathological change. Together, the bacteroides and the anaerobic cocci are by far the commonest cause of anaerobic bacterial disease, whose frequent occurrence as significant pathogens is often overlooked by the clinician and missed by the microbiologist.

In the present short text attention is focused on non-clostridial anaerobic infections. For more detailed accounts of these and other aspects of anaerobic bacterial disease reference should be made to Willis (1969, 1977), Shapton and Board (1971), Balows et al (1974), Gorbach and Bartlett (1974), Phillips and Sussman (1974), Smith (1975), and Finegold (1977a).

INFECTIONS DUE TO NON-CLOSTRIDIAL ANAEROBES

The non-sporing anaerobic bacteria, and especially the bacteroides, are a common cause of infective disease in man. The term 'bacteroides' is used here to refer to the group comprised of the genera *Bacteroides* and *Fusobacterium*; much the commonest species involved in human infections are *B. fragilis*, *B. melaninogenicus*, *F. nucleatum* and *F. necrophorum*. Infections due to the non-clostridial anaerobes are endogenous because most of these organisms are obligate parasites that form part of the normal bacterial flora of the oropharynx, and of the alimentary and female genital tracts. While strains of *Bacteroides* are normally present in all these situations, species of *Fusobacterium* are most commonly encountered in the oropharynx; and anaerobic cocci are prevalent in the upper respiratory and genital tracts, but are relatively sparse in the intestinal tract.

Pathogenesis of infection

Although the development of anaerobic conditions in the tissues must clearly pave the way for their invasion by anaerobic bacteria, many of which are intolerant of even traces of oxygen, the conditions necessary for the development of many of these endogenous infections are not understood. When the local resistance of the tissues is lowered by inadequate diet or by unrelated infections such as measles and pertussis, or by immunosuppressive drugs, rapidly progressive synergistic fusospirochaetal infections such as acute ulcerative gingivitis, gangrenous stomatitis, and pulmonary abscess and gangrene may result. Infection of the female genital tract is greatly favoured by blood loss and tissue damage, as may occur in septic abortion, in prolonged labour and in postpartum haemorrhage. The trauma of abdominal surgery, especially colonic and gynaecological surgery, provides conditions favourable to the development of bacteroides infections. Malignant disease and diabetes appear to be general predisposing causes. The use of neomycin for the preoperative 'sterilization' of the large bowel may also be a predisposing factor in colonic surgery, since anaerobes are insensitive to this drug. Both the anaerobic cocci and the bacteroides induce thrombophlebitis much more readily than aerobic species, a factor which explains some common characters of these infections, namely local extension, bacteraemia and metastatic abscess formation.

The bacteroides, fusobacteria and anaerobic cocci cause a variety of infections of virtually all types which are most commonly initiated in the vicinity of their normal habitats. In addition, the anaerobic cocci, classically, but also the bacteroides play an important part in three rare synergistic wound infections—anaerobic streptococcal myositis, Meleney's synergistic gangrene and anaerobic necrotizing fasciitis. In these infections, anaerobic bacteria are associated with pyogenic aerobic organisms such as *Staphylococcus aureus*. These conditions are distinguished from gas gangrene by the absence of severe toxaemia, and on the microscopic appearance of the wound exudate (Tehrani and Ledingham, 1977).

The march of events in infections due to non-clostridial anaerobes may be illustrated by reference to the female genital tract. Almost any condition that causes bleeding and tissue damage in the female genital tract predisposes to invasion of the pelvic viscera by non-sporing anaerobes. Important among these are malignant disease, gynaecological surgery including hysterectomy, curettage and cervical cauterization, child birth including delivery by caesarean section, and incomplete abortion. A variety of localized vulvovaginal infections may be caused by these organisms—incisional abscess, periurethral abscess, Bartholinitis, peri-rectal abscess and labial abscess (Parker and Jones, 1966). Much the most dangerous obstetrical and gynaecological infections, however, are those that commence in the uterus. Septic thrombophlebitis originating in the uterine sinusoids may extend via venous and lymphatic routes into the broad ligaments and retroperitoneal spaces in the pelvic floor. Adnexal abscesses thus formed may rupture into the peritoneal cavity producing general peritonitis or multiple intra-abdominal abscesses. Septic thrombophlebitis of the pelvic veins results in a continuous bacteraemia, endocarditis may develop, and there may be metastatic abscess formation in the lungs, brain, liver, bones and joints, and other organs.

Types of infection

Like the staphylococcus, these organisms are able to produce a great diversity of infections (Table 14.1). Those most frequently encountered in civilian practice include anorectal and vulvovaginal suppurative infections; pelvic, intra-abdominal and wound sepsis following appendicectomy, and gynaecological and colonic surgery; periodontal infection and aspiration pneumonia. Those listed under 'other infections' in Table 14.1 are also not infrequently encountered. It is of special interest to note that abdominal wound dehiscence and herniation is commonly due to wound infection (Irvin et al, 1977), a form of postsurgical sepsis that is almost always caused by non-sporing anaerobic bacteria.

Clinical diagnosis

The diagnosis of the various synergistic infections is usually not difficult; acute ulcerative gingivitis and stomatitis, Meleney's synergistic gangrene, anaerobic streptococcal myositis and anaerobic necrotizing fasciitis each presents its own fairly typical clinical picture; and in all of these conditions the appearances of direct Gram-stained films are characteristic.

The more general forms of non-clostridial anaerobic infection (Table 14.1)

Table 14.1   A summary of some endogenous non-clostridial anaerobic infections (After Willis, 1977)

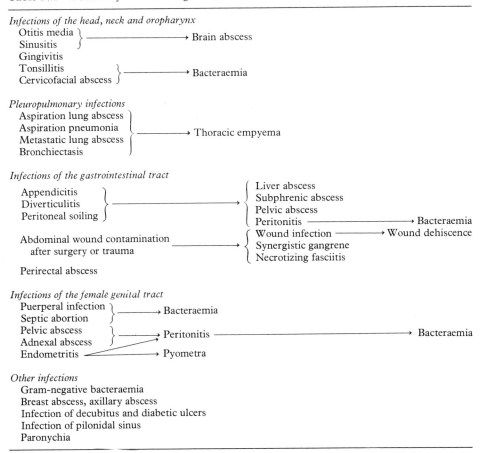

Infections of the head, neck and oropharynx
Otitis media ⎫
Sinusitis   ⎬ ─────────────→ Brain abscess
Gingivitis
Tonsillitis   ⎫
Cervicofacial abscess ⎬ ─────────→ Bacteraemia

Pleuropulmonary infections
Aspiration lung abscess   ⎫
Aspiration pneumonia   ⎬ ────────→ Thoracic empyema
Metastatic lung abscess   ⎪
Bronchiectasis   ⎭

Infections of the gastrointestinal tract
Appendicitis   ⎫   ⎧ Liver abscess
Diverticulitis ⎬ ──────────────────→ ⎨ Subphrenic abscess
Peritoneal soiling ⎭   ⎪ Pelvic abscess
                                      ⎩ Peritonitis ─────────────→ Bacteraemia
Abdominal wound contamination   ⎧ Wound infection ────→ Wound dehiscence
    after surgery or trauma ──────────⎨ Synergistic gangrene
                                      ⎩ Necrotizing fasciitis
Perirectal abscess

Infections of the female genital tract
Puerperal infection ⎫ ──────→ Bacteraemia
Septic abortion   ⎭
Pelvic abscess ⎫
Adnexal abscess ⎬ ──→ Peritonitis ──────────────────→ Bacteraemia
Endometritis ───────→ Pyometra

Other infections
Gram-negative bacteraemia
Breast abscess, axillary abscess
Infection of decubitus and diabetic ulcers
Infection of pilonidal sinus
Paronychia

share many of the clinical features that are common to most types of pyogenic sepsis. There are, however, a number of features that help to distinguish non-clostridial anaerobic sepsis from other types of bacterial infection:

1. The proximity of the infection to a mucosal surface—oropharyngeal, gastro-intestinal or vaginal—reflects the portal of entry of endogenously derived organisms.

2. Pre-existing states that compromise the integrity of the mucosal surfaces, such as accidental trauma, surgery, appendicitis, perforation of ulcer, prolonged or difficult labour, and malignant disease.

3. Infections that are related to the use of aminoglycosides; and those that follow human or animal bites.

4. Copious foul-smelling discharge is the hallmark of non-clostridial anaerobic infections. It may take the form of frank pus from superficial or deep seated abscesses (including brain abscess), and from such infections as thoracic empyema, chronic otitis media, sinusitis and mastoiditis. Alternatively the discharge may be an offensive lochia, a purulent sputum or a serosanguinous exudate from infections

such as peritonitis, abdominal wound cellulitis and decubitus ulcer. Contrary to popular belief *Enterobacteriaceae* pus is never foul smelling and is usually odour-less; however, the discharge from some non-clostridial anaerobic infections is also odourless.

5. Failure of antimicrobial therapy directed against aerobic organisms.

6. Untreated non-clostridial anaerobic infections are prone to progress to a bacteraemic state, and may also be complicated by septic thromboembolic phenomena. Consequntly, bacteraemia, especially when associated with icterus, septic thrombophlebitis or metastatic abscess formation, is an important pointer to an underlying anaerobic infection. Gunn (1956) summarized the common clinical sequence of events in bacteroides bacteraemia as follows: i. Symptoms and signs of the primary lesion, e.g. appendicitis; ii. a period of apparent recovery; iii. symptoms and signs of a spreading infection at the site of the original lesion; iv. abrupt onset of septicaemia with rigors, profuse sweating, anaemia and icterus; and v. symptoms and signs of metastatic infective lesions.

Although the development of a bacteraemia may be the first declaration of the presence of an underlying 'silent' bacteroides infection, e.g. liver abscess, bacteroides bacteraemias most commonly follow from a failure to recognize the likely anaerobic aetiology of obvious pre-existing sepsis. Not uncommonly the preceding infection is mistakenly attributed to facultatively anaerobic bacteria. There can be little doubt that most anaerobic bacteraemias are preventable, and that established bacteraemias may be recognized by fostering a high index of suspicion and a knowledge of the natural history and pathogenesis of bacteroides infections.

Bacteriological diagnosis

The specimen

Non-clostridial anaerobes are prevalent throughout the body, especially in associa-tion with mucosal surfaces, and this 'normal bacterial presence' must be borne in mind when considering the microbiology of pathological specimens. It is this problem that has led some workers to take the view that clinical specimens for anaerobic culture must be collected by methods that avoid contamination with the normal bacterial flora (Sutter and Finegold, 1973; Gorbach and Bartlett, 1974). Ellner, Granato and May (1973) have gone so far as to recommend that 'only specimens from normally sterile areas should be cultured anaerobically'.

Clearly, contamination of specimens with the normal flora of the colon (faeces) is likely to render them useless because pathologically significant organisms will be overwhelmed by the sheer diversity and weight of numbers of the faecal flora. In most other cases, however, including pulmonary and uterine infections, contamination of samples by normal bacterial floras causes much less technical difficulty than is generally supposed. There is usually little difficulty in interpreting direct plate cultures of expectorated sputum provided that the inoculum is carefully chosen from the sample, and that multiple cultures are incubated in parallel so that direct comparative assessment can be made of the anaerobic, facultatively anaerobic and carbon dioxide-dependent flora. It is unlikely that clinicians will spontaneously submit transtracheal aspirations, and it seems unreasonable for microbiologists to request them. The same sorts of considerations apply to specimens collected from the female genital tract, although a 'perineal wipe' is not a substitute for a properly taken high vaginal or cervical swab.

Because many non-sporing anaerobes are intolerant of oxygen it is important that specimens in which they are to be sought are not exposed unnecessarily to the atmosphere. Close liaison between the clinician and the microbiologist helps to ensure that the appropriate specimen, freshly collected, is transmitted to the laboratory without delay for immediate culture. Many workers consider that special precautions should be taken to protect 'anaerobic' bacteriological specimens from the toxic effects of oxygen, and a variety of specimen transport systems have been designed for this purpose. These include double stoppered tubes containing oxygen-free carbon dioxide or nitrogen (gassed-out tubes) into which fluid specimens are injected at the bedside, prereduced and anaerobically sterilized (PRAS) semisolid tranport medium for the transport of swabs, and a disposable 'mini' anaerobic jar for the transport of samples of tissue (Sutter, Vargo and Finegold, 1975; Holdeman and Moore, 1975). There is, however, some evidence to suggest that many exacting anaerobes will tolerate at least short periods of exposure to atmospheric oxygen, and in my own experience there is rarely much difficulty in recovering exacting species from pathological material on swabs provided that the interval between collection of the specimen and its culture is short—say 20–30 minutes (Collee et al, 1974; Tally et al, 1975). Alternatively, swabs may be sent to the laboratory in a non-nutrient transport media, such as Stuart's medium, provided that the swab is not held longer than about six hours. Recently Smith and Ferguson (1977) described a haemoglobin-impregnated swab upon which non-sporing anaerobes survive for prolonged periods when exposed to atmospheric oxygen at ambient temperature.

A successful transport system implies that specimens at culture contain the same viable microorganisms in the same proportions as in the infected lesion; thus, the viability of oxygen-intolerant species must be maintained, and their overgrowth by more robust anaerobes, or by facultative anaerobes must be prevented. *Under no circumstances should specimens be transported in nutrient media.*

Quite the best specimens for anaerobic bacteriological examination are volumes of pus or other exudate, and pieces of tissue. Exudates are conveniently collected and transported in disposable plastic syringes; soiled dressings from infected wounds may be sealed in plastic bags; samples of excised tissue should be placed in small screw-capped bottles. Early culture of these materials is not so urgent as for swabs, but should, nevertheless, be effected without undue delay.

Specimens that must be examined for non-clostridial anaerobes include material from most infective lesions of the gastrointestinal, female genital and lower respiratory tracts; blood for culture; pus from any deep-seated abscess; peritoneal and pleural exudate; joint effusions; discharge from middle ear, chronic sinus and mastoid infections; and cerebrospinal fluid in cases of meningitis, especially those associated with middle-ear infections, brain abscess and fractured base of skull. A surprising number of superficial abscesses and other infections commonly contain anaerobes—breast abscess, axillary abscess, ischiorectal abscess, infected pilonidal sinus, paronychia, infected abdominal and episiotomy wounds and so on.

In addition, any specimen that is sterile or shows only a minimal aerobic flora without a satisfactory explanation is suspect.

Direct microscopy

Bacteroides and related organisms are often easy to recognize in Gram-stained films of pathological material. They may present as small faintly stained Gram-negative bacilli, similar in appearance to *Haemophilus influenzae*, as fusiform-shaped rods or spheroids. Marked pleomorphism and irregular staining are characteristic of the Gram-negative anaerobes. It is worth remembering, however, that Gram-negative organisms may sometimes not be seen in direct films of specimens, even when present in large numbers.

Ultraviolet light fluorescence

Pathological specimens that contain *B. melaninogenicus* commonly show a brick-red fluorescence under ultraviolet light (Myers et al, 1969). All suspect swabs, exudates, samples of pus, wound dressings and pieces of tissue should be 'screened' under a Wood's lamp. Examination of unstained smears of pathological specimens by ultraviolet light microscopy may show the presence of individual red-fluorescing bacilli.

Direct gas liquid chromatography

Gas liquid chromatographic analysis of samples of pus provides a rapid and reliable means for the presumptive differentiation of anaerobic from aerobic infections (Phillips, Tearle and Willis, 1976; Eykyn and Phillips, 1976). An aliquot of the specimen is processed in the same way as a bacterial culture, an extract of it being examined for the presence of volatile fatty acids. The detection of volatile acids other than acetic, is strong presumptive evidence of the presence of significant numbers of anaerobes in the specimen. Exudates from sepsis due exclusively to facultatively anaerobic bacteria usually contain no volatile acids or acetic acid only.

Culture

Although non-sporing anaerobes are not infrequently mixed with facultative anaerobes in clinical material, there is rarely any difficulty in determining their likely significance. This is accomplished by conventional methods of direct plating of the specimen on to media for anaerobic and aerobic incubation, and for incubation in air plus 10 per cent carbon dioxide. These cultures are subsequently examined for the identity of isolates and are compared with one another for the relative proportions of aerobic, facultatively anaerobic and carbon dioxide-dependant growth. For the purpose of making this 'value judgment', selective agents should not be added to plating media, and enrichment cultures should not be used. Selective and enrichment techniques may be used subsequently for purification of cultures prior to specific identification. The mere presence of non-sporing anaerobes in a lesion does not necessarily imply that they are causing an infection.

Any one of a number of cultural methods may be used successfully for the isolation of non-clostridial anaerobes from clinical material (Ellner et al, 1973; Dowell and Hawkins, 1974; Sutter et al, 1975; Duerden et al, 1976). These vary in their complexity, and it is important that the method chosen by any particular laboratory is one that can be fitted into the normal daily routine. Sophisticated methods are not necessarily the best; and the best methods may not take account of other laboratory commitments.

Anaerobiosis. For the establishment of an oxygen-free atmosphere for the culture of clinical specimens, anaerobic jars provide the method of choice. It has been shown that more sophisticated methods such as the pre-reduced anaerobically sterilized (PRAS) roll-tube technique, and the anaerobic cabinet or glove box are not superior to the anaerobic jar for the recovery of clinically significant anaerobes from pathological specimens (Watt, Collee and Brown, 1974; Balows et al, 1974; Wren, 1977).

In modern anaerobic jars pellets of alumina coated with finely divided palladium (Dexo Catalyst–Englehard Industries) catalyse the combination of oxygen and hydrogen to form water. This may be achieved by generation of hydrogen within the jar, or by partial evacuation of air from the jar and its replacement with hydrogen from an external source. The GasPak anaerobic system (Becton, Dickinson) is designed specifically for internal gas generation, although the GasPak anaerobic jar may be adapted for use by the evacuation/replacement method. Other anaerobic jars, such as the Whitley (Don Whitley Scientific) and BTL (Baird and Tatlock, London) jars, may be used with either gas supply method. The two internal gas generators at present available are the GasPak H_2/CO_2 generator (Becton, Dickinson) and the GasKit H_2/CO_2 generator (Oxoid Ltd), in both of which water reacts with tablets of sodium borohydride and citric acid/sodium bicarbonate to produce hydrogen and carbon dioxide respectively.

In the GasPak gas generator the reaction of borohydride with water results in a highly alkaline residue which commonly prevents activation of the bicarbonate tablet, so that only a fraction of the available carbon dioxide is released. Moreover, the alkaline residue is likely to absorb any carbon dioxide that is present in the atmosphere of the jar. The proportion of carbon dioxide in the GasPak jar under these circumstances must therefore be regarded as random, variable and unknown, and may lead to reduced isolation rates (Ferguson, Phillips and Tearle, 1975).

The GasKit generator does not have these disadvantages, since the alkalinity of the borohydride reaction is neutralized, thus ensuring that poisoning of the carbon dioxide tablet does not occur and that the pH of the final reaction is slightly acidic (Ferguson, Phillips and Willis, 1976).

Internal gas generation on the one hand, and evacuation/replacement on the other each have advantages and disadvantages, but both provide effective means of producing an anaerobic environment. The outstanding features of the disposable gas generator envelope are that it does away with the need for a vacuum pump, monometer and cylinders of compressed gas, so that operation of the jar is quick and simple. On the other hand, the internal production of hydrogen makes it difficult to test the apparatus for catalyst activity and impossible to do so in the standard GasPak jar, which is not vented. Further, as internal gas generation does not require pre-evacuation of the jar a relatively large volume of water is formed during catalysis.

When hydrogen is provided from an external source a vented jar is clearly essential, the valves incidentally providing a facility for assessing catalyst activity and for testing the jar for leaks. Schrader valves, as supplied with the Whitley jar, are very reliable. Anaerobiosis is achieved somewhat more rapidly when preliminary evacuation of the jar is practiced, so that a higher isolation rate of demanding organisms may be expected. Moreover, the cost of disposable gas generators is high compared with that of compressed gas.

For laboratories in which experience with strict anaerobes is likely to be limited or sporadic internal gas generation is probably the anaerobic method of choice. For laboratories that deal with anaerobes on a larger scale, a method employing evacuation and an external hydrogen/carbon dioxide source is preferred.

Evaluations of anaerobic jar methodology have been published by Collee et al (1972); Jarvis and Bruten (1972); and Burt and Phillips (1977).

Culture procedure. Standard horse blood agar prepared from a good quality basal medium is appropriate for the primary isolation of non-clostridial anaerobes. Plates should be freshly prepared, or prereduced by storage in an anaerobic jar until required. Since the growth of many anaerobes is improved by the addition to the medium of a reducing agent such as cysteine hydrochloride, it is a sound practice to do this routinely. Although some strains of anaerobes, notably *B. melaninogenicus*, require vitamin K and/or haemin as growth factors, these organisms can usually be cultured from pathological material without difficulty on the routine horse blood agar medium. However, it is usually necessary to add these growth factors to plating media for the subsequent isolation of these organisms in pure culture.

Each specimen is inoculated onto three horse blood agar plates for incubation in the three different atmospheres—aerobic, anaerobic with 10 per cent carbon dioxide, and aerobic with 10 per cent carbon dioxide. It is convenient to include a fourth culture on a blood plate containing 100 μg/ml neomycin sulphate for anaerobic incubation; this culture facilitates the subsequent isolation of anaerobes in pure culture by suppressing the growth of aerobic organisms.

As a guide to the differentiation of the growth of facultative anaerobes from that of obligate anaerobes, metronidazole and gentamicin discs may be placed on the non-selective blood agar plate culture for anaerobic incubation. After incubation, a zone of inhibition about the metronidazole disc indicates the presence of obligate anaerobes; inhibition of growth about the gentamicin disc indicates the presence of facultatively anaerobic bacteria.

All cultures are examined at the end of 24 and 48 hours' incubation; the incubation of primary anaerobic plates is continued for 96 hours. Recognition of the growth of obligate anaerobes is facilitated by direct comparison of the aerobic and anaerobic cultures, and by noting the effects of gentamicin and metronidazole on the anaerobic plate. Carbon dioxide-dependent facultative bacteria (sometimes incorrectly referred to as 'micro-aerophilic' organisms), show growth on plates incubated both anaerobically and in air plus carbon dioxide, but not on those incubated in the absence of added carbon dioxide. Carbon dioxide-dependent, facultatively anaerobic bacteria are uniformly resistant to metronidazole, but show variable sensitivity to gentamicin.

The presence of *B. melaninogenicus* is often overlooked if cultures are discarded too early, since pigmentation of colonies may not become obvious until the third day or later. Not infrequently young colonies of *B. melaninogenicus* (24 hours) fluoresce brick-red in ultra-violet light; some colonies that fail to fluoresce in situ produce a red fluorescent solution when extracted with methanol. Fluorescent colonies of *B. melaninogenicus* may induce fluorescence in adjacent colonies of other bacterial species.

The extent to which specific identification of anaerobic isolates is undertaken is governed, not only by the requirements of the particular clinical case, but also by the facilities of the investigating laboratory. Every clinical laboratory should be capable of broadly interpreting primary anaerobic plate cultures, and most should have little difficulty in identifying such common isolates as *B. fragilis* and *B. melaninogenicus*. Most anaerobic cultures can be interpreted within 24 hours, although it may take some days to attach specific names to isolated strains; the early 'interpretation' is of much greater clinical value than a definitive taxonomic report five days later.

Management

Surgical treatment

Copious pus, often with the formation of large abscesses, is a common denominator of almost all non-clostridial anaerobic infections, for which the treatment of first importance is surgical drainage. It is clear that in many instances establishment of drainage alone may be sufficient to effect a cure, as for example in tooth extraction for periapical abscess, and in surgical incision of superficial abscesses such as ischiorectal abscess, Bartholin's cyst abscess and axillary abscess. In more serious infections such as thoracic empyema, subphrenic abscess, septic abortion and brain abscess, it is a common practice to institute antibiotic therapy in addition to surgical drainage. In accordance with accepted surgical principles, however, it is clear that antimicrobial therapy can in no way replace surgical drainage when pus has accumulated in the tissues.

Antibiotic therapy

Antimicrobial agents active against anaerobes. There is developing a fairly considerable literature concerning the activity of antimicrobial agents against the non-clostridial anaerobes, much of which was usefully reviewed by Hamilton-Miller (1975) and Finegold (1977b). Chloramphenicol, lincomycin, clindamycin, metronidazole and rifampicin are the drugs most widely active against the non-clostridial anaerobes, and for the empirical treatment of anaerobic infections the choice must lie with one or another of these. From this choice, however, we may for the time being exclude rifampicin, the use of which is quite properly restricted to the treatment of tuberculosis.

Benzylpenicillin and other β-lactam antibiotics are active against most anaerobes, *B. fragilis* being an important exception. Thus, for those anaerobic infections that are known to be due to organisms other than *B. fragilis*, benzyl-penicillin may be regarded as a drug of choice. In this connection it is important to note that although many of the anaerobic infections that occur 'above the diaphragm' are due to penicillin-sensitive organisms derived from the mouth and upper respiratory tract, this is by no means always the case: a significant proportion is due to *B. fragilis*.

Chloramphenicol is active against virtually all anaerobes, and some workers have recommended it as the drug of choice for infections due to *Bacteroides* species. The great disadvantage of chloramphenicol is its potential activity as a bone marrow depressant.

Lincomycin and clindamycin are active against the whole range of non-clostridial anaerobes and are regarded by some as the drugs of choice for infections due to these organisms. Therapy with these drugs is commonly associated with a marked disturbance of the gut flora, and with looseness of the bowels or frank diarrhoea. Pseudomembranous colitis is a much more serious side effect that has been attributed to lincomycin and clindamycin therapy, although there are conflicting reports about its frequency.

Metronidazole has for some years been the drug of choice for the treatment of trichomoniasis, giardiasis and amoebiasis. The first indication that this nitro-imidazole compound might be of value in the treatment of anaerobic infections followed from the chance observation of Shinn (1962) that the drug was highly effective in the treatment of Vincent's stomatitis. Subsequently the in vitro susceptibility to metronidazole of a wide range of clinically important anaerobes has been determined, and it is clear that the drug has a universally bactericidal effect on anaerobic organisms, that aerobic and facultatively anaerobic bacteria are universally resistant to it, and that the in vitro minimum inhibitory and minimum bactericidal concentrations of the drug are equivalent. The antimicrobial activity and uses of metronidazole have been reviewed by Ingham, Selkon and Hale (1975) and Roe (1977).

Although the potential of metronidazole in the treatment of anaerobic infections has been recognized for some time, it is only recently that serious attention has been paid to its use in the management of anaerobic infections in man. Recent studies have shown that oral metronidazole is highly effective in the treatment and prophylaxis of a wide variety of non-clostridial anaerobic infections, and that the drug can also be administered effectively and safely by the intravenous and rectal routes. A recent study of Salem, Jackson and McFadzean (1975) showed that metronidazole is compatible with most other antimicrobial agents in common use.

Antimicrobial agents in treatment. For many non-clostridial anaerobic infections there is a clear requirement for antimicrobial therapy. Absolute indications include bacteraemia, endocarditis, meningitis and brain abscess, pneumonia, pulmonary abscess, septic thrombophlebitis and embolic phenomena, unresolving cellulitis, acute ulcerative gingivitis and stomatitis, anaerobic streptococcal myositis, and anaerobic necrotizing fasciitis and related infections. In addition, it is a common and acceptable practice to combine antibiotic therapy with surgical evacuation of pus from localized infections at sites that are known to carry a special risk of bacteraemia or of thromboembolic complications; of particular importance in this respect are intra-abdominal infections, and pelvic sepsis associated with the female genital tract.

Because the response of the non-clostridial anaerobes to the various first line drugs is fairly predictable, there should rarely be any difficulty in choosing the most appropriate antimicrobial agent in particular circumstances. Chloramphenicol, lincomycin, clindamycin and metronidazole are all active against the whole range of non-clostridial anaerobes, so that these drugs may be used empirically. The choice of drug will be influenced by such factors as its toxicity, the required route of administration, the severity of the infection, and the presence of concomitant aerobic infection.

For patients with severe Gram-negative sepsis, in particular those with bacteraemia, in whom antimicrobial therapy must begin before a bacteriological diagnosis is made, it is necessary to cover the possibilities that the infection may be due to either anaerobic or to facultatively anaerobic bacteria. Under these circumstances it is a common practice to initiate combined antimicrobial therapy, which may then be modified in the light of the bacteriological findings. One such regimen is lincomycin or clindamycin combined with gentamicin. Another, which has proved equally successful, is metronidazole combined with gentamicin. Although many non-clostridial anaerobic infections contain facultatively anaerobic bacteria in addition to the predominant anaerobic flora, it is rarely necessary or desirable to use antimicrobial therapy against the facultative components. Treatment of the facultatively anaerobic flora *only*, invariably fails; but antimicrobial therapy directed against the anaerobic bacteria is consistently successful.

Since non-clostridial anaerobic infections of the head-and-neck and thoracic regions are often due to organisms that are sensitive to penicillin, high cure rates with benzylpenicillin may be expected in many pleuropulmonary and oropharyngeal infections. It will be recalled, however, that in a proportion of these infections, the presence of *B. fragilis* necessitates the use of a drug other than penicillin.

As in many other types of bacterial infection it is helpful to control antimicrobial therapy by in vitro sensitivity testing; this is especially important when drugs such as erythromycin and tetracycline are in use, whose activity against different strains of anaerobic bacteria is erratic. When first line drugs are used, however, in vitro sensitivity testing usually provides essential confirmatory information— that the empirically selected drug, which has led to an improvement in the patient's clinical condition, is, indeed, active against the incriminated anaerobic bacteria.

Metronidazole therapy. Metronidazole is regarded as the drug of choice for all those anaerobic infections that require antimicrobial therapy. The drug may be given orally, rectally (or per colostomy) or intravenously, according to the following schedules (*see* Drug and Therapeutics Bulletin, 1976):

Oral route. Loading dose of 1 g, then 200 to 400 mg 8-hourly for 5 to 7 days. For children up to the age of 12 years, 7 mg per kg body weight 8-hourly.

Rectal (or colostomy) route. 1 g metronidazole by suppository 8-hourly for 3 days, then 12-hourly for 4 days if necessary. For children aged 5–11 years, half this dosage schedule; for children under 5 years appropriate reductions in the dosage should be made.

Intravenous route. One hundred ml of the intravenous preparation of metronidazole (equivalent to 500 mg metronidazole) is infused over a period of 20 minutes. This dose is repeated 8-hourly until oral medication becomes possible. The paediatric dosage is calculated on the basis of 21 mg per kg body weight per day. (There are 20 mg metronidazole in each 4 ml of the intravenous preparation.)

Accounts of metronidazole therapy for treatment of anaerobic sepsis have been published by Tally, Sutter and Finegold (1975); Study Group (1974, 1975, 1976, 1977); Ingham et al, 1975a, b, 1977; Eykyn and Phillips, 1976; Giamarellou et al, 1977; McGowan et al, 1977; Sharp et al, 1977.

Antimicrobial agents in prophylaxis. The common occurrence of sepsis as a complication of gastrointestinal and gynaecological surgery has been a continuing problem for many years. The incidence of postappendicectomy sepsis, for example, varies from 4 per cent for normal appendices to 77 per cent for gangrenous or perforated appendices. Similarly, infection remains the principle complication of colonic surgery, and it is also an important cause of morbidity following hysterectomy. Over the years, efforts to reduce the incidence of post-appendicectomy sepsis have led surgeons to employ a variety of topical and systemic prophylactic antibacterial agents; and various prophylactic oral antibiotic regimens have been used in the preoperative preparation of patients for elective colonic surgery. The large number of suggested regimens attests to the fact that none has been entirely successful (*see* Report, 1977). Many of the studies on the chemoprophylaxis of these postoperative infections have been concerned solely with clinical aspects of infection, and have not considered the nature of the infecting agents. This is unfortunate, because in these clinical settings, where a great variety of bacteria is likely to be present, the effectiveness of any prophylactic antibiotic must clearly depend on its spectrum of antibacterial activity. Despite an increasing awareness of the importance of the non-clostridial anaerobes as common causes of postoperative infection, it is still widely believed that postsurgical abdominal infections are usually caused by the Enterobacteriaceae (e.g. *E. coli*) and enterococci. Indeed, conventional procedures for the preoperative 'sterilization' of the gut utilize antimicrobial agents such as neomycin and kanamycin, which act only upon the facultatively anaerobic inhabitants of the colon; obligate anaerobes, which outnumber the aerobic faecal flora by 1000 to 1, are universally resistant to these drugs. Under these circumstances, it may not be an over-statement to suggest that this selective suppression of the aerobic flora may actually increase the risk of infection by anaerobes. In any event, it is clear that any prophylactic regimen aimed at preventing infection following surgery upon the gastrointestinal and female genital tracts, must take account of both the aerobic and anaerobic components of the indigenous bacterial flora. There is no doubt that carefully chosen short term antibiotic prophylaxis in surgery significantly reduces the incidence of postoperative sepsis. The prophylactic use of metronidazole in gastrointestinal and female genital tract surgery has been conspicuously successful in the prevention of postsurgical anaerobic infections (Study Group, 1974, 1975, 1976, 1977; Goldring et al, 1975; Feathers et al, 1977; Taylor and Cawdery, 1977; Leading Article, 1976, 1977).

In appendicectomy and hysterectomy patients on the one hand, and in patients submitted to major colonic surgery on the other, the use of prophylactic metronidazole may be confidently expected to reduce anaerobic sepsis rates of around 20 per cent and 50 per cent respectively, to nil. Because aerobes and facultative anaerobes (including carbon dioxide-dependant organisms) are universally resistant to metronidazole, the drug can have no direct effect on the relatively low incidence of postoperative infection due to these organisms.

Metronidazole prophylaxis. Metronidazole is regarded as the drug of choice if protection against the development of anaerobic infections is required, and may be administered according to one of the following schedules:

Elective surgical patients (e.g. hysterectomy and colonic surgery)
Preoperatively. On the last preoperative day, 1 g metronidazole orally, then 200 mg 8-hourly until preoperative starvation. With premedication, 1 g metronidazole by suppository per rectum (or per colostomy).
Postoperatively. Per rectum (or per colostomy) 1 g metronidazole by suppository 8-hourly for 3 days, then 12-hourly for 4 days if necessary: or orally, 200–400 mg metronidazole 8-hourly over the same period.

Acute surgical patients (e.g. appendicectomy; gastrointestinal perforation)
Preoperatively. 1 g metronidazole by suppository per rectum with the premedication.
Postoperatively. As for elective surgical patients (above).

Paediatric dosages
1. Oral paediatric dosage is 7 mg per kg body weight 8-hourly up to the age of 12 years.
2. Rectal paediatric dosage is one half of the adult dosage for children aged 5–11 years; this dosage is appropriately reduced for children under 5 years.

Intravenous prophylaxis may be given to patients in whom the oral and rectal routes are not available. The dosage is as outlined for intravenous treatment, the first dose being given at the time of premedication.

Campylobacter enteritis
During the last decade *Cl. perfringens* has been recognized as the commonest single cause of food poisoning in the United Kingdom. Now, as a result of the recent pioneer studies of Skirrow (1977) in Worcester, another group of anaerobes —the campylobacters—has emerged as a frequent cause of infectious diarrhoea.

The primary source of human infections with *Campylobacter jejuni* and *Campylobacter coli* is probably poultry in which these organisms cause vibrionic hepatitis; in man the infection occurs as an enteritis. The organism spreads readily among young children, and from infected children to their mothers, but seldom between adults. The onset of the infection may be sudden with severe colicky abdominal pain, nausea and malaise followed by copious foul smelling diarrhoea which is often bile-stained and sometimes contains frank blood. In some patients there is a prodromal febrile period lasting a few hours to several days. The acute diarrhoeal phase lasts for 1–3 days but may be remittent.

Bacteriological diagnosis is readily made by direct culture of light faecal suspensions on Skirrow's campylobacter selective agar—a 7 per cent lysed horse blood medium containing vancomycin, polymyxin B and trimethoprim. Cultures are incubated overnight at 43°C in an atmosphere of hydrogen containing about 5 per cent oxygen and 10 per cent carbon dioxide. Campylobacters, which are small, highly motile, spiral or S-shaped, weakly-staining Gram-negative bacilli, are easily recognized by their characteristic effuse, coalescing growth which has a shiny, almost metallic appearance.

The organisms are sensitive to aminoglycosides, macrolides and nitroimidazole compounds, but are resistant to penicillin and ampicillin. For patients in need of antimicrobial therapy Skirrow recommended erythromycin stearate. Metronidazole is another logical choice in view of the efficacy of nitroimidazoles in the prevention and treatment of campylobacter dysentery in pigs (Fernie, Ware and Park, 1977).

ACKNOWLEDGEMENT

I am indebted to Butterworth and Co (Publishers) Ltd for permission to use some copyright material.

REFERENCES

Balows, A., De Haan, R. M., Dowell, V. R. & Guze, L. B. (1974) *Anaerobic Bacteria : Role in Disease*, Springfield: Thomas.

Burt, R. & Phillips, K. D. (1977) A new anaerobic jar. *Journal of Clinical Pathology*, **30**, 1082–1084.

Collee, J. G., Watt, B., Fowler, E. B. & Brown, R. (1972) An evaluation of the GasPak system in the culture of anaerobic bacteria. *Journal of Applied Bacteriology*, **35**, 71–82.

Collee, J. G., Watt, B., Brown, R. & Johnstone, S. (1974) The recovery of anaerobic bacteria from swabs. *Journal of Hygiene, Cambridge*, **72**, 339–347.

Dowell, V. R. & Hawkins, T. M. (1974) *Laboratory methods in anaerobic bacteriology. CDC Laboratory Manual*. Atlanta: US Department of Health, Education & Welfare.

Drug & Therapeutics Bulletin (1976) Metronidazole in anaerobic infections, **14**, 25–27.

Duerden, B. I., Holbrook, W. P., Collee, J. G. & Watt, B. (1976) The characterization of clinically important Gram-negative anaerobic bacilli by conventional bacteriological tests. *Journal of Applied Bacteriology*, **40**, 163–188.

Ellner, P. D., Granato, P. A. & May, C. B. (1973) Recovery and identification of anaerobes: a system suitable for the routine clinical laboratory. *Applied Microbiology*, **26**, 904–913.

Eykyn, S. J. & Phillips, I. (1976) Metronidazole and anaerobic sepsis. *British Medical Journal*, **4**, 1418–1421.

Feathers, R. S., Lewis, A. A. M., Sagor, G. R., Amirak, I. D. & Noone, P. (1977) Prophylactic systemic antibiotics in colorectal surgery. *Lancet*, **2**, 4–8.

Ferguson, I. R., Phillips, K. D. & Tearle, P. V. (1975) An evaluation of the carbon dioxide component of the GasPak anaerobic system. *Journal of Applied Bacteriology*, **39**, 167–173.

Ferguson, I. R., Phillips, K. D. & Willis, A. T. (1976) An evaluation of the GasKit disposable hydrogen and carbon dioxide generator for the culture of anaerobic bacteria. *Journal of Applied Bacteriology*, **41**, 433–437.

Fernie, D. S., Ware, D. A. & Park, R. W. A. (1977) The effect of the nitroimidazole drug dimetridazole in microaerophilic campylobacters. *Journal of Clinical Microbiology*, **10**, 233–240.

Finegold, S. M. (1977a) *Anaerobic Bacteria in Human Disease*. New York: Academic Press.

Finegold, S. M. (1977b) Clinical experience with clindamycin in anaerobic bacterial infections. I. Therapy for infections due to anaerobic bacteria: an overview. *Journal of Infectious Diseases*, **135**, S25–S29.

Giamarellou, H., Kanellakopoulou, K., Pragastis, D., Tagaris, N. & Daikos, G. K. (1977) Treatment with metronidazole of 48 patients with serious anaerobic infections. *Journal of Antimicrobial Chemotherapy*, **3**, 347–353.

Goldring, J., Scott, A., McNaught, W. & Gillespie, G. (1975) Prophylactic oral antimicrobial agents in elective colonic surgery. *Lancet*, **2**, 997–1000.

Gorbach, S. L. & Bartlett, J. G. (1974) Anaerobic infections. *New England Journal of Medicine*, **290**, 1177–1184, 1237–1245, 1289–1294.

Gunn, A. A. (1956) Bacteroides septicaemia. *Journal of the Royal College of Surgeons of Edinburgh*, **2**, 41–50.

Hamilton-Miller, J. M. T. (1975) Antimicrobial agents acting against anaerobes. *Journal of Antimicrobial Chemotherapy*, **1**, 273–289.

Holdeman, L. V. & Moore, W. E. C. (1975) *Anaerobe Laboratory Manual*. Blacksburg: Virginia Polytechnic Institute Anaerobe Laboratory.

Ingham, H. R., Selkon, J. B. & Hale, J. H. (1975) The antibacterial activity of metronidazole. *Journal of Antimicrobial Chemotherapy*, **1**, 355–361.

Ingham, H. R., Selkon, J. B., So, S. C. & Weiser, R. (1975a) Brain abscess. *British Medical Journal*, **4**, 39–40.

Ingham, H. R., Rich, G. E., Selkon, J. B., Hale, J. H., Roxby, C. M., Betty, M. J., Johnson, R. W. G. & Uldall, P. R. (1975b) Treatment with metronidazole of three patients with serious infections due to *Bacteroides fragilis*. *Journal of Antimicrobial Chemotherapy*, **1**, 235–242.

Ingham, H. R., Hood, F. J. C., Bradnum, P., Tharagonnet, D. & Selkon, J. B. (1977) Metronidazole compared with penicillin in the treatment of acute dental infections. *British Journal of Oral Surgery*, **14**, 264–269.

Irvin, T. T., Stoddard, C. J., Greaney, M. G. & Duthie, H. L. (1977) Abdominal wound healing: a prospective clinical study. *British Medical Journal*, **2**, 351–352.

Jarvis, J. D. & Bruten, D. M. (1972) Observations in the use of anaerobic jars and the methods of their control. *Medical Laboratory Technology*, **29**, 325–328.

Leading Article (1976) Preventing infection at the operation site. *British Medical Journal*, **4**, 773–774.

Leading Article (1977) Pelvic sepsis after hysterectomy. *British Medical Journal*, **2**, 1239–1240.

MacLennan, J. D. (1951) *Recent Advances in Bacteriology*, 3rd edition, p. 207. London: Churchill.

McGowan, D. A., Murphy, K. J. & Sheiham, A. (1977) Metronidazole in the treatment of severe acute pericoronitis. *British Dental Journal*, **142**, 221–223.

Myers, M. B., Cherry, G., Bornside, B. B. & Bornside, G. H. (1969) Ultraviolet red fluorescence of *Bacteroides melaninogenicus*. *Applied Microbiology*, **17**, 760–762.

Parker, R. T. & Jones, C. P. (1966) Anaerobic pelvic infections and developments in hyperbaric oxygen therapy. *American Journal of Obstetrics and Gynaecology*, **96**, 645–658.

Phillips, I. & Sussman, M. (1974) *Infection with non-sporing Anaerobic Bacteria*. Edinburgh: Churchill Livingstone.

Phillips, K. D., Tearle, P. V. & Willis, A. T. (1976) Rapid diagnosis of anaerobic infections by gas-liquid chromatography of clinical material. *Journal of Clinical Pathology*, **29**, 428–432.

Report (1977) Prophylactic antimicrobial drug therapy at five London teaching hospitals. *Lancet*, **1**, 1351–1353.

Roe, F. J. C. (1977) Metronidazole: review of uses and toxicity. *Journal of Antimicrobial Chemotherapy*, **3**, 205–212.

Salem, A. R., Jackson, D. D. & McFadzean, J. A. (1975) An investigation of interactions between metronidazole ('Flagyl') and other antimicrobial agents. *Journal of Antimicrobial Chemotherapy*, **1**, 387–391.

Shapton, D. A. & Board, R. G. (1971) Isolation of anaerobes. *Society for Applied Bacteriology Technical Series No. 5*. London: Academic Press.

Sharp, D. J., Corringham, R. E. T., Nye, E. B., Sagor, G. R. & Noone, P. (1977) Successful treatment of bacteroides bacteraemia with metronidazole, after failure with clindamycin and lincomycin. *Journal of Antimicrobial Chemotherapy*, **3**, 233–237.

Shinn, D. L. S. (1962) Metronidazole in acute ulcerative gingivitis. *Lancet*, **1**, 1191.

Skirrow, M. B. (1977) Campylobacter enteritis: a 'new' disease. *British Medical Journal*, **2**, 9–11.

Smith, L. D. S. (1975) *The Pathogenic Anaerobic Bacteria*, 2nd edition. Springfield: Thomas.

Smith, L. L. & Ferguson, I. R. (1977) Modified bacteriological swabs for the transport of anaerobes in clinical specimens. *Medical Laboratory Sciences*, **34**, 247–258.

Study Group (1974) Metronidazole in the prevention and treatment of bacteroides infections in gynaecological patients. *Lancet*, **2**, 1540–1543.

Study Group (1975) An evaluation of metronidazole in the prophylaxis and treatment of anaerobic infections in surgical patients. *Journal of Antimicrobial Chemotherapy*, **1**, 393–401.

Study Group (1976) Metronidazole in the prevention and treatment of bacteroides infections following appendicectomy. *British Medical Journal*, **1**, 318–321.

Study Group (1977) Metronidazole in prevention and treatment of bacteroides infections in elective colonic surgery. *British Medical Journal*, **1**, 607–610.

Sutter, V. L. & Finegold, S. M. (1973) Anaerobic bacteria: their recognition and significance in the clinical laboratory. *Progress in Clinical Pathology*, **5,** 219–238.

Sutter, V. L., Vargo, V. L. & Finegold, S. M. (1975) *Anaerobic Bacteriology Manual*, 2nd edition. Los Angeles: University of California.

Tally, F. P., Sutter, V. L. & Finegold, S. M. (1975) Treatment of anaerobic infections with metronidazole. *Antimicrobial Agents and Chemotherapy*, **7,** 672–675.

Tally, F. P., Stewart, P. R., Sutter, V. L. & Rosenblatt, J. E. (1975) Oxygen tolerance of fresh clinical anaerobic bacteria. *Journal of Clinical Microbiology*, **1,** 161–164.

Taylor, S. A. & Cawdery, H. M. (1977) The use of metronidazole in the preparation of the bowel for surgery. *Proceedings of the Royal Society of Medicine*, **70,** 481–482.

Tehrani, M. A. & Ledingham, I. McA. (1977) Necrotizing fasciitis. *Postgraduate Medical Journal*, **53,** 237–242.

Watt, B., Collee, J. G. & Brown, R. (1974) The isolation of strict anaerobes: the use of an anaerobic cabinet compared with a conventional procedure. *Journal of Medical Microbiology*, **7,** 315–324.

Willis, A. T. (1969) *The Clostridia of Wound Infection*. London: Butterworths.

Willis, A. T. (1977) *Anaerobic bacteriology. Clinical and Laboratory Practice*, 3rd edition. London: Butterworths.

Wren, M. D. W. (1977) The culture of clinical specimens for anaerobic bacteria: a comparison of three regimens. *Journal of Medical Microbiology*, **10,** 195–201.

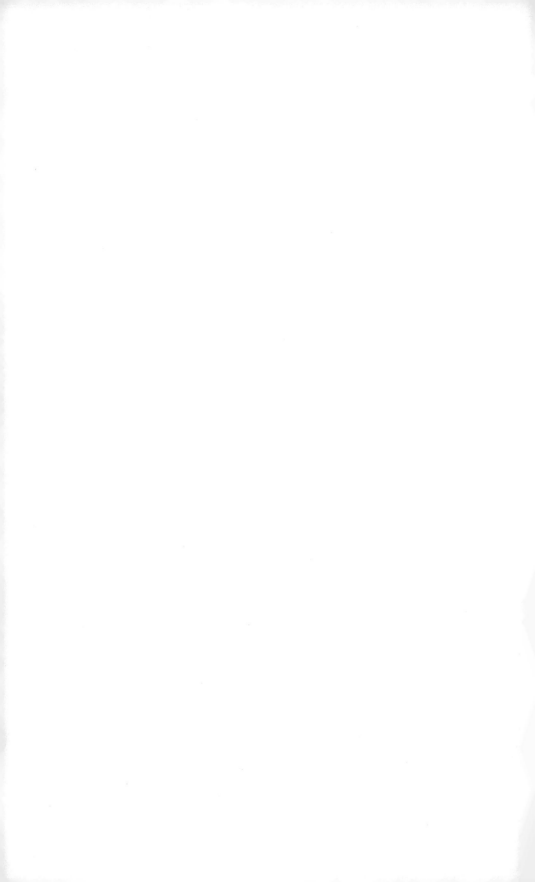

Index